Challenging Cases in Palliative Care

Published and forthcoming titles in the Challenging Cases in series

Anaesthesia (Edited by Dr Phoebe Syme, Dr Robert Jackson, and Dr Timothy Cook)

Cardiovascular Medicine (Edited by Dr Aung Myat, Dr Shouvik Haldar, and Professor Simon Redwood)

Congenital and Acquired Heart Disease in the Young (Edited by Dr Salim Jivanji and Dr Michael Rigby)

Critical Care (Edited by Dr Christopher Gough, Dr Justine Barnett, Professor Tim Cook, and Professor Jerry Nolan)

Emergency Medicine (Edited by Dr Sam Thenabadu, Dr Fleur Cantle, and Dr Chris Lacy)

Infectious Diseases and Clinical Microbiology (Edited by Dr Amber Arnold and Professor George E. Griffin)

Interventional Radiology (Edited by Dr Irfan Ahmed, Dr Miltiadis Krokidis, and Dr Tarun Sabharwal)

Neurology (Edited by Dr Krishna Chinthapalli, Dr Nadia Magdalinou, and Professor Nicholas Wood)

Neurosurgery (Edited by Mr Robin Bhatia and Mr Ian Sabin)

Obstetrics and Gynaecology (Edited by Dr Natasha Hezelgrave, Dr Danielle Abbott, and Professor Andrew Shennan)

Oncology (Edited by Dr Madhumita Bhattacharyya, Dr Sarah Payne, and Professor Iain McNeish)

Oral and Maxillofacial Surgery (Edited by Mr Matthew Idle and Group Captain Andrew Monaghan)

Paediatric Critical Care (Edited by Dr Hari Krishnan, Dr Miriam R. Fine-Goulden, Dr Sainath Raman, and Dr Akash Deep)

Respiratory Medicine (Edited by Dr Lucy Schomberg, Dr Elizabeth Sage, and Dr Nick Hart)

Urological Surgery (Edited by Dr Karl Pang and Dr James Catto)

Challenging Cases in Palliative Care

Cases with Expert Commentary

Edited By

Felicity Dewhurst
Consultant in Palliative Medicine, St Oswald's Hospice,
NIHR Advanced Fellow, Senior Clinical Lecturer, Population Health Sciences Institute,
Newcastle University, Newcastle, UK

Polly Edmonds
Consultant in Palliative Care, King's College Hospital NHS Foundation Trust,
Cicely Saunders Institute, London, UK

Suzie Gillon
Consultant in Palliative Medicine, Leeds Teaching Hospitals NHS Trust, Leeds, UK

Amy Hawkins
Consultant in Palliative Medicine, Royal Trinity Hospice, London, UK

Mary Miller
Oxford University Hospitals NHS Trust, Oxford, UK

Sarah Yardley
Associate Professor in Palliative Medicine, Marie Curie Palliative Care Research Department,
University College London, London, UK

Series editors

Aung Myat
Medical Director for Cardiology and Academic Interventional Cardiologist, Medpace Inc., London, UK

Shouvik Haldar
Consultant Cardiologist and Electrophysiologist, Heart Rhythm Centre,
Royal Brompton and Harefield NHS Foundation Trust,
and Honorary Clinical Senior Lecturer, Imperial College London, London, UK

OXFORD
UNIVERSITY PRESS

OXFORD
UNIVERSITY PRESS

Great Clarendon Street, Oxford, OX2 6DP,
United Kingdom

Oxford University Press is a department of the University of Oxford.
It furthers the University's objective of excellence in research, scholarship, and education by publishing worldwide. Oxford is a registered trade mark of Oxford University Press in the UK and in certain other countries

Published in the United States of America by Oxford University Press
198 Madison Avenue, New York, NY 10016, United States of America

British Library Cataloguing in Publication Data

Data available

Library of Congress Control Number is on file at the Library of Congress

ISBN 978–0–19–286474–1

DOI: 10.1093/med/9780192864741.001.0001

Printed and bound by
CPI Group (UK) Ltd, Croydon, CR0 4YY

PREFACE

This case-based guide to managing challenging cases in Palliative Care has been developed to help palliative care doctors, physician associates, nurse specialists, allied health professionals and advanced practitioners, develop their knowledge to manage complex situations. Each case is accompanied by 'Learning points', 'Clinical tips', 'Evidence base', and 'Future advances' boxes, highlighting critical information, facilitating learning and aiding revision. The 'Expert commentary' gives a unique insight into how today's opinion leaders confront and deal with these complex cases.

The cases chosen for Challenging Cases in Palliative Care have been chosen to cover a wide range of challenging scenarios encountered in everyday clinical practice. The book encompasses cases considering complex pain and symptom management; transfer of care between settings; advance care planning; uncertainty and prognostication; escalation decisions; palliative care for specific conditions (including serious physical and psychiatric illness); psychosocial care; care of the dying person and bereavement; supportive oncology; desire for hastened death and compassionate communities. The cases take a multiprofessional approach, considering the holistic palliative care approach, evidence base, and the application of national and international guidelines. This case series brings together the most up-to-date evidence, management strategies, guidelines, and controversies, to provide doctors, physicians associates and advanced practitioners with a unique insight on how the experts approach and deal with real-world clinical scenarios.

Challenging Cases in Palliative Care is suitable as a revision tool for doctors preparing for the UK specialty certificate examination, for physician associates working in palliative care and for nurses and allied health professionals undertaking advanced study.

CONTENTS

ABBREVIATIONS

ACE	Adverse childhood experiences
ACP	Advance care planning
ACT	Acceptance and commitment therapy
ADRT	Advance decision to refuse treatment
AED	Antiepileptic drugs
AKI	Acute kidney injury
AKPS	Australia-modified Karnofsky Performance Scale
ALP	Alkaline phosphatase
AMP	Approved mental health practitioner
AMU	Acute Medical Unit
ATS	American Thoracic Society
BAM	Bile acid malabsorption
BD	Twice daily
BMA	British Medical Association
BP	Blood pressure
BPI	Brief Pain Inventory
BPS	British Pain Society
BPSD	Behavioural and psychological symptoms of dementia
BRISQ	Bereavement Risk Inventory and Screening Questionnaire
CAH	Clinically assisted hydration
CAM	Confusion Assessment Method
CANH	Clinically Assisted Nutrition and Hydration
CBT	Cognitive behavioural therapy
CGA	Comprehensive Geriatric Assessment
CGM	Continuous Glucose Monitoring
CIPN	Chemotherapy-induced peripheral neuropathy
CKD	Chronic kidney disease
CKS	Clinical Knowledge Summary
CMM	Comprehensive medical management
CN	Community nursing
CNCP	Chronic non-cancer pain
CNS	Clinical nurse specialist
COPD	Chronic obstructive pulmonary disease
CPCT	Community palliative care team
CPIC	Clinical Pharmacogenetics Implementation Consortium
CPR	Cardiopulmonary resuscitation
CRP	C-reactive protein
CSNAT	Carer Support Needs Assessment Tool
CT	Computerised tomography
CTC	Common Toxicology Criteria
CXR	Chest X-ray
DDRS	Desire to Die Rating Scale
DisDAT	Distress and Discomfort Assessment Tool
DN	District nursing
DNACPR	Do not attempt cardio-pulmonary resuscitation
DOPPS	Dialysis Outcomes and Practice Patterns Study
DRE	Digital rectal examination
DVT	Deep vein thrombosis
EAPC	European Association of Palliative Care
ED	Emergency department
EMT	Emergency medical teams
ENT	Ear, nose and throat
EoL	End of life
EOLC	End of life care
EPaCCS	Electronic Palliative care Coordination System
ERAS	Enhanced Recovery for Surgery
ESAS	Edmonton symptom assessment scale
ESC	Enhanced supportive care
ESGE	European Society of Gastrointestinal Endoscopy
ESKD	End-stage kidney disease
FOLFOX	Folinic acid, fluorouracil, and oxaliplatin
FPM	Faculty of Pain Medicine
GAIN	Guidelines and Audit Implementation Network
GI	Gastrointestinal
GLIM	Global Leadership Initiative on Malnutrition
GMC	General Medical Council
GP	General Practice or Practitioner
GSF	Gold Standards Framework
HIC	High-income countries
HPA	Hypothalamic-pituitary-adrenal
HPCT	Hospital palliative care team
IASP	International Association for the Study of Pain
IBACS	Indicator of Bereavement Adaptation-Cruse Scotland

ICNARC	Intensive Care National Audit & Research Centre
ICU	Intensive care unit
IDDS	Implantable drug delivery system
IMCA	Independent Mental Capacity Advocate
IPOS	Integrated Palliative Care Outcome Scale
IPU	Inpatient unit
IR	Immediate release
LANSS	Leeds Assessment of Neuropathic Symptoms and Signs
LAS	London Ambulance Service
LCP	Liverpool Care Pathway
LFT	Liver Function Tests
LMIC	Low- and middle-income countries
LTOT	Long-term oxygen therapy
MAAR	Medication authorization and administration record
MASCC	Multinational Association of Supportive Care in Cancer
MAT	Medication assisted treatment
MBO	Malignant Bowel Obstruction
MCA	Mental Capacity Act
MCE	Mass Casualty Events
MDM	mobile device management
MDM	Multidisciplinary meeting
MHA	Mental Health Act
MHLT	Mental Health Liaison Team
MLTC	Multiple long-term conditions
MMSE	Mini-Mental State Examination
MND	Motor neurone disease
MoCA	Montreal Cognitive Assessment
MR	Modified release
MRC	Medical Research Council
MRI	Magnetic resonance imaging
MSA	Multiple system atrophy
MSCC	Malignant spinal cord compression
NBS	Narcotic bowel syndrome
NGO	Non-governmental organization
NICE	National Institute for Clinical Excellence
NIV	Non-invasive ventilation
NNH	Number needed to harm
NNPC	Neighbourhood Network in Palliative Care
NNT	Number needed to treat
NRS	Numerical rating scale
NSAID	Nonsteroidal anti-inflammatory drugs
NSCLC	Non-small-cell lung cancer
OCEBM	Oxford Centre for Evidence-Based Medicine
OD	Once daily
OGT	Oxygenated glycerol trimester
OIBD	Opioid-induced bowel dysfunction
OIC	Opioid-induced constipation
OME	Oral morphine equivalent
ONS	Oral nutritional supplements
OT	Occupational therapy
OTC	Over the counter
PAMORA	Peripherally acting mu-opioid receptor antagonists
PaP	Palliative Prognostic
PAS	Physician Assisted Suicide
PC	Palliative care
PCA	Patient controlled analgesia
PCC	Percutaneous cervical cordotomy
PCF	Palliative Care Formulary
PD	Parkinson's disease
PEG	Percutaneous endoscopic gastrostomy
PET	Positron emission tomography
PFA	Psychological first aid
PFM	Preservative free morphine
PGD	Prolonged grief disorder
PiPS	Prognosis in Palliative Care Study
PN	Parenteral nutrition
PPI	Palliative Prognostic Index
PPI	Proton-pump inhibitor
PPC	Preferred place of care
PPV	Positive Predictive Value
PRN	Pro re nata (as required)
PSA	Prostate-specific antigen
PSP	Progressive supranuclear palsy
QDS	Four times daily
QOL	Quality of life
RCT	Randomized control trial
ReSPECT	Recommended Summary Plan for Emergency Care and Treatment
RR	Respiratory rate
RRT	Renal replacement therapy
SABR	Stereotactic ablative radiotherapy
SACT	Systemic anti-cancer therapy
SAHD	Schedule of Attitudes towards Hastened Death
SALT	Speech and language therapy team
SCC	Squamous cell carcinoma
SCI	Spinal cord injury
SeHCAT	Selenium-Homo-Taurocholic Acid Test
SIGN	Scottish Intercollegiate Guidelines Network

SINS	Spinal Instability Neoplastic Score
SMI	Severe Mental Illness
SNRI	Serotonin-noradrenaline reuptake inhibitors
SPICT	Supportive and Palliative Care Indicators Tool
SQUID	Single Question in Delirium
SRE	Skeletal-related events
SUS	Substance use services
SW	Social worker
TDS	Three times daily
TEE	Total energy expenditure
TENS	Transcutaneous electrical nerve stimulation
TEP	Treatment escalation plans or planning
TIGDS	Terminally Ill Grief or Depression Scale
TRP	Transient receptor potential
US	Ultrasound
VAS	Visual analogue scale
VBG	Venous blood gas
VIP	Vasoactive intestinal peptide
WBC	White blood cell
WHO	World Health Organization
WTHD	Wish to hasten death

CONTRIBUTORS

Stephanie Ainley, Palliative Medicine Registrar, London, UK

Manraj Bhamra, Psychiatrist, South London and Maudsley NHS Foundation Trust, London, UK

Anna Bradley, Palliative Medicine Consultant, West Middlesex University Hospital, Isleworth, UK

Charlotte Chamberlain, Consultant in Palliative Medicine, University Hospitals Bristol and Weston NHS Foundation Trust and Honorary Senior Lecturer at the University of Bristol, Bristol, UK

Max Charles, Specialty Trainee in Palliative Medicine, North East England, Health Education England, UK

Alice Copley, Palliative Medicine Registrar, Leeds Teaching Hospitals NHS Trust, Leeds, UK

Lara Datta-Paulin, Palliative Medicine Registrar, North West, UK

Kirsty Douglas, Palliative Medicine Registrar, Roxburghe House, NHS Grampian, UK

Felicity Dewhurst, Consultant in Palliative Medicine, St Oswald's Hospice, NIHR Advanced Fellow, Senior Clinical Lecturer, Population Health Sciences Institute, Newcastle University, Newcastle, UK

Simon Noah Etkind, Assistant Professor in Palliative Care, University of Cambridge, Cambridge, UK

Mairi Finlay, Department of Palliative Medicine, NHS Tayside, UK

Simeon Senders-Galloway, Specialty Registrar in Palliative Medicine Sue Ryder Duchess of Kent Hospice, Reading, UK

Rebecca Gemmell, Palliative Medicine Registrar, London, UK

Alice Gray, Palliative Medicine Registrar, West Midlands, UK

Philippa Guppy, Palliative Care SpR, Senior Lecturer, St. Georges University, London, UK

Gurpreet Gupta, Consultant in Palliative Medicine, St Luke's Hospice, Harrow, UK

Nathaniel Luke Hatton, Academic Clinical Oncology Registrar, University of Leeds, Leeds, UK

Lucy Hetherington, Consultant in Palliative Medicine and Interventional Cancer Pain Management, Beatson West of Scotland Cancer Centre, Glasgow, UK

Stephanie Hicks, Consultant in Palliative Medicine, Guy's and St Thomas' NHS Foundation Trust, London, UK

Rosanna Hill, Palliative Medicine Registrar, Leeds Teaching Hospitals NHS Trust, Leeds, UK

Daniel Hughes, Consultant Psychiatrist Camden and Islington NHS Foundation Trust, UK

Lucy Ison, Consultant in Palliative Medicine, Imperial College Healthcare NHS Trust, London, UK

Catriona Jackson, Palliative Medicine Registrar, Leeds Teaching Hospitals NHS Trust, Leeds, UK

Kitty Jackson, NIHR Academic Clinical Fellow in Palliative Medicine, Hull York Medical School/Wolfson, Palliative Care Research Center, UK

Oliver Jackson, Specialty Registrar in Clinical Oncology, Leeds Cancer Centre, St James University Hospital, Leeds, UK

Gemma Lewis-Williams, Consultant in Palliative Medicine Betsicadwaladr University Health Board, Wales

Stephanie Lister-Flynn, Palliative Medicine Registrar, Guys and St. Thomas' NHS Foundation Trust, London, UK

Sarah Longwell, Specialist Registrar in Palliative Medicine, Leeds Teaching Hospitals NHS Trust, Leeds, UK

Natasha Lovell, Consultant in Palliative Medicine, North Bristol NHS Foundation Trust, Bristol, UK

Sarah Maan, Palliative Medicine Registrar, Barts Health, London, UK

Jaspal Kaur Mann, Specialist Registrar in Palliative Medicine, St Christopher's Hospice, London, UK

Athul Manuel, Department of Pain and Palliative Care, General Hospital Ernakulam, Kerala, India

Robert McConnell, Specialty Trainee in Palliative Medicine, Health Education England, UK

Holly McGuigan, Consultant in Palliative Medicine, Ardgowan Hospice, Inverclyde, Scotland

Toni Mortimer, Specialist Registrar in Palliative Medicine, Marie Curie Hospice, Hampstead, London, UK

Matt Mulvey, Research Associate, University of Leeds, Leeds, UK

Rose O'Duffy, Palliative Medicine Trainee, South Yorkshire, UK

Georgina Osborne, Consultant in Palliative Medicine, Barts Health NHS Trust, UK

Tammy Oxley, Specialist Registrar in Palliative Medicine, St Gemma's Hospice, Leeds, UK

Rebecca Payne, Specialty Doctor in Palliative Medicine, Royal Trinity Hospice, London, UK

Constantina Pitsillides, Consultant in Palliative Medicine, Sheffield Teaching Hospitals, Sheffield, UK

Maggie Presswood, Palliative Care Consultant, North Bristol NHS Trust, Bristol, UK

Shaun Peter Qureshi, Lecturer in Medical Education, Centre for Medical Education, University of Dundee, Dundee, UK

Emily Rea, Consultant in Palliative Medicine, Aneurin Bevan University Health Board, Wales

Jamie Richardson, Consultant Psychiatrist for People with Learning Disabilities, Leeds and York Partnership NHS Foundation Trust, Leeds, UK

Marie-Claire Rooney, Palliative Medicine Specialty Registrar, Royal Marsden Hospital, London, UK

Grace Rowley, Consultant in Palliative Medicine, North Cumbria Integrated Care Trust, UK

Joseph Sawyer, Consultant in palliative care, St Elizabeth Hospice, Ipswich, London, UK

Anna Schuberth, Consultant in Palliative Medicine, Mid Yorkshire Hospitals NHS Trust and Wakefield Hospice, Wakefield, UK

Lauri Simkiss, Consultant in Palliative Medicine, North Tees and Hartlepool NHS Foundation Trust, UK

Rebecca Tiberini, Palliative Care Physiotherapist, Clinical Educator and Consultant, UK/Switzerland

Kirsty Tolmie, Specialist Trainee in Palliative Medicine, NHS Greater Glasgow and Clyde, Glasgow, UK

Mark Warren, Operational Lead and Clinical Nurse Specialist, Specialist Supportive Care Team, The Christie NHS Foundation Trust, Manchester, UK

Sarah Webster, Palliative Care Trainee, Bristol, UK

Geoffrey Wells, Senior Lecturer in Medical Education, Brighton and Sussex Medical School and Honorary Consultant in Palliative Medicine, East Sussex Healthcare NHS Trust, UK

EXPERTS

Sabrina Bajwah, Clinical Senior Lecturer, King's College London, London, UK

Richard Berman, Consultant in Supportive Care and Palliative Medicine, The Christie NHS Foundation Trust, Manchester, UK

Maggie Bisset, (Retired) Nurse Consultant in Palliative Care, Central and North West London NHS Foundation Trust, London, UK

Jason Boland, Senior Clinical Lecturer and Honorary Consultant in Palliative Medicine Wolfson Palliative Care Research Centre, Hull York Medical School, University of Hull, UK

Ben Bowers, Wellcome Post-Doctoral Fellow and Honorary Nurse Consultant in Palliative Care, University of Cambridge, UK

Rachel Burman, Consultant in Palliative Care, King's College Hospital NHS Foundation Trust, London, UK

Leona Butterly, Clinical Nurse Specialist in Palliative Care, Portiuncula University Hospital, Ballinasloe, Galway, Ireland

Michael Connolly, Joint Associate Professor of Clinical Nursing, University College Dublin and Our Lady's Hospice and Care Services, Ireland

Sunitha Daniel, Consultant in Palliative Medicine, York and Scarborough Teaching Hospitals NHS Foundation Trust, York, UK

Karen Harrison Dening, Head of Research and Publications, Dementia UK, London, UK

Jo Elverson, Consultant in Palliative Medicine, Newcastle Upon Tyne Hospitals NHS Foundation Trust and St Oswald's Hospice, Newcastle, UK

Christopher Farnham, Consultant in Palliative Medicine William Harvey Hospital Ashford Kent, UK

Andrew Goodhead, St Christophers Hospice, London, UK

Anna Gorringe, Palliative Medicine Consultant, Whittington Health, London, UK

Adam Hurlow, Leeds Teaching Hospitals NHS Trust, Leeds, UK

Emma Husbands, Consultant Palliative Medicine, Gloucestershire Hospitals NHS Foundation Trust, Gloucester, UK

Khalida Ismail, Institute of Psychiatry, Psychology, and Neuroscience, King's College London, London, UK

Iain Jones, Consultant in Anaesthesia and Pain Management Royal Victoria Infirmary Newcastle upon Tyne, UK

Jonathan Koffman, Professor of Palliative Care Wolfson Palliative Care Research Centre. Hull York Medcial School, UK

Joanna Laddie, Consultant in Paediatric Palliative Medicine, Evelina London Children's Hospital, London, UK

Barry Laird, Edinburgh Palliative and Supportive Care Group, Institute of Genetics and Cancer, Edinburgh Cancer Research, Edinburgh, UK

Philip Lodge, Consultant in Palliative Medicine, Royal Free Hospital and Marie Curie Hospice, Hampstead, London, UK

Alastair Lumb, Oxford University Hospitals NHS Foundation Trust, Oxford, UK

Samantha Lund, Medical Director, Royal Trinity Hospice, London, UK

Catherine Malia, Nurse Consultant St Gemma's Hospice Leeds, UK

Jonathan Martin, Consultant in Palliative Medicine, National Hospital for Neurology & Neurosurgery, University College London Hospitals NHS Foundation Trust, Central and North West London NHS Foundation Trust, London, UK

Emma Murphy, Associate Professor in Nephrology Nursing, University Hospitals Coventry and Warwickshire NHS Trust, Centre for Care Excellence, Coventry UK, Coventry University, Coventry, UK

Alison Mitchell, Consultant in Palliative Medicine Beatson West of Scotland Cancer Centre, NHS Greater Glasgow and Clyde, UK

Craig Montgomery, Consultant in Anaesthesia and Pain Medicine, The Leeds Teaching Hospitals NHS Trust, Leeds, UK

Jane Neerkin, Consultant in Symptom Control and Palliative Medicine, University College Hospital London, UK

Caroline Nicholson, Professor of Palliative care and Ageing, University of Surrey, Guildford, UK

Valerie Potter, Consultant in Palliative Medicine, St Bartholomew's Hospital, Bart's Health NHS Trust, London, UK

Melinda Presland, Consultant Pharmacist, Palliative and End of Life Care, Oxford University Hospitals NHS Trust, Oxford, UK

Annabel Price, Department of Public Health and Primary Care, University of Cambridge, Cambridge, UK

Rasha Al-Qurainy, Clinical Lead and Consultant in Palliative Medicine, University College London Hospital, London, UK

Libby Sallnow, Honorary Senior Clinical Lecturer, Marie Curie Palliative Care Research Group, University College London, London, UK

Lucy Selman, Associate Professor in Palliative and End of Life Care, University of Bristol, Bristol, UK

Caroline Shulman, University College London, London, UK

Richard Skipworth, Consultant Surgeon and Honorary Reader, Royal Infirmary of Edinburgh and University of Edinburgh, UK

Paddy Stone, Head of Marie Curie Palliative Care Research Department, University College London, London, UK

Anna Sutherland, Consultant in Palliative Medicine, Strathcarron Hospice, Denny and Forth Valley Royal Hospital, Larbert; and Honorary Senior Lecturer, Glasgow University, Glasgow, UK

Mark Taubert, Consultant and Clinical Director in Palliative Medicine, Professor in Palliative Medicine, Velindre University NHS Trust, Cardiff University School of Medicine, Cardiff, Wales

Mark Teo, Consultant Clinical Oncologist, Leeds Cancer Centre, St James University Hospital, Leeds, UK

Bee Wee, Consultant in Palliative Medicine, Oxford University Hospitals NHS Foundation Trust and Harris Manchester College, Oxford University, Oxford, UK

Lou Wiblin, Neurology Consultant with Special Interest in Movement Disorder and Palliative Care, James Cook Hospital, Middlesbrough, UK

Felicity Wood, Consultant Liaison Psychiatrist, Leeds and York Partnership NHS Foundation Trust, Leeds, UK

Lucy Wyld, Consultant in Palliative Medicine, Bradford Teaching Hospitals NHS Trust, Bradford, UK

Sarah Yardley, Associate Professor in Palliative Medicine Marie Curie Palliative Care Research Department, University College London, London, UK

SECTION 1

Pain management

CASE

1 Cancer-related Bone Pain

Anna Schuberth

Expert: Matt Mulvey

Case history

Michael, a 69-year-old retired accountant presented to his GP with new onset pain in his left thigh. The pain was 'aching' in nature and worse on weight bearing. Paracetamol and ibuprofen were not adequately controlling the pain. There was no history of trauma.

Eighteen months earlier, Michael had been diagnosed with adenocarcinoma of the prostate, Gleason 7, T3b. He underwent a radical prostatectomy. Subsequently Michael's prostate-specific antigen (PSA) rose, and he commenced bicalutamide followed by leuprorelin.

Expert Comment

Bone metastases are common in patients with advanced cancer. Epidemiological data suggest that approximately 70% of patients with breast and prostate cancer have bone metastases, 30–40% with lung cancer and other solid tumours. Bone metastases are less likely to be associated with gastrointestinal cancers.[2] Cancer-related bone pain is reported by 92% of patients with bone metastases.[3] Complications affecting bone integrity are known as skeletal-related events (SREs). These include the need for radiation to bone (to manage pain or prevent a fracture), pathological fractures, surgery to bone, and spinal cord compression, all of which can be pain-producing.

Clinical Tip Clinical Features of Cancer-related Bone Pain

'Annoying, gnawing, aching, and nagging'[1] are words commonly used to describe cancer-related bone pain. Pain is felt where bone metastases are present, most commonly, vertebrae, pelvis, long bones, and ribs. Patients with cancer-related bone pain may experience background pain, spontaneous pain, and movement-induced pain.

On examination Michael had swelling and focal tenderness on palpation of his left femur. He had full range of movement of his hip and knee. Neurological and vascular examination of his lower limbs were normal, as were his vital signs.

Learning Point Mechanisms of Cancer-related Bone Pain

The mechanisms of cancer-related bone pain are complex and involve inflammatory and neuropathic components.

Clinical Tip Imaging Modalities

The advantages and disadvantages of imaging modalities used in cancer-related bone pain are outlined in Table 1.1.

Table 1.1 Imaging modalities used in the investigation and diagnosis of cancer-related bone pain

Imaging modality	Advantages	Disadvantages
Plain radiograph	Widely available Relatively low cost	Sensitivity relatively low 30–50% bone mineral loss required for metastasis to be radiographically visible
CT	High sensitivity Enables soft tissues to be assessed Can be used to guide percutaneous biopsy for definitive diagnosis	Metastases have to involve the cortical bone to be detectable Relatively high cost

Learning Point Clinical Assessment

The European standards[4] for cancer pain management provide a helpful pain assessment process. Pain screening can be achieved by asking the patient whether they 'have experienced pain that interferes with daily activities' or via the use of a numerical rating scale (NRS) or visual analogue scale (VAS).

A detailed pain assessment should determine the intensity, aetiology, temporal characteristics, and underlying pain mechanism. The characteristics of cancer-related bone pain may change over time, so regular assessment is required.

Imaging modality	Advantages	Disadvantages
MRI	Enables bone marrow and soft tissues to be comprehensively assessed High sensitivity	Limited access Relatively high cost Some patients find MRI scanning claustrophobic
Bone scintigraphy (using technetium 99m methylene disphophonate)	Widely available Whole skeleton imaging Helpful for determining extent of metastatic bony disease	Sclerotic metastases can be poorly demonstrated Specificity relatively low
Positron Emission Tomography (PET)	High sensitivity Whole body imaging	Limited access Relatively high cost Reduced sensitivity in sclerotic metastases

Plain radiographs showed a lytic lesion in Michael's left femur (Figure 1.1). He was told this was likely to be a metastasis from his prostate cancer.

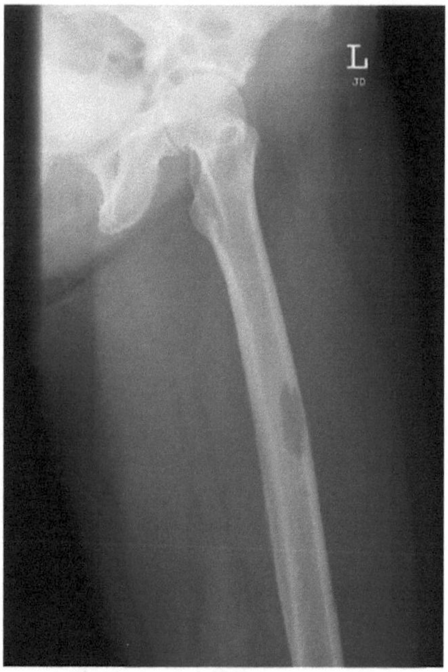

Figure 1.1 Radiograph showing bone metastasis to left femur.

Reproduced with permission from Sutcliffe, Robert P. et al., 'Biliary diseases', *Liver and Pancreatobiliary Surgery: with Liver Transplantation*, Oxford Specialist Handbooks (Oxford, 2009; online edn, Oxford Academic, 1 Oct. 2011), https://doi.org/10.1093/med/9780199205387.003.10, accessed 8 Apr. 2023.

Expert Comment

In cases of suspected neuropathic pain, imaging of a cancer lesion can provide useful evidence of a tumour-mass causing neural compression or destruction at the site of pain. When combined with the distribution of pain, and the presence/absence of sensory abnormalities, a rapid diagnosis of the likelihood of neuropathic pain can be made at the bedside. Application of the IASP NeupSIG neuropathic pain grading tool can be a quick and efficient method for ruling in or out neuropathic mechanisms.[5]

A pain assessment revealed predominantly nociceptive and inflammatory mechanisms of pain, therefore Michael was commenced on modified release (MR) morphine sulphate 10 mg BD.

Learning Point Non-pharmacological Interventions

Non-pharmacological interventions may provide pain relief with relatively few side effects. The use of heat, cold, and relaxation may be helpful for some patients with cancer-related bone pain.

A feasibility study indicated that movement-induced cancer-related bone pain may be helped by Transcutaneous Electrical Nerve Stimulation (TENS).[6] A recent systematic review and meta-analysis found moderate-certainty evidence that TENS results in lower pain intensity during or immediately after TENS compared to placebo,[7] for pain in adults, irrespective of their diagnosis.

Acupuncture may make pain more manageable by modulating emotional responses to pain. There have been studies showing some benefit, however, overall there is insufficient evidence to determine whether acupuncture is an effective treatment for cancer-related bone pain.[8]

Physiotherapy and occupational therapy have an important role in providing strategies to manage disability and promote, maintain, or restore function. The provision of aids and adaptations may also improve a patient's quality of life when living with cancer-related bone pain.

Learning Point Pharmacological Interventions

The World Health Organization (WHO) cancer pain treatment ladder is used to guide cancer pain management. The updated WHO guidance advises that when initiating analgesia, non-steroidal anti-inflammatory drugs (NSAIDs), paracetamol, and opioids alone or in combination can be used, depending on the assessment and severity of pain. If pain is moderate or severe, paracetamol and NSAIDs should not be used alone.[9]

There has been an assumption due to the role of inflammation in cancer-related bone pain that NSAIDs should be beneficial. Some evidence indicates that NSAIDs may be helpful for managing cancer pain, achieving benefit within one to two weeks.[10] In palliative care celecoxib is overall the oral NSAID of choice. Parecoxib, diclofenac, and ketorolac can be used subcutaneously, the gastrointestinal risks are significantly more for ketorolac. NSAIDs can have gastrointestinal, renal, and cardiovascular toxicity, so consideration needs to be given to the potential risks and benefits of their use.

Strong opioids often provide effective analgesia in moderate to severe cancer-related pain, and are usually the main treatment for background pain in cancer-related bone pain. National Institute for Health and Care Excellence (NICE) recommend oral sustained-release morphine first line for patients with advanced and progressive disease if they require a strong opioid[11]. Pain on movement can be more difficult to manage than background pain. Immediate-release morphine is usually trialled first, however if this is not effective, transmucosal (fast-acting) fentanyl is an option for movement-induced pain in patients on background opioids. Fast-acting fentanyl can be administered via sublingual, nasal, buccal, or oral routes.

Antidepressants and anticonvulsants can be used as adjuncts to strong opioids and may be helpful for managing a neuropathic aspect to the pain. Methodologically strong randomized controlled trial evidence did not find any benefit of gabapentin or pregabalin in cancer-related bone pain. However less robust evidence found a reduction in pain scores for pregabalin and gabapentin.[12] Clinically, the use of concurrent opioid and gabapentinoid therapy needs to be weighed against the increased risk of adverse effects and the uncertain research evidence.

The evidence for the use of corticosteroids for cancer-related bone pain is weak, with a lack of randomized controlled trial (RCT) level evidence, despite their widespread use.

Clinical Tip Mirels' Score and Surgery

Mirels proposed a scoring system to determine the risk of sustaining a pathological fracture in long bones affected by a metastasis.[13] The site, size, nature of the metastasis, and the presence of pain are the scoring criteria. A score of 8 or more indicates that prophylactic internal fixation is indicated.

Michael declined prophylactic surgical fixation, and underwent radiotherapy to his femur, which relieved his pain. He had restaging scans, which showed disease progression. Michael was offered further oncological treatment; however, he opted for best supportive care, and remained at home until his death three months later.

Learning Point Surgical Intervention

Prophylactic stabilization through surgical internal fixation may be considered for high-risk lesions, in patients with a good performance status. However, this is not always possible, due to the location of the lesion, for example if metastases affect the pelvis, scapulae, or ribs. High-risk vertebral lesions may be managed using the less invasive treatment of vertebroplasty or kyphoplasty. Both methods have been found to significantly and rapidly improve pain intensity and reduce disability.[14]

Pathological fractures can be managed surgically. Internal fixation is the management of choice for pathological long bone fractures to try and improve pain and function. If surgery is not possible or appropriate, radiotherapy can be useful for pain management, to reduce tumour bulk and restore bone integrity.

Expert Comment

The use of bone-targeting agents, such as bisphosphonates, can ameliorate pain complications associated with SREs. These agents can improve pain outcomes in patients with metastatic bone disease, although the time to analgesic effect can often be delayed.

Learning Point Radiotherapy

External beam radiotherapy should be considered if pain due to bone metastases is difficult to manage using pharmacological options. A meta-analysis of RCTs found that approximately 60% of patients obtained pain relief.[15] It may take up to 6–8 weeks for the full effect of radiotherapy to be achieved.

Overall and complete response rates have been found to be similar for single and multiple fraction schedules. Therefore, a single fraction is recommended for most patients with uncomplicated symptomatic bone metastases. Patients receiving single fraction radiotherapy are more likely to require retreatment. Retreatment with a further single fraction of radiotherapy can usually be undertaken, with an overall response rate for retreatment of 58–68%, and complete response rate of 20%.[16]

Some patients will experience a 'pain flare' following radiotherapy, where an increase in pain at the site of irradiation occurs, after 1–4 days. Prophylactic or adjuvant dexamethasone to prevent a pain flare is not supported by robust evidence.

Clinical Tip Side Effects of Bisphosphonates

Side effects include acute systemic inflammatory reactions, adverse renal effects, hypocalcaemia, ocular toxicity, and osteonecrosis affecting the jaw and external auditory canal. Renal function should be considered and monitored. Calcium and vitamin D supplements may be required. Dental screening and treatment is recommended prior to commencing bisphosphonates.

NICE recommends denosumab for patients with bone metastases due to solid tumours, except prostate cancer, for the prevention of SREs.

Learning Point Bisphosphonates

Bisphosphonates, such as zolendronic acid, pamidronate and ibandronate, are used to manage cancer-induced bone pain not responding to other treatment modalities and to prevent SREs. Bisphosphonates are usually used in cancer-related bone pain if analgesics and/or radiotherapy have not provided adequate analgesia. Due to the time of onset of analgesia, bisphosphonates should be considered if prognosis is more than two weeks. A systematic review found that bisphosphonates may delay the onset of pain rather than providing an analgesic effect.[17] However, a trial found that a single infusion of ibandronate provided a comparable outcome compared to a single fraction of radiotherapy.[18] A Cochrane review found evidence to support the use of bisphosphonates for bone pain, with a number needed to treat of 11 at 4 weeks and 7 at 12 weeks.[19]

Expert Comment

Denosumab may prevent pain worsening and delay the need for treatment with strong opioids. In patients with no or mild pain at baseline, denosumab reduced the risk of increasing pain severity and delayed pain worsening along with the time to increased pain interference compared with zolendronic acid, suggesting that use of denosumab before patients develop bone pain may improve outcomes.

Evidence Base Radiotherapy or Ibandronate (RIB) Trial

The RIB trial was a Phase 3, multicentre, randomized non-blind two-arm trial.[18] The primary end point was pain response at 4 weeks, reported using self-assessed pain scores and analgesic use. A single infusion of Ibandronate IV (6 mg) was compared to single-dose radiotherapy (8 Gy) in patients with prostate cancer and metastatic bone pain.

There was no difference for worst pain response (WHO criteria) at 4 weeks (ibandronate 49.5% vs. radiotherapy 53.1%, difference = 3.7%, CI −12.4% to 5.0%, P = 0.49) or 12 weeks using WHO criteria (ibandronate 56.1% vs. radiotherapy 49.4%, difference = 6.7%, CI −2.6–16%, P = 0.24). Radiotherapy was slightly more effective in the first 4 weeks. Quality of life was similar at 4 and 12 weeks.

Discussion

Michael's case illustrates how a patient may present with cancer-related bone pain, and the assessment and management options available. Cancer-related bone pain often remains a challenging symptom to manage due to the complex pathophysiological mechanisms, components of pain including background, spontaneous, and movement-induced pain, as well as the effects it can have on physical and psychological health and social functioning. Increased use of standardized classification tools (such as International classification of diseases (ICD) 11 classification of chronic cancer pain), assessment, and management guidelines to provide individualized treatment plans help optimize pain outcomes for patients.

Management focuses on preservation of function and pain management to optimize quality of life. Patients are managed using a multimodal approach with pharmacological therapies, namely opioids and NSAIDs. Radiotherapy has a significant role in the management of cancer-related bone pain, but consideration needs to be given as to whether a patient's prognosis is long enough for them to benefit. Other management options can be used if these measures are inadequate for controlling a patient's cancer-related bone pain.

Learning Point Radioisotopes

Radioisotopes can provide effective pain relief in patients with multiple osteoblastic bone metastases. Radium-223 is effective in improving bone pain and reducing SREs in patients with castrate-resistant prostate cancer. Radioisotope treatment using strontium, samarium or rhenium have shown a small positive effect on pain control in the short to medium term (1–6 months), however they are associated with bone marrow toxicity.

Future Advances

Well-designed pragmatic trials are needed to evaluate the benefits and harms of existing treatments, to build a reliable evidence base.

The use of biomarkers to identify patients who have a high risk of SREs, bone lesion progression, and patients who are more likely to benefit from treatments are being developed. For example, the biomarker MAF, which is amplified is approximately 20% of bone metastases has been used to determine patients who may benefit from zolendronic acid. Patients with normal MAF status predicted disease benefit with zolendronic acid, whereas patients with MAF amplification were more likely to suffer harm.[20]

Targeted therapies are also under development, such as targeted radionuclide therapy, for example Lutetium-177 labelled prostate-specific membrane antigen. Developments in treatment may be individualized to take into account the primary tumour site, and possibly other factors such as the characteristics of the pain.

Learning Point Interventional Analgesia

Referral to a pain team and interventional procedures should be considered if cancer-related bone pain is not responding to oral analgesia, radiotherapy, or bisphosphonates.

A Final Word from the Expert

Cancer-related bone pain remains the most common form of cancer-related pain. Better understanding of the underlying aetiology and pathophysiological mechanisms of cancer-related bone pain will improve the use and application of existing treatment options and drive further advances in novel treatment targets.

Opioids remain the mainstay analgesic treatment option for patients with cancer-related bone pain. Clinical trial data support the use of regular assessment of pain in patients with cancer-related bone pain using standardized tools to optimize patient outcomes by delivering tailored treatment plans to reduce the burden of cancer pain.

References

1. Laird BJA, Walley J, Murray GD, et al. Characterization of cancer-induced bone pain: an exploratory study. *Support Care Cancer* 2011; 19(9): 1393–1401.
2. Coleman RE. Clinical features of metastatic bone disease and risk of skeletal morbidity. *Clin Cancer Res* 2006; 12: 6243s–6249s.
3. Vieira C, Fragoso M, Pereira D, et al. Pain prevalence and treatment in patients with metastatic bone disease. *Oncol Lett* 2019; 17: 3362–3370.

4. Bennett MI, Eisenberg E, Ahmedzai SH, et al. Standards for the management of cancer-related pain across Europe: a position paper from the EFIC Task Force on Cancer Pain. *Eur J Pain* 2019; 23: 660–668.
5. Mulvey MR, Rolke R, Klepstad P, et al. Confirming neuropathic pain in cancer patients: applying the NeuPSIG grading system in clinical practice and clinical research. *Pain* 2014; 155: 859–863.
6. Bennett MI, Johnson MI, Brown SR, et al. Feasibility study of transcutaneous electrical stimulation (TENS) for cancer bone pain. *J Pain* 2009; 11(4): 251–359.
7. Johnson MI, Paley CA, Jones G, et al. Efficacy and safety of transcutaneous electrical nerve stimulation (TENS) for acute and chronic pain in adults: a systematic review and meta-analysis of 381 studies (the meta-TENS study). *BMJ Open* 2022; 12. Available at: https://bmjopen.bmj.com/content/bmjopen/12/2/e051073.full.pdf
8. Paley CA, Johnson MI, Tashani OA et al. Acupuncture for Cancer Pain in Adults. 2015. *Cochrane Database Syst Rev*. Available at: https://www.cochranelibrary.com/cdsr/doi/10.1002/14651858.CD007753.pub3/full
9. World Health Organization. WHO Guidelines for the Pharmacological and Radiotherapeutic Management of Cancer Pain in Adults and Adolescents. 2018. Available at: https://www.who.int/publications/i/item/9789241550390
10. Derry S, Wiffen PJ, Moore RA, et al. Oral non-steroidal anti-inflammatory drugs (NSAIDs) for cancer pain in adults. *Cochrane Database Syst Rev* 2017. Available at: https://www.cochranelibrary.com/cdsr/doi/10.1002/14651858.CD012638.pub2/full
11. National Institute for Health and Care Excellence. Palliative care for adults: strong opioids for pain relief. 2016. Available at: https://www.nice.org.uk/guidance/cg140/chapter/1-Recommendations
12. Miller S. Effectiveness of gabapentin and pregabalin for cancer-induced bone pain: a systematic review. *BMJ Support Palliat Care* 2017; 7(A46–A47).
13. Mirels H. Metastatic disease in long bones: a proposed scoring system for diagnosing impending pathologic fractures. *Clin Orthop Relat Res*1989; 249: 256–264.
14. Pron G, Holubowich C, Kaulback K. Vertebral augumentation involving vertebroplasty or kyphoplasty for cancer-related vertebral compression fractures: a systematic review. *Ont Health Technol Assess Ser* 2016; 16(11): 1–202.
15. Chow E, Zeng L, Salvo N, et al. Update on the systematic review of palliative radiotherapy trials for bone metastases. *Clin Oncol* 2012; 24(2): 112–124.
16. Wong E, Hoskin P, Bedard G et al. Re-irradiation for painful bone metastases—a systematic review. *Radiother Oncol* 2013; 110(1): 61–70.
17. Porta-Sales J, Garzon-Rodriguez C, Llorens-Torrome S, et al. Evidence on the analgesic role of bisphosphonates and denosumab in the treatment of pain due to bone metastases: a systematic review within the European Association for Palliative Care Guidelines Project. *Palliative Med* 2017; 31(1): 5–25.
18. Hoskin P, Sundar S, Reczko K, et al. A multicenter randomized trial of ibandronate compared with single-dose radiotherapy for localized metastatic bone pain in prostate cancer. *J Natl Cancer Inst* 2015; 107(10): djv197.
19. Wong RKS, Wiffen PJ. Bisphosphonates for the Relief if Pain Secondary to Bone Metastases. *Cochrane Database Syst Rev* 2002. Available at: https://www.cochranelibrary.com/cdsr/doi/10.1002/14651858.CD002068/full
20. Coleman R, Hadji P, Body J-J, Aapro M, Jordan K. Bone health in cancer: ESMO clinical practice guidelines. *Ann Oncol* 2020; 31(12): 1650–1663.

CASE

2 Cancer-related Neuropathic Pain

Rebecca Gemmell

Expert: Craig Montgomery

Case history

Ezra, a 55-year-old man, with locally advanced mesothelioma was referred to the community palliative care team. His disease had progressed despite chemotherapy and immunotherapy. Ezra had a Karnofsky performance status of 80 and continued to work. He was troubled by persistent pain at and around the site of his disease (pleura overlying the left lower lobe with direct invasion into the adjacent chest wall). Ezra's pain was constant, and he described it as burning in nature. The pain was felt in the left side of his chest, radiating around his chest in a radicular manner. On examination, there was mottling of Ezra's skin in the area where he described pain, numbness of that area, and allodynia. Ezra's sleep was frequently disrupted by pain. He had no other symptoms.

Learning Point

Neuropathic pain is defined by the International Association for the Study of Pain (IASP) as 'pain caused by a lesion or disease of the somatosensory nervous system'.[1]

Neuropathic pain may have many causes, arising from the peripheral nervous system and/or central nervous system. Neuropathic pain syndromes may range from peripheral neuropathy, radiculopathy, or plexopathy to central abnormalities such as those caused by leptomeningeal disease. Common causes include tumour infiltration; chemotherapy-induced neuropathy; post-herpetic neuralgia; diabetic neuropathy; and trauma.

Chemotherapy-induced peripheral neuropathy (CIPN) is increasingly important given cancer survivorship. CIPN is usually dose-dependent and typically appears in a glove and stocking distribution. Patients may also note increased sensitivity to hot or cold temperatures. Chemotherapy such as platinum drugs, taxanes, and thalidomide are most likely to cause CIPN.[2] Patients with diabetes or pre-existing neuropathy are more likely to develop CIPN.

Pain is often described as burning, tingling, shooting, or like an electric shock.

Neuropathic pain has both negative (e.g. sensory loss, numbness) and positive (e.g. tingling, allodynia, hyperalgesia) features. Neuropathic pain may be experienced alongside nociceptive pain, e.g. spinal metastatic disease causing both bone pain and radicular pain.

Clinical Tip

The Leeds Assessment of Neuropathic Symptoms and Signs (LANSS) pain scale is used to help diagnose neuropathic pain.[3] Data are derived from a questionnaire and an examination. A score of 12 or higher (out of a possible total of 24) indicates that pain is likely to be neuropathic in origin.

Descriptors such as prickling or tingling may suggest a neuropathic cause of pain. Observing skin mottling in the area of pain and determining the presence of allodynia on examination may also suggest a neuropathic cause for pain. Determining the distribution of positive and negative symptoms (e.g. dermatomal or a glove and stocking distribution), as well as other neurological signs (e.g. unilateral loss of power, tone or hyperreflexia) support the diagnosis.

At the time of referral to the palliative care team, Ezra was taking a low dose of immediate release (IR) oral morphine solution as required for pain. He had been using IR morphine 5 mg up to four times daily, which had been partially effective, providing some analgesia for 3 to 4 hours after each dose. Modified release (MR) morphine 10 mg twice daily was started to provide a background analgesia, with some improvement in pain. Ezra continued to work and preferred to minimize opioid use in order to minimize cognitive side effects of opioids.

Evidence Base

In 2013, Cochrane reviewed opioid use in neuropathic pain,[4] examining 31 studies evaluating the effect of opioids on neuropathic pain from any cause. Cochrane reported most studies were likely to overestimate the effectiveness of opioids due to small study size or short study duration. Evidence was equivocal regarding short term opioids, with opioids providing better analgesia than placebo in the intermediate term.

Due to side effects and potential for addiction and abuse, opioid use in neuropathic pain should be restricted to use by specialists.

Clinical Tip

The Neuropathic Pain Scale[5] is used to determine intensity of pain that has already been determined to be neuropathic in nature. It may be used to assess response to treatment or change in intensity of pain over time.

Ezra was keen to explore topical and non-pharmacological options to minimize tablet burden. A lidocaine patch was applied over the affected area of mottled skin. The patch was discontinued after a week's trial failed to have any significant effect on his pain. TENS (transcutaneous electrical nerve stimulation) was trialled with limited benefit and Ezra found it cumbersome. Capsaicin 0.075% cream produced an unpleasant intense burning sensation on application, with minimal impact on pain.

Learning Point

First line adjuvant medications for neuropathic pain include:

- amitriptyline
- duloxetine
- pregabalin
- gabapentin.[10]

The choice of drug is decided by factors including concurrent comorbidities, tablet burden, side-effect profile, and cost.

Patients preferring once-daily medications may prefer duloxetine or amitriptyline. Patients with concomitant depression may benefit from an antidepressant medication. Consideration should be given to renal impairment, cardiac disease, seizure threshold, and the availability of oral solution where this might be needed at a future point.

Clinical Tip

When managing neuropathic pain, topical interventions may be more acceptable to patients than medications. Use in neuropathic pain caused by cancer may be off-licence. Capsaicin cream is licensed for post-herpetic neuralgia and peripheral polyneuropathy. Lidocaine plasters are licensed for post-herpetic neuralgia.[6] Non-pharmacological interventions, such as TENS and acupuncture, may be trialled. The evidence base for their use is not strong.[7,8] Both topical and non-pharmacological management have side effects and may be poorly tolerated.

Lidocaine patches are expensive, and use is discouraged. Use should only be continued for patients receiving significant benefit from their application.[9]

Having optimized Ezra's opioids, balancing efficacy and adverse effects, adjuvant medications were discussed with Ezra. He had no significant comorbidities. He preferred to take as few tablets as possible. Ezra's pain was most troublesome at night and affected his sleep. Given these considerations, amitriptyline at night was selected as the initial treatment of choice, the common side-effect of drowsiness being beneficial for Ezra.

Evidence Base

Neuropathic pain has several potential underlying mechanisms, as reflected in its multiple potential pharmacological treatments.[12] Tricyclic antidepressants (TCAs) such as amitriptyline, or serotonin-noradrenaline reuptake inhibitors (SNRIs) such as duloxetine increase inhibitory descending pathways to reduce pain sensation. Their multiple sites of action mean that they are likely to reduce neuropathic pain through other mechanisms, such as blocking NMDA receptors in the spinal cord and modulating the immune system. However, their action on multiple receptors also causes side effects, largely relating to their anticholinergic activity. Anticholinergic side effects of tricyclic antidepressants include urinary retention, dry mouth, constipation, and orthostatic hypotension.

The action of tricyclic antidepressants on neuropathic pain is independent of their effect on depression, and the effective dose for neuropathic pain is much lower than the dose needed to treat depression.

Clinical Tip

Steroids may improve neuropathic pain by reducing inflammation surrounding the tumour e.g. where there is pain and weakness suggesting spinal cord compression.[10] Long-term steroid use should be avoided; steroid dose should be reduced to the lowest effective dose and used for the shortest possible duration.

A starting dose of amitriptyline 10 mg was partially effective for Ezra's pain. The dose was titrated to 50 mg over a four-week period. Ezra was still experiencing pain and an unacceptable level of drowsiness. Given the partial analgesic effect of an antidepressant, duloxetine was prescribed for Ezra. A dose of 30 mg once daily was commenced and titrated to 60 mg after 2 weeks. However, Ezra described intolerable drowsiness throughout the day.

Following unsuccessful trials of antidepressants, Ezra was started on antiepileptic medication. Pregabalin was started at a dose of 75 mg twice daily and titrated to 300 mg daily over 2 weeks, with a significant improvement in Ezra's pain. This dose was continued alongside the MR morphine. Ezra maintains a good quality of life and judges that he has an acceptable level of analgesia at present.

Expert Comment

The 2019 MHRA* safety update described the reclassification of gabapentanoids (gabapentin and pregabalin) to class C controlled drugs (under the UK Misuse of Drugs Act 1971) due to the risk of abuse and dependence. It recommends patient evaluation for a history of drug abuse before prescription, observation for signs of abuse and, most importantly in a palliative care setting, warning patients about potentially fatal drug interactions with other medicines that cause central nervous system (CNS) depression, including strong opioids.[11]

* Medicines and Healthcare products Regulatory Agency, UK

Evidence Base

Pregabalin and gabapentin bind to and inhibit the action of voltage-gated calcium channels, preventing the release of neurotransmitters causing pain. They also have an antagonistic effect at NMDA receptors, and may have other pharmacological sites of action.[12,13] Pregabalin is known to be beneficial in treating anxiety disorders and may be particularly useful for patients with coexisting anxiety.

The most extensive evidence base for gabapentinoids is in the management of post-herpetic and peripheral diabetic neuropathy, with less evidence for other forms of neuropathic pain.[14] Common side effects include drowsiness and dizziness.

Evidence Base

First- and second-line treatments for neuropathic pain may be compared by their number needed to treat (NNT) and number needed to harm (NNH). These values may have been determined in the context of specific neuropathic pain syndromes (e.g. diabetic neuropathy) and at particular doses of medications, which may not reflect real-life scenarios. Examples are shown in Table 2.1.[15]

Table 2.1 Number needed to treat and Number needed to harm

Medication	Number needed to treat (number of patients who would need to receive treatment to achieve 50% pain reduction for one patient)	Number needed to harm (number of patients who would need to receive treatment for one patient to withdraw from the study due to adverse effects)
Tricyclic antidepressants	3.6	28
Serotonin and norepinephrine reuptake inhibitors	6.4	11.8
Gabapentin	6.3	25.6
Pregabalin	7.7	13.9
Morphine	2.1 to 5.1 for 30% pain reduction	17.1

Source: data from Bates, D. et al. (2019). A comprehensive algorithm for management of neuropathic pain. *Pain Med.* 20(Suppl 1): S2–12. DOI: 10.1093/pm/pnz075.

Clinical Tip

Drug combinations can be trialled if one approach is well-tolerated but only partially effective.[10] Drug combinations should offer different mechanisms of action, for example, a combination of antidepressant and antiepileptic medications.

Clinical Tip

Due to the potential for abuse of gabapentinoids, patients should be evaluated for previous history of drug abuse before prescribing gabapentinoids, and once started, should be monitored for signs of drug abuse.[9]

Expert Comment

Patients who continue to have significant pain despite best medical management should be considered for interventional pain management treatments. Interventional treatments may include local nerve blocks with local anaesthetic or neurolytic agents such as alcohol or phenol, neuromodulation in the form of peripheral nerve or spinal cord stimulators, intrathecal pumps, or percutaneous cordotomy. The choice of technique is complex and depends upon a number of factors, such as location and character of pain, patient life expectancy, patient choice, and operator expertise. Communication with cancer pain management specialists and centres is important and ideally decisions are made in a multidisciplinary setting with patient involvement.

Expert Comment

Cervical percutaneous cordotomy is a highly specialist interventional pain management technique that can be utilized to provide unilateral pain relief below the shoulder (C4 dermatome). It can be particularly useful for the management of uncontrolled pain in lung mesothelioma. It is performed by creating a destructive lesion in the anterior spinothalamic tract under conscious sedation at the level of C1/2 with fluoroscopic or CT guidance. It can be considered in patients with an expected life expectancy of less than 1 year and unilateral pain below C4.

Learning Point

Under palliative medical specialist supervision, there may be a role for methadone, ketamine, systemic lidocaine, or antiepileptics such as oxcarbazepine or valproate.[10]

Methadone is a strong opioid with agonist action at μ opioid receptors. It also acts as an antagonist at NMDA receptors and inhibits presynaptic serotonin and noradrenaline uptake. Because of its risk of fatal cardiac arrythmias and difficulty with initiation and titration it is restricted to specialist use only.[10] There is some evidence for its use as a third line opioid, in particular where neuropathic pain is poorly responsive to opioids.[16]

Ketamine is an NMDA receptor blocker and is used off-licence in specialist palliative care for pain that has not responded to other treatments. The evidence base for its use is limited, with one study finding it as effective as placebo.[17] Ketamine may be more effective in patients with central sensitization, where central nervous system receptors are more sensitive to stimuli. Future studies may further explore the use of ketamine in this patient population.

Learning Point

Input from the multidisciplinary team should be considered alongside medication and anaesthetic interventions. Support from physiotherapy, occupational therapy, psychotherapists, and social workers should be included in the holistic management of patients with neuropathic pain. A multidisciplinary approach has been shown to benefit patients.[18]

A Final Word from the Expert

Pain management in palliative care settings can be complex, and patients often require trials of a range of medications to achieve satisfactory pain control. In those who do not achieve relief with medication and multidisciplinary team (MDT) interventions, consideration should be given to referral for specialist intervention. Ideally, multidisciplinary discussions should select appropriate patients. To help achieve this, the Framework for Provision of Pain Services for Adults Across the UK with Cancer or Life-limiting Disease has been written by several medical colleges as a collaborative document.[19] This covers the level of assessment and intervention expected of each healthcare group from group 1 (all healthcare professional) through to group 4 (specialist cancer pain medicine consultants).

References

1. International Association for the Study of Pain. Terminology | International Association for the Study of Pain [Internet]. International Association for the Study of Pain (IASP). 2011. Available at: https://www.iasp-pain.org/resources/terminology/
2. Brown TJ, Sedhom R, Gupta A. Chemotherapy-induced peripheral neuropathy. *JAMA Oncol* 2019; 5(5): 750.
3. Bennett M. The LANSS Pain Scale: the Leeds assessment of neuropathic symptoms and signs. *Pain* 2001; 92(1): 147–157.
4. McNicol ED, Midbari A, Eisenberg E. Opioids for neuropathic pain. *Cochrane Database Syst Rev* 2013; 8: CD006146.
5. Galer BS, Jensen MP. Development and preliminary validation of a pain measure specific to neuropathic pain: the neuropathic pain scale. *Neurology* 1997; 48(2): 332–338.
6. NICE. BNF treatment summary—neuropathic pain. *NICE*. Available at: https://bnf.nice.org.uk/treatment-summaries/neuropathic-pain/
7. Ju ZY, Wang K, Cui HS, et al. Acupuncture for neuropathic pain in adults. *Cochrane Database Syst Rev* 2016; 12(12): CD012057.
8. Gibson W, Wand BM, O'Connell NE. Transcutaneous electrical nerve stimulation (TENS) for neuropathic pain in adults. *Cochrane Database Syst Rev* 2017; 9(9): CD011976.
9. NICE. NICE CKS Neuropathic pain—drug treatment [Internet]. *NICE*. 2022. Available at: https://cks.nice.org.uk/topics/neuropathic-pain-drug-treatment/
10. Wilcock A. *Palliative Care Formulary*. 8th ed. London: Pharmaceutical Press; 2022.
11. Medicines and Healthcare products Regulatory Agency. Drug safety update latest advice for medicines users—the monthly newsletter from the Medicines and Healthcare products Regulatory Agency and its independent advisor the Commission on Human. 2019. Available at: https://assets.publishing.service.gov.uk/government/uploads/system/uploads/attachment_data/file/795950/April-2019-PDF-final.pdf
12. Fornasari D. Pharmacotherapy for neuropathic pain: a review. *Pain Ther* 2017; 6(S1): 25–33.
13. Finnerup NB, Attal N, Haroutounian S. Pharmacotherapy for neuropathic pain in adults: a systematic review and meta-analysis. *J Vasc Surg* 2015; 62(4): 1091.
14. Wiffen PJ, Derry S, Bell RF, et al. Gabapentin for chronic neuropathic pain in adults. Cochrane Database Syst Rev. 2017;(6). Available at: https://www.cochrane.org/CD007938/SYMPT_gabapentin-chronic-neuropathic-pain-adults
15. Bates D, Schultheis BC, Hanes MC, et al. A comprehensive algorithm for management of neuropathic pain. *Pain Med* 2019; 20(Supplement_1): S2–12.
16. Ding H, Song Y, Xin W, et al. Methadone switching for refractory cancer pain. *BMC Palliative Care* 2022; 21(1): 191.
17. Fallon MT, Wilcock A, Kelly CA, et al. Oral ketamine vs placebo in patients with cancer-related neuropathic pain. *JAMA Oncol* 2018; 4(6): 870.
18. Shaygan M, Böger A, Kröner-Herwig B. Predicting factors of outcome in multidisciplinary treatment of chronic neuropathic pain. *J Pain Res* 2018; 11: 2433–2443.
19. Faculty of Pain Medicine, Association for Palliative Medicine, Association of Cancer Physicians, The Royal College of Radiologists (Faculty of Clinical Oncology), Independent Chair. Framework for provision of pain services for adults across the UK with cancer or life-limiting disease. 2019. Available at: https://fpm.ac.uk/sites/fpm/files/documents/2019-07/Framework%20for%20pain%20services%20cancer%20and%20life%20limiting%20disease%202019.pdf

CASE

3 Interventional Pain Management

Lucy Hetherington

Expert: Alison Mitchell

Case history

A 63-year-old female, Marie, was referred by her local palliative care team to the interventional cancer pain service with a six-month history of right hip pain. She had metastatic breast cancer and an un-displaced pathological fracture of the right acetabulum. Surgical management had been considered but was not feasible. Marie had been treated with radiotherapy to her right hip. This was initially effective for one month after the fracture, but when repeated due to increasing pain there was no benefit. She was receiving weekly paclitaxel chemotherapy and had a prognosis of around two years.

Marie described pain deep in her right hip and right groin. Rest pain had been controlled by analgesia but she was still experiencing severe pain on movement. She was only able to mobilize a few metres using a stick and this resulted in unbearable pain. Stairs were particularly problematic. Marie was taking oxycodone modified release 15 mg twice daily, pregabalin 75 mg twice daily, paracetamol 1 g four times a day and oxycodone immediate release 5 mg as required, on average using it four times per day. Attempts to titrate opioid and adjuvant analgesia had been unsuccessful in managing the pain and had resulted in confusion and lethargy. The degree of pain experienced was significantly limiting her quality of life and she felt her overall function was declining as a result.

Expert Comment When to Consider Interventional Pain Management

Consider interventional cancer pain management when pain is not responding or amenable to conventional measures.[1,2] Usually, surgical options will have been considered and radiotherapy may have been trialled if appropriate. Attempts to titrate opioid and adjuvant analgesia may have been limited by inefficacy or by intolerable side effects such as toxicity or decline in function.

Discussion

Marie was referred to the interventional cancer pain service where she underwent a multi-professional assessment incorporating consultants in Palliative Medicine and Anaesthetics, a specialist nurse, a specialist physiotherapist, and a clinical psychologist. Time was taken to ascertain Marie's goals. These were to maintain her independence, in particular to be able to stand in the kitchen to cook a meal and to take her granddaughter to the park. Continuing chemotherapy was very important to her. She reported Brief Pain Inventory (BPI) scores of 10 at worst, 6 at least, 8 on average, and 7 during the assessment.[3] Her worst pain was on descending stairs.

Expert Comment Multi-professional Assessment

Careful patient selection for an interventional approach is essential and includes a multi-professional assessment of symptoms, disease status, psychological, and social factors, current and previous treatments and consideration of other treatment options.[1,2]

The multidisciplinary team (MDT) considered Marie's case and possible interventions. Intrathecal drug delivery (ITDD) and percutaneous cervical cordotomy (PCC) were both discussed as possible options and a decision was made to offer ITDD based on the patient's prognosis being near the maximum of two years that would be deemed appropriate for PCC. As well as Marie's goals, the team also set goals. These were to reduce the pain score on mobilizing by 2 points, to enable her to manage stairs more comfortably and to reduce the side effects from analgesia.

Learning Point **Intrathecal Drug Delivery (ITDD)**

Intrathecal catheters allow continuous drug delivery into the cerebrospinal fluid (CSF), delivering opioid and local anaesthetic mixture directly to dorsal horn/spinal nerves.

Temporary, external pumps can be used as a short-term intervention or a trial of intrathecal drug delivery.

Fully implanted pumps can be used for ongoing drug delivery and refilled via a subcutaneous needle port at regular intervals (see Figure 3.1).

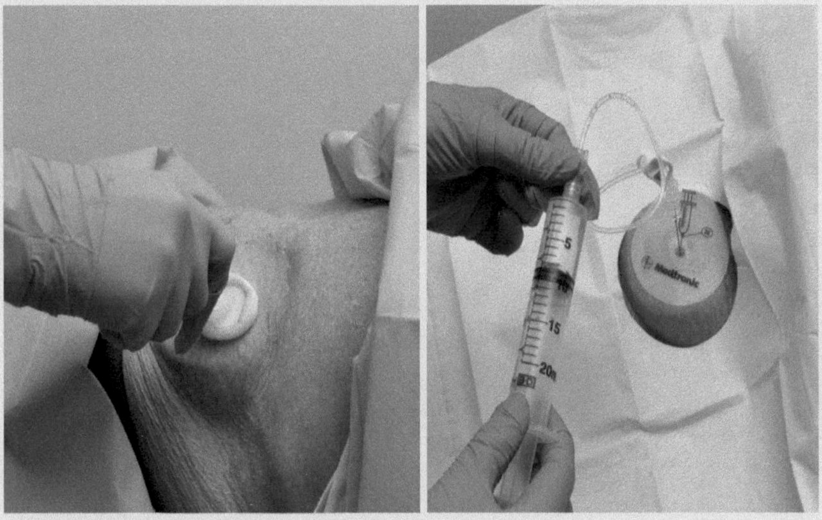

Figure 3.1 Refill of an implanted intrathecal pump.

Intrathecal Opioids:

- Inhibit pain transmission at dorsal horn
- Effective dose is around 1/300 of oral dose
- Can provide effective analgesia with very few side effects

Intrathecal Local Anaesthetic:

- No alternative oral option
- LA delivered directly to site of action
- Offers segmental analgesia -below the waist
- Sodium channel blockade
- Sensory/motor nerve blockade
- Effect is reversible

Expert Comment **Goal-setting**

Goal setting is an essential step in interventional cancer pain management. It is of vital importance that the patient has clear, achievable goals that are realistic and align with those set by the clinical team. If a patient has unrealistic goals and is unable to modify them, then an interventional procedure may not be appropriate. Reflecting on goals and evaluating the outcome against goals can help assess the outcome and guide decision-making.[1,2]

Evidence Base **Intrathecal Drug Delivery**

ITDD can improve quality of life, pain control, and reduce drug toxicity compared to comprehensive medical management.[4-6]

ITDD has been found to be a cost-effective alternative to systemic, intravenous, or external infusion devices for cancer patients who require pain management for three months or more.[7,8]

The British Pain Society (BPS) supports the use of ITDD for cancer pain where this is not controlled by systemic analgesia or where systemic analgesia causes intolerable side effects.[1] BPS also believes ITDD to be a cost-effective method in this circumstance, with the cost per quality adjusted life year falling within the NICE willingness to pay threshold.[1]

Clinical Tip Intrathecal Drug Delivery

ITDD can be helpful for:

- Bilateral pain, below the waist
- Sacral, pelvic pain
- Patients with an uncertain prognosis (can be continued indefinitely)
- Patients who can attend for refills

ITDD can be titrated as disease progresses.

ITDD can be continued at the end of life.

Learning Point Percutaneous Cervical Cordotomy (PCC)

PCC is a specialized injection to the side of the neck, performed with the patient awake, through which the spinothalamic tract is located and lesioned, using a radiofrequency electrode, in order to relieve one-sided pain below the neck (see Figure 3.2).

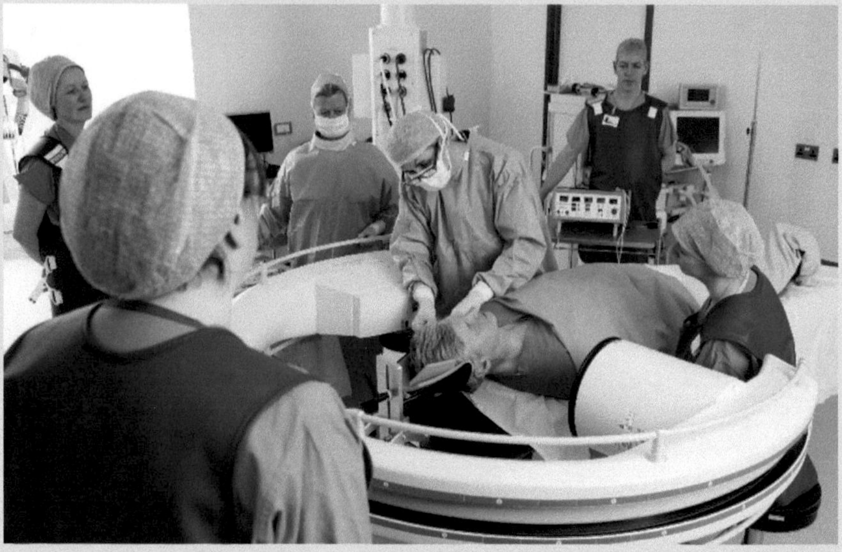

Figure 3.2 Performing a percutaneous cervical cordotomy (PCC).

- Selective radiofrequency destruction of the spinothalamic tract, on one side of the spinal cord. Performed at the level C1–C2.
- Results in selective loss of pain and temperature, unilaterally, below the neck on the contralateral side, with no other sensory or motor deficit.
- Is irreversible.
- Can be very effective for unilateral chest wall pain such as from mesothelioma, lung, or breast cancer.

Evidence Base Percutaneous Cervical Cordotomy

The evidence base for PCC in cancer pain is small but demonstrates good initial pain relief in most patients (80-98%).[9] There is some evidence of ongoing benefit at six-month follow-up, but data on duration of effect is limited by short follow-up periods and the prognosis of patients selected for treatment.[9] Life-threatening complications occur in 1%, but minor side effects are common (transient headache, mirror pain, temporary weakness, and mild dysaesthesia).[10]

Following PCC for mesothelioma pain, a study of 52 patients found 83% of patients had a reduction in pain such that their dose of opioid could be halved. Of these, 38% were able to stop their opioid completely.[11]

A systematic review of PCC for mesothelioma related pain found the available evidence to be of limited quantity and quality but concluded it to be a safe and effective procedure for patients with intractable pain due to mesothelioma.[12]

A review of UK national data found PCC to be an effective treatment for unilateral cancer pain; however, PCC referrals tended to be late in patients' disease trajectories.[13]

Clinical Tip Percutaneous Cervical Cordotomy

Useful for unilateral, localized pain below the neck and above the knees.

- Can only be performed on one side due to risk of hypoventilation with bilateral interruption of reticulospinal fibres.
- Reduced respiratory reserve, particularly lung disease affecting the ipsilateral lung, would be a relative contraindication requiring further consideration of the risks and benefits of cordotomy.[9]
- In time, nerve fibre regeneration may result in pain as, or more, severe than the original pain.[9] As a result, PCC would not normally be used where life expectancy is greater than two years.
- The patient needs to be alert, cooperative, and able to lie flat and still for 60 minutes.

Future Advances Cordotomy Registry

Much of the published evidence on cordotomy has been limited to case series data and individual clinical experience. Steps have been taken to collect cordotomy data nationally in the UK which has helped to further understanding of its role and utility, although this has been limited by the small number of procedures performed.[13] Ongoing data collection on a national level may help further understanding and promote advances in the field. Data collection internationally would be ideal in order to collect data from a larger number of procedures, since the number done in any one country is likely to be low.

Marie proceeded to a trial of intrathecal drug delivery (opioid and local anaesthetic) via an intrathecal catheter and external pump. Within 24 hours she was able to mobilize more and pain was less problematic. Intrathecal drugs were titrated over a few days, as an inpatient, and regular opioids and pregabalin were discontinued. The team met with Marie and her husband and it was agreed that Marie had met her goals. She had a permanent implanted pump fitted prior to discharge.

Expert Comment Intrathecal Drug Delivery Trial Period

A trial of ITDD allows the patient and the multi professional team to evaluate the efficacy of ITDD as an analgesic treatment modality. There are several ways of conducting a trial:

- Intrathecal infusion
- Epidural infusion
- Bolus injections

A trial of a continuous intrathecal infusion most closely simulates the effect of a permanent implanted pump and therefore will give the most realistic assessment of the potential benefits of an implanted intrathecal pump prior to committing to it.

An implanted intrathecal pump requires refilling up until and including end of life so it is imperative to be clear that the patient is benefitting prior to committing the patient to this process.

At assessment one month following her implanted pump Marie attended clinic review with well controlled pain. She reported that she was comfortably managing the stairs with 1/10 pain. She reported BPI scores of worst 2, least 0, average 2, and at assessment 1. Marie was managing to spend quality time with her granddaughter and attend for ongoing chemotherapy. She was no longer on adjuvant analgesia and was requiring occasional 2 mg oxycodone for breakthrough pain. Marie's energy levels had improved and medication related toxicity resolved.

Learning Point Ongoing Oncological Treatment and Imaging

Patients can continue to receive systemic anticancer treatment with an implanted intrathecal pump. There is no contraindication to computerized tomography (CT) scanning. Magnetic resonance imaging (MRI) is also possible but this should be discussed with an expert so that the pump can be interrogated immediately after scanning to ensure the pump is running safely and effectively.

Marie continued to attend two-weekly for intrathecal pump refills. She developed bone metastasis to her left shoulder resulting in new pain. This pain was outside of the area covered by her intrathecal. It was managed initially with radiotherapy and naproxen. Shoulder pain later progressed and a low dose of modified release oxycodone was introduced in addition to intrathecal drug delivery, with good effect. Marie lived with her pump for 16 months before dying from metastatic breast cancer. For months she walked into clinic with help of her stick and was significantly more active than before intervention. Marie was able to spend most of her remaining time at home with her family and even managed to go abroad on holiday. As her cancer progressed, she became less mobile due to fatigue and general deterioration. Escalation of pain towards the end of life was managed with titration of her intrathecal pump.

Expert Comment Selection and Titration of Intrathecal Medication

There are a small number of medications with evidence for use in cancer pain via the intrathecal route. These include:

- Opioids including preservative free morphine (PFM) and fentanyl.
- Local anaesthetics.
- Clonidine (an alpha-2 agonist).
- Ziconitide (a calcium channel blocker).

There is pharmacy stability data supporting the use of a combination of PFM and bupivacaine.[14]

The 1 to 300 conversion is used for converting the 24-hour oral morphine equivalent (OME) of the existing opioid to a 24-hour dose of intrathecal PFM.

For example:

- Morphine sulphate modified release 60 mg twice daily is equivalent to 0.4 mg intrathecal PFM over 24 hours.

With titration of intrathecal local anaesthetic, a balance must be struck between improved pain control and retention of motor function. The desired balance will vary depending on the patients' goals and stage of disease. As a patient's overall condition declines with advancing disease, they may spend increasing periods in bed, such that maintaining motor function is of lower importance to them.

Marie was admitted to hospice for her end of life care as per her wish. A continuous subcutaneous infusion was commenced to deliver additional medication at the end-of-life while her intrathecal pump continued. After her death Marie's family wrote to the team to express gratitude. They described how the intervention had transformed Marie's life and helped her to live viewing every day as a blessing.

Learning Point Other Interventional Procedures

Coeliac plexus block, using 100% alcohol neurolysis.[15]

- Useful for visceral pain related to upper gastrointestinal (GI) malignancy.
- Block is performed under X-ray or ultrasound guidance, or may have been performed at laparotomy (check operative notes).
- Patient can be awake or sedated.
- Patient must be able to lie prone for around 30 minutes.

Phenol intrathecal neurolysis

- Useful for pelvic and sacral pain
- There is a high risk of loss of bladder, bowel, and lower limb motor control so reserved for end-of-life or use in those with poor baseline function.

Alcohol intrathecal neurolysis

- Helpful for chest wall pain.
- Less effective than cordotomy and shorter duration of action.
- Potential to perform procedure bilaterally (on different days).
- Can be repeated as needed.

A Final Word from the Expert

Pain is a common symptom in patients with cancer. Standard pain management, following the WHO three step analgesic ladder provides effective pain management in approximately 70–90% of cancer patients. However, cancer pain may be refractory to treatment if the standard approach is ineffective, or there are intolerable adverse side effects from the analgesic medication. An interventional approach is indicated in an estimated 5-15% of patients with cancer pain and is underused.[1] The Framework for Provision of Pain Services for Adults Across the UK with Cancer or Life Liming disease is a collaborative document that sets out operational guidance for managing cancer pain, including access to specialist cancer pain interventions where the patient is assessed by a multi-professional team and interventions are offered by pain management consultants with relevant expertise.[2]

An awareness of the role of interventions and equitable access to these services on a regional level is essential for comprehensive cancer pain management.[1,2]

References

1. Duarte R, Raphael J, Eldabe S. Intrathecal drug delivery for the management of pain and spasticity in adults: an executive summary of the British Pain Society's recommendations for best clinical practice. *Br J Pain* 2016; 10(2): 67–69.
2. Faculty of Pain Medicine. Framework for provision of pain services for adults across the UK with cancer or life-limiting disease. 2019; 1–14. Available at: https://fpm.ac.uk/sites/fpm/files/documents/2019-07/Framework%20for%20pain%20services%20cancer%20and%20life%20limiting%20disease%202019.pdf
3. Cleeland CS. *Brief Pain Inventory User Guide*. Available at: https://www.mdanderson.org/documents/Departments-and-Divisions/Symptom-Research/BPI_UserGuide.pdf
4. Smith TJ, Coyne PJ, Staats PS, et al. An implantable drug delivery system (IDDS) for refractory cancer pain provides sustained pain control, less drug-related toxicity, and possibly better survival compared with comprehensive medical management (CMM). *Ann Oncol* 2005; 16(5): 825–833.
5. Smith TJ, Coyne PJ. Implantable drug delivery systems (IDDS) after failure of comprehensive medical management (CMM) can palliate symptoms in the most refractory cancer pain patients. *J Palliat Med* 2005; 8(4): 736–742.
6. Mitchell A, McGhie J, Owen M, McGinn G. Audit of intrathecal drug delivery for patients with difficult-to-control cancer pain shows a sustained reduction in pain severity scores over a 6-month period. *Palliat Med* 2015; 29(6): 554–563.
7. Hassenbusch SJ, Paice JA, Patt RB, Bedder MD, Bell GK. Clinical realities and economic considerations: economics of intrathecal therapy. *J Pain Symptom Manage* 1997; 14(3 Suppl): S36–48.
8. Mueller-Schwefe G, Hassenbusch SJ, Reig E. Cost effectiveness of intrathecal therapy for pain. *Neuromodulation* 1999; 2(2): 77–87.
9. Javed S, Viswanathan A, Abdi S. Cordotomy for intractable cancer pain: a narrative review. *Pain Physician* 2020; 23(3): 283–292.

10. Feizerfan A, Antrobus JHL. Role of percutaneous cervical cordotomy in cancer pain management. *Cont Educ Anaesth Crit Care Pain* 2014; 14(1): 23–26.
11. Jackson MB, Pounder D, Price C, Matthews AW, Neville E. Percutaneous cervical cordotomy for the control of pain in patients with pleural mesothelioma *Thorax* 1999; 54: 238–241.
12. France BD, Lewis RA, Sharma ML, Poolman M. Cordotomy in mesothelioma-related pain: a systematic review. *BMJ Support Palliat Care* 2014; 4: 19–29.
13. Poolman M, Makin M, Briggs J. Percutaneous cervical cordotomy for cancer-related pain: national data. *BMJ Support Palliat Care* 2020; 10: 429–434.
14. Deer TR, Pope JE, Hayek SM, et al. The Polyanalgesic Consensus Conference (PACC): Recommendations on Intrathecal Drug Infusion Systems Best Practices and Guidelines. *Neuromodulation* 2017; 20(2): 96–132.
15. Arcidiacono PGG, Calori G, Carrara S, McNicol ED, Testoni PA. Celiac plexus block for pancreatic cancer pain in adults. *Cochrane Database Syst Rev* 2011(3): CD007519.

CASE

4 Pain in People with Substance Use Disorder

Lucy Hetherington

Expert: Christopher Farnham

Case history

A 49-year-old lady, Lydia, was admitted to hospital having been found unresponsive at home. She reported a six-month history of weight loss, increasing breathlessness and back pain. Investigations revealed a new diagnosis of lung cancer with pulmonary, nodal, and bone metastases.

Lydia had a history of substance use disorder, with previous use of heroin intravenously. She took methadone medication-assisted treatment (MAT), 50 mg daily, dispensed weekly. Past medical history included chronic obstructive pulmonary disease (COPD), anxiety, and depression. Lydia had a good rapport with her substance use services (SUS) key worker but despite concerns about her weight loss and breathlessness, she had declined medical review.

The admitting team suspected that Lydia may have taken non-prescribed substances resulting in a reduced level of consciousness. They were concerned about prescribing methadone and analgesia. Lydia was referred to the hospital palliative care team (HPCT) for assistance with symptom control.

Evidence Base Drug Use Trends and An Ageing Population

There is a high prevalence of substance use in the UK (9.4% in England and Wales, 12% in Scotland and 5.9% in Northern Ireland).[1] The age of people using drugs in the UK continues to trend upwards such that 56% of people in treatment are over 40 years old.[2] This growing, ageing cohort is at increased risk of developing life-limiting illness, both drug and non-drug-related. They are frequently from deprived communities with consequent health inequalities and comorbidity. Substance use may lead to an earlier age of death and a greater burden of disease and ill health.[3]

Over recent years there has been an increase in polydrug use, especially benzodiazepine co-use.[4] Benzodiazepines may potentiate the effects of prescribed and non-prescribed substances, increasing the risk of respiratory depression when taken alongside opioids, particularly in older people. Patients may experience withdrawal from benzodiazepines on admission to hospital.

Provision of palliative care for those with substance use disorder is of high and growing importance, and can be particularly complex.

Clinical Tip Multiple Complex Needs/Severe Multiple Disadvantage

Substance use is often driven by complex life challenges, a history of poverty, childhood adversity, and trauma. Furthermore, there is a high association with physical and mental ill health, poor housing or homelessness, contact with the criminal justice system and gender-based violence. Health and social care models struggle to comprehensively meet these multiple needs, and patients are often passed from one service to another.[5] This experience, combined with a possible history of trauma and subsequent distrust, fear of stigma, and fear of inappropriate management of substance use disorder, can result in healthcare avoidance and delayed presentation.

Pharmacology of symptom control can be complex, challenging social circumstances are common, and providing continuity of care can be difficult.

It is vital that these patients are offered compassionate, coordinated, trauma-informed, non-judgemental care.[6]

The HPCT recognized the complex situation and arranged an early review. They offered Lydia reassurance that they would work jointly with SUS to prescribe the appropriate medication for symptom control, alongside the ongoing use of methadone MAT.

After discussing the shock of her new diagnosis, Lydia confided that she used street benzodiazepine in addition to methadone. She found it helpful for her pain. Lydia had taken benzodiazepines on the day of admission, as her pain was very severe. She reported that she had not taken additional street opioids but had occasionally taken some of her partner's methadone when the pain was particularly troublesome.

History and examination revealed lumbar spinal pain, which increased with movement and on palpation. There was radicular radiation around her flanks. Neurological examination was normal. Lydia was troubled by shortness of breath on exertion and constipation. She was anxious about being in hospital and about her diagnosis. Lydia was worried she might experience withdrawal from benzodiazepines.

After discussion with SUS, methadone MAT was continued at Lydia's normal dose (see Figure 4.1). For analgesia, Morphine sulphate modified release (MR) 20 mg BD was commenced and morphine sulphate immediate release (IR) 7 mg, orally, as required for breakthrough pain. In this hospital setting, a minimum interval of hourly was set, with clear instruction to contact the palliative care team if frequent breakthrough was required. Lydia was also commenced on diazepam 2 mg QDS and laxatives.

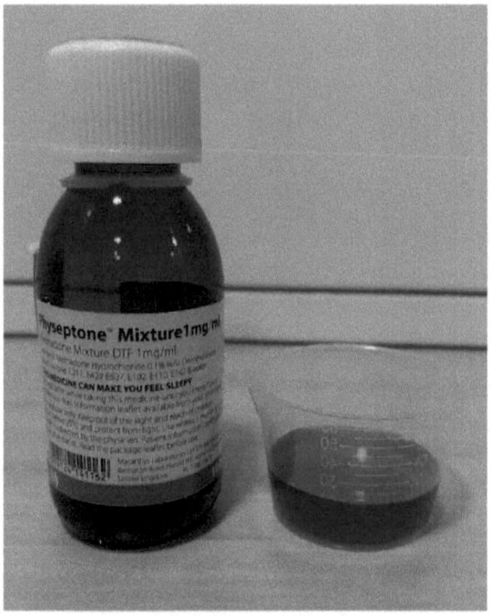

Figure 4.1 Oral methadone liquid.

Expert Comment Compassionate Joined-up Care

Compassionate communication is essential in order to build trust and encourage disclosure of substance use. Once reassured that the information is required to provide optimal treatment, and that MAT will be continued, patients may be more willing to speak honestly. A punitive approach should not be taken as this is likely to reduce the chance of disclosure.

It is of vital importance that decisions are made jointly with SUS and that patients are treated holistically. A joint review with SUS may be beneficial where possible. In some circumstances, a case conference may be of value. This is particularly valuable when planning complex discharges.

Try to familiarize yourself with your local SUS provision, including access to SUS out of hours.

Learning Point Prescribing Opioids

Healthcare professionals can be reluctant to prescribe opioids where there is a history of substance use.[7,8] Under-prescribing could influence the patient to seek non-prescribed substances for symptom management. A patient with a history of substance use may have reservations about starting opioids. This will require careful and sensitive discussion.

- MAT should continue as advised by SUS and would not usually be titrated for palliative symptom control.[9]
- MAT should be treated as a separate prescription and not counted in breakthrough dose calculations.
- Whilst the patient may have a degree of opioid tolerance, this is variable and difficult to predict. Opioids should therefore be started as they normally would for symptom control. Regular review and responsive titration are paramount.
- Aim to proactively titrate the background MR opioid in order to minimize reliance on immediate-release opioid preparations.
- Frequent breakthrough use may be a sign of inappropriate use or uncontrolled pain.[10]

Clinical Tip Methadone Medication Assisted Treatment in Palliative Care

- Ensure joint working between services and clarity as to who will provide which scripts.[7]
- If a patient has missed doses of their methadone, or may not have been taking it as prescribed, discuss with SUS for advice around the reintroduction.
- If the oral route is not available, methadone can be administered as a continuous subcutaneous infusion (CSCI) at 50% of the daily oral dose. This should be diluted in 0.9% saline and administered in a syringe without any other drugs over 24 hours.[11] The site should be monitored as local irritation is common.
- Where a CSCI is not practicable, Methadone MAT could be administered at 50% of the daily oral dose split into twice daily subcutaneous bolus injections.[11]
- Methadone can prolong the QT interval. Care should be taken when adding other QT-prolonging drugs.
- Methadone dose may require 50% reduction where eGFR falls below 10 ml/min or in hepatic failure.[11]

Clinical Tip Buprenorphine Medication Assisted Treatment in Palliative Care

Buprenorphine has partial opioid agonist (mu opioid receptors and opioid-receptor-like) and partial antagonist properties (kappa opioid and delta opioid receptors).[7] Antagonism of the kappa opioid receptor means it provides less euphoric and less sedating effects compared to methadone. Because of its higher affinity for opioid receptors, it reduces the effect of additional opioids.[12]

- For MAT, buprenorphine may be combined with an opioid antagonist (e.g. naloxone or naltrexone) as a misuse deterrent. Analgesia in this circumstance is particularly challenging.

- Buprenorphine MAT is usually prescribed at higher doses than buprenorphine in the palliative care setting. Even without an opioid antagonist this can result in antagonism when other opioids are required, typically with doses of 16 mg per day or higher.[13]
- A switch to methadone MAT, guided by SUS, could be considered where additional opioids are required and antagonism is a concern.
- There is increasing use of long-acting subcutaneous buprenorphine preparations for MAT such as Buvidal®. These last for up to 4 weeks.[14] This poses additional challenges when analgesia is required.
- Where opioid analgesia is required alongside buprenorphine MAT, opioids with a high mu opioid receptor affinity, such as fentanyl and alfentanil, may be more effective.[14, 15]
- Titration of short-acting opioids to the desired analgesic effect in those treated with buprenorphine may require higher doses.[15]
- If the oral route is lost when using oral buprenorphine MAT discussion with SUS may help in selecting an alternative opioid or route.
- Buprenorphine is well tolerated in renal failure. In severe hepatic impairment, smaller doses and cautious titration would be advised.[16]

Morphine sulphate MR was titrated over subsequent days with improved pain control. An MRI spine confirmed lumbar metastases and ruled out cord compression. Lydia's case was discussed at the lung multidisciplinary team meeting. Oncology follow-up was arranged for lumbar spinal radiotherapy and consideration of systemic anti-cancer therapy (SACT).

Lydia's goal was to improve pain control and spend time with her 20-year-old daughter. She had recently secured her own flat after a period of living in hostels and was re-forging a relationship with her daughter. She was discharged home with community palliative care follow-up. Lydia's case was discussed directly with her GP, pharmacy, and SUS including discussions around the safe provision of controlled drugs.

Expert Comment Provision of Controlled Drugs in the Community

Decide who will issue controlled drug prescriptions—this is normally the GP. Be clear with the patient, carers, hospice, and hospital providers about who is prescribing, what, and how often. Allow SUS to continue their own separate prescribing.

Note the circumstances in which the patient is living—for example, is it safe for them to have opioids in the house/accommodation—many hostels are 'dry' and it may be difficult to enable access to pain relief. Consider topical, longer-acting preparations that require less or easier storage.

Consider how the prescriber will respond to 'lost' or missing prescriptions and requests for reissues—these can be genuine, or the result of diversion, and difficult choices have to be made balancing risk and harm to the patient and pain control.

Visiting a patient at home can entail risks—other inhabitants may see a visiting healthcare professional as 'easy access' to substances. Discarded needles in duvets and sofas pose risks, and unattended syringe pumps can disappear or start to behave oddly with loss of medication.

Once home, Lydia initially met with the community team and attended for her oncology appointment. Soon after this, she stopped responding to phone calls and did not attend subsequent appointments. A number of weeks later, Lydia was readmitted to hospital, unable to walk. After hearing of Lydia's diagnosis, her partner left, and friends who were actively using drugs became involved in her life again. Lydia restarted using heroin, feeling it provided an escape from the 'hopelessness' she was experiencing. At the point of readmission, she had a declining performance status, further weight loss, and lower back pain with radiation down her legs. Mobility had rapidly declined and an MRI scan confirmed spinal cord compression. Radiotherapy was arranged but it was concluded that SACT would not be of benefit at this point due to Lydia's poor performance status.

The HPCT worked with SUS to re-establish methadone MAT and manage her symptoms of pain and anxiety. Gabapentin was added for neuropathic pain.

Expert Comment Service Provision

We are used to offering set appointments for our patients at home or clinic. We expect patients to be present when we arrive. We expect them to sit patiently in a crowded waiting room, for our convenience. In other words, we expect them to fit in. Substance use may make 'fitting in' harder to achieve. Perhaps being homeless with poor access to washing facilities makes being with others harder—either from judging stares or frank hostility—or needing to find the next drink or substance might mean sitting for hours is unbearable.

Such patients can be labelled as not attending or engaging with the service and discharged. It is important that exceptions are made to accommodate their needs. Meeting them whilst they attend SUS may be effective and aid communication between services. Trying to understand how a service can help and explaining what can be offered, where and when, can go a long way to meeting their needs as well as service needs.

Learning Point Use of Adjuvants and Non-pharmacological Interventions

- There may be a temptation to opt for non-opioid medication for pain control. Adjuvants should be considered when appropriate, but strong opioids should not be withheld where they would be of benefit.
- Many of the medications used in palliative care have street value. Benzodiazepines and gabapentinoids can be particularly sought after, so too are opioids, including patches.
- Amitriptyline has less potential for misuse but can be dangerous if taken in excess.
- Radiotherapy, surgery, transcutaneous electrical nerve stimulation (TENS), and regional anaesthetic techniques should be considered.

Lydia was transferred to a hospice in-patient unit for ongoing symptom management. She settled in well and was pleased that her daughter was able to visit her in a safe place. Lydia confided that she felt vulnerable at home, concerned that people may try to break into her flat to steal her medication.

Pain control improved with titration of morphine and gabapentin. Methadone was continued unaltered as per SUS. Unfortunately, Lydia did not regain mobility and her clinical condition deteriorated such that her prognosis was thought to be one of short weeks. Lydia did not wish to be at home and did not have friends or family who were able to provide 24-hour care. Due to the complexities of managing Lydia's symptoms and the limited prognosis, she continued to be cared for in the hospice. On two occasions, staff expressed concern that friends may have brought non-prescribed substances to the hospice as Lydia had been particularly sleepy after their visit. This was escalated, hospice policy and the legal standpoint were clearly discussed, and the possible risks explained.

As Lydia deteriorated two CSCIs were commenced. One contained morphine and midazolam to replace the oral morphine and diazepam. A second contained methadone at 50% of her oral dose. The morphine and midazolam were titrated as required. Lydia later experienced terminal agitation requiring escalation of midazolam and the addition of levomepromazine. She died in the hospice with her daughter present as per her wish.

Expert Comment Terminal Agitation and Substance Use

Anecdotally there is a high incidence of terminal agitation in those with a history of substance use. This is not surprising given that agitation may be a manifestation of spiritual and psychological distress, especially given the well-established links between substance use, mental ill health, and trauma. In this case it is also possible that gabapentin withdrawal could have contributed to agitation at the end of life.

Clinical Tip Naloxone

- There have been programmes to increase provision of naloxone in the community to be used in the event of drug overdose and reduce the risk of drug related deaths.
- When a patient is nearing the end of life, naloxone may no longer be appropriate. If administered it could result in severe exacerbation of pain. This should be clearly communicated with patients, carers, and other healthcare professionals.
- In some circumstances naloxone may be removed from the house but this would not be recommended if other members of the household are at risk of overdose.

A Final Word from the Expert

We, as a palliative care community, have evolved over the last 50 years to support the symptom control needs of people with non-malignant life limiting or life-threatening conditions. People who use substances are no different in this respect—however, the hidden nature of their 'needs' and often challenging circumstances, make it easy for them to be forgotten.

Little research has been done looking at how multiple substances affect the ageing brain, the frail lung, or the atheromatous heart. Add to this blood borne viruses, consequent iatrogenic immune suppression and presumably a higher incidence of malignancy and we have a population that will need our care to manage complex and difficult symptoms, be they social, physical, or mental. We need to embrace these opportunities to make real differences and bring our skills to those who might not have had the benefit of palliative care previously.

References

1. United Kingdom Government. United Kingdom Drug Situation 2019: Summary. March 2021. Available at: https://www.gov.uk/government/publications/united-kingdom-drug-situation-focal-point-annual-report/uk-drug-situation-2019-summary
2. United Kingdom Government. National statistics. Adult Substance Misuse Treatment Statistics 2020 to 2021: Report. Available at: https://www.gov.uk/government/statistics/substance-misuse-treatment-for-adults-statistics-2020-to-2021/adult-substance-misuse-treatment-statistics-2020-to-2021-report
3. Vogt I. Life situations and health of older drug addicts: a literature report. *Suchttherapie* 2009; 10(1): 17–24.
4. Sarangi A, McMahon T, Gude J. Benzodiazepine misuse: an epidemic within a pandemic. *Cureus* 2021; 13(6): e15816.
5. Bramley G, Fitzpatrick S, Wood J, et al. *Hard Edges Scotland: New Conversations About Severe and Multiple Disadvantage*. London: Lankelly Chase Foundation, 2019, p. 189.
6. NES Trauma Informed. Available at: https://:transformingpsychologicaltrauma.scot
7. NHS Scotland. *Scottish Palliative Care Guidelines* Available at: https://www.palliativecareguidelines.scot.nhs.uk/guidelines/pain/individuals-with-substance-use-disorder.aspx
8. Rupp T, Delaney KA. Inadequate analgesia in emergency medicine. *Ann Emerg Med* 2004; 43(4): 494–503.
9. Scimeca MM, Savage SR, Portenoy R, Lowinson J. Treatment of pain in methadone-maintained patients. *Mt Sinai J Med* 2000; 67(5–6): 412–422.

10. Human S, Walker G, Sykes J (2015). Palliative care prescribing for patients who are substance misusers. *Rowcroft Hospice*. Available at: https://rowcrofthospice.org.uk/wp-content/uploads/Rowcroft-Hospice-Palliative-Care-Prescribing-For-Substance-Misusers.pdf
11. Twycross R, Wilcock A, Howard P (eds). Methadone. In: *Palliative Care Formulary* 5. Nottingham: Palliativedrugs.com Ltd, 2015, pp. 433–439.
12. Greenwald MK, Johanson CE, Moody DE, et al. Effects of buprenorphine maintenance dose on mu-opioid receptor availability, plasma concentrations, and antagonist blockade in heroin-dependent volunteers. *Neuropsychopharmacology* 2003; 28(11): 2000–2009.
13. Mattick RP, Breen C, Kimber J, Davoli M. Buprenorphine maintenance versus placebo or methadone maintenance for opioid dependence. *Cochrane Database Syst Rev* 2014; (2): CD002207.
14. Electronic Medicines Compendium. Buvidal 8 mg *Prolonged-release Solution for Injection*. Available at: https://www.medicines.org.uk/emc/product/9705/smpc#gref
15. Savage SR, Kirsh KL, Passik SD. Challenges in using opioids to treat pain in persons with substance use disorders. *Addict Sci Clin Pract* 2008; 4(2): 4–25.
16. Twycross R, Wilcock A, Howard P (eds). Buprenorphine. In: *Palliative Care Formulary* 5. Nottingham: Palliativedrugs.com Ltd, 2015, pp. 392–400.

CASE

5 Chronic Non-cancer Pain

Lauri Simkiss

Expert: Iain Jones

Case summary

Mark, a 66-year-old man with severe left ventricular failure, was admitted to an inpatient palliative care unit as he was unable to care for himself at home and his pain was uncontrolled. Following a recent echocardiogram, his diuretics, antianginal medications, and antihypertensives had been optimized. His prognosis was expected to be 6 months. He was known to community palliative care and heart failure nurse specialists.

Mark had a traumatic back injury, aged 43, when he fell from a ladder. He required surgical stabilization and fusion of his spine from T11 to L2. Back pain worsened at 51, and an MRI showed multilevel spinal degenerative changes, with stenosis affecting his right L3 nerve root.

In recent weeks, Mark experienced a flare of his usual back pain, his mobility deteriorated, and he was unable to carry out personal care. Mark experienced orthopnoea, but physical functioning was limited by pain rather than breathlessness or angina secondary to cardiac disease. His daughter raised concerns with Mark's community team, they were unable to manage pain effectively at home and Mark was admitted.

On admission, pain was assessed using a numerical pain rating scale; Mark's lumbar back pain scored 7/10 at rest, 10/10 on movement. He described sharp right leg pain, numbness, and weakness consistent with an L3 radiculopathy. Mark reported that pain had caused loss of employment as a labourer, subsequent financial difficulties, and breakdown in relationships, including with his daughter who now assisted with his care.

Analgesics included oxycodone modified release (MR) 30 mg BD with 3–4 doses of oxycodone immediate release (IR) 10 mg daily. Mark reported little improvement since commencing opioids 10 years ago. Although concerned about the duration of oxycodone use, he feared withdrawal symptoms and pain worsening without it. Mark was taking pregabalin 300 mg BD and regular paracetamol. Amitriptyline and gabapentin had been trialled unsuccessfully. Mark had used cannabis as suggested by friends.

A cautious trial of reducing the oxycodone MR was collaboratively discussed and agreed. Other pharmacological strategies were considered however Mark was reluctant for fear of adverse effects.

An MRI showed no new pathology. Review by the orthopaedic team concluded that further surgery would not be beneficial and there were significant concerns about perioperative risk given Mark's cardiac disease. A nerve root block had been helpful in the past, but the effect was short-lived. Mark was reviewed by a pain consultant and a further nerve block was successful.

The physiotherapist found that Mark was deconditioned and worked to improve posture and movements limited by stiffness and pain. Occupational therapists discussed strategies and adjustments to his daily living to build Mark's independence. By exploring his feelings of anxiety and depression with a psychologist, Mark was able to share that his pain experience had led to isolation, loss of relationships, and meant he could not fly-fish, an interest of value to Mark. He disclosed some unresolved childhood trauma arising from an abusive relationship with his father.

Recognizing limitations in ability to reduce pain scores, the team focussed on strategies to enable Mark to manage his pain. A referral for a pain management programme was considered once a course of individual psychology sessions was completed. Mark was discharged with multidisciplinary (MDT) outpatient follow up led by the palliative medicine consultant. Community teams were advised not to escalate opioids if pain increased with increasing frailty.

Learning Point Definition of Chronic Pain

The International Classification of Diseases (ICD)-11 defines chronic pain as that which 'lasts or recurs for longer than 3 months'.[1] Chronic pain is sub-divided into seven types, including chronic primary pain, where there is no clear underlying condition, or pain is disproportionate to the injury or disease (see Figure 5.1). Chronic pain is often complex and may present with combined nociceptive and neuropathic elements. Chronic primary pain may coexist with chronic secondary pain.[2]

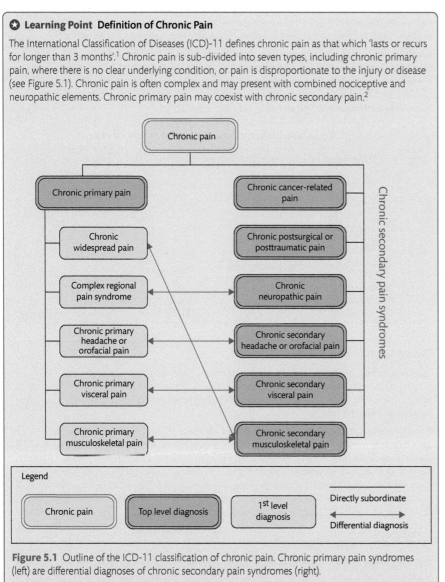

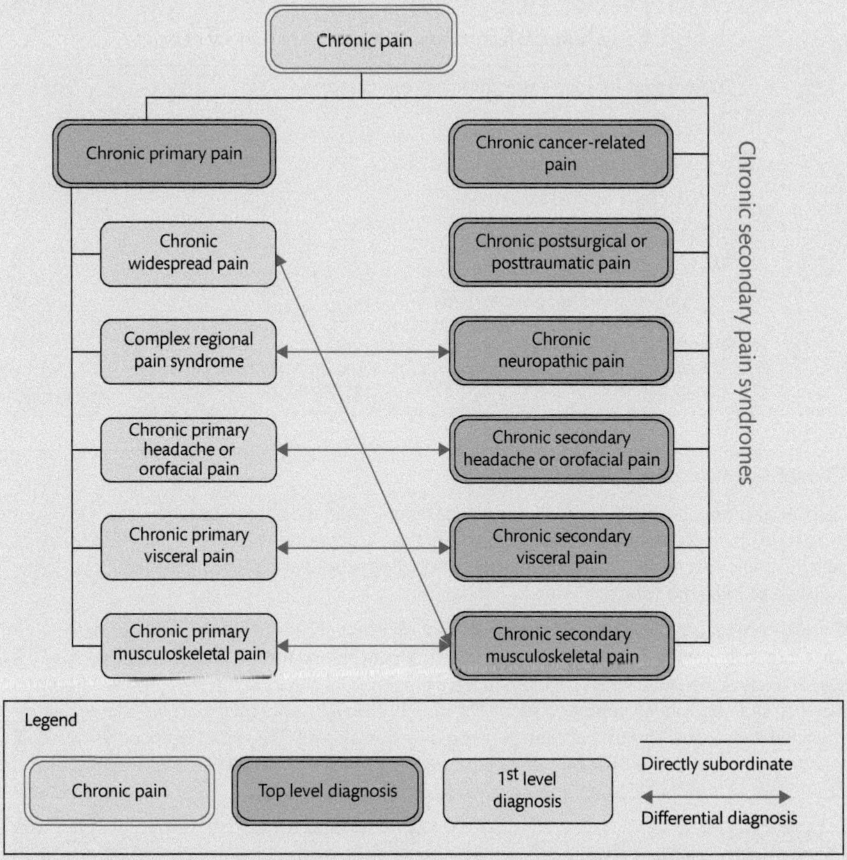

Figure 5.1 Outline of the ICD-11 classification of chronic pain. Chronic primary pain syndromes (left) are differential diagnoses of chronic secondary pain syndromes (right).

Reproduced with permission from Treede R. et al. (2019). Chronic pain as a symptom or a disease: the IASP classification of chronic pain for the international classification of diseases (ICD-11). *Pain*. 160(1): pp.19-27. DOI: 10.1097/J.PAIN.0000000000001384.

Expert Comment

Pain serves an important evolutionary function and is essential for survival, directing attention to the situation and promoting reflexive withdrawal, active defence, or instigating actions to prevent further damage in order to facilitate healing. Pain and nociception are different phenomena. Nociception is the activation of sensory transduction in nerves by thermal, mechanical, or chemical stimuli on specialized nerve endings. Central summation of stimulation from non-nociceptive receptors are involved in the sensory processing of nociception. Pain is defined as an unpleasant sensory and emotional experience associated with, or resembling that associated with, actual or potential tissue damage.

Sensitization may occur peripherally and centrally with changes in the primary receptor, in the spinal cord and at the supraspinal level. Chronic pain arises as a consequence of these pathological changes where pain is uncoupled from tissue damage.

Neuroimaging techniques such as functional MRI have helped our understanding of neural mechanisms and specific regions of the brain that are activated in the presence of chronic pain. These include areas associated with memory and emotional regulation such as the hippocampus and amygdala.[3]

However, clinical studies have shown a poor correlation between radiological evidence of joint degeneration and pain. MRI scans demonstrate that spinal abnormalities can be found in 40–60% of asymptomatic patients. Susceptibility to developing pain following surgery, injury, or disease varies considerably.[3] There are several physiological mechanisms by which psychological and affective factors may contribute to the experience of pain (see Table 5.1).

Table 5.1 Psychosocial factors that may predict chronicity of pain[4]

Yellow flags for long-term chronicity and disability
Catastrophic thinking
A belief that pain and activity are harmful
Avoidance of normal activity
Depression or anxiety
Withdrawal from social activity
Occupational or financial problems

Source: data from Nicholas MK. *et al*. (2011). Early Identification and Management of Psychological Risk Factors ("Yellow Flags") in Patients With Low Back Pain: A Reappraisal. *Phys Ther*. 91(5):737-53. DOI: 10.2522/ptj.20100224.

Learning Point Key Statistics

Globally, approximately 20% of people experience chronic pain, the proportion who present to healthcare professionals is unknown.[1,2] Up to 5% of the UK population experience chronic primary pain.[5] Chronic pain is more common in women, socially deprived populations, some ethnic minority groups, and with advancing age.[6]

Chronic non-cancer pain (CNCP) impacts quality of life in a number of ways. Patients feel that it subsumes their identity. Depression is noted in 49% of patients and there is an increased risk of suicide. Patients are more likely to choose to leave employment and 25% lose their jobs. Relationships are often strained, with an impact on socializing in 50%. The wider physical impact includes impaired cognition and fatigue, and 65% of patients report difficulty sleeping. The impact beyond the individual is also profound, with low back pain alone estimated to cost the economy £12.3 billion annually.[5]

Clinical Tip General Approach

The management of CNCP differs from the management of acute pain, or from where there is a prognosis of weeks or short months because of differences in pathophysiology and the lack of effect of opioids.

CNCP is difficult to treat, and no single intervention is highly successful. Useful approaches include[2]:

- Acknowledging pain and associated distress
- Ascertaining the meaning of the pain to the patient

- Explaining the limitations of treatments, helping the patient to understand that complete relief of pain should not be the goal
- Empowering the patient
- Working collaboratively with patients
- Promoting self-management, with aims to improve function and develop coping skills
- Working alongside an integrated interdisciplinary team to ensure a biopsychosocial approach

Expert Comment

NICE guidelines for the management of spinal pain recommend that when there are radiological findings consistent with symptoms of sciatica spinal decompressive surgery may be considered when non-surgical treatment has not improved pain or function.[7] However, the guidelines do not recommend spinal fusion surgery or disc replacement surgery for people with low back pain.

Chronic post-surgical pain is a risk of any surgical procedure. Risk factors for developing chronic pain following surgery include younger age in adults, female sex, pre-existing pain in the area of surgery, and psychological factors, including anxiety and fear of having surgery. Review with a pain specialist to discuss pain management options may be helpful for patients at greater risk of developing post-surgical pain or for whom the benefits of surgery are uncertain.

Clinical Tip Effectiveness of Opioids

The efficacy of opioids for acute, cancer pain or at the end of life is well evidenced. The research base for patients with CNCP is limited. Evidence has demonstrated a short or medium-term benefit of opioids in the management of chronic pain; however, evidence for the longer term is limited and of very low quality.[8] There is no advantage of an opioid over a placebo for pain management, functional status, or quality of life in CNCP when trials adjust for dropout rates. The Faculty of Pain Medicine (FPM) suggest that when a clinician undertakes a trial of opioids they do so for a short period of time, closely evaluating benefits and adverse effects, understanding that opioids are unlikely to result in long-term benefit.[8]

Learning Point Long-term Effects of Opioids

Hypogonadism and adrenal insufficiency[9]: This leads to amenorrhoea, reduced libido, infertility, osteopaenia, depression, and fatigue. Effects are likely dose-related.

Increased risk of falls and fractures: Solomon et al. compared opioid management of arthritic pain to selective cyclooxygenase-2 (COX-2) inhibitors in a cohort of 12,840 patients with a mean age of 80 years.[10] The incidence of fractures in opioid users was 101 per 1,000 person-years compared to 19 per 1,000 in those using selective COX2 inhibitors.

Opioid-induced hyperalgesia[11]: OIH is experienced by the patient as increased pain sensitivity and may cause diffuse allodynia. It may develop through similar neuroimmune mechanisms to chronic pain.

Immunosuppression[12]: Pain can cause immunosuppression via effects on the hypothalamic-pituitary-adrenal axis. Opioids have immunosuppressive properties via the μ-opioid receptor and indirectly through the hypothalamic-pituitary-adrenal axis and sympathetic nervous system. Different opioids have different effects; morphine and fentanyl cause most immunosuppression in animal models. The effect of oxycodone, hydromorphone, buprenorphine, and methadone on immunosuppression in humans is yet to be determined.

Increased mortality: Solomon et al. also demonstrated increased all-cause mortality compared with other analgesics in older people.[10]

Expert Comment

The opioid epidemic has altered approaches to opioid prescribing globally. There are concerns about rising prescribed opioid use for CNCP in the UK, especially in areas of high deprivation. The risk of harm increases substantially at doses above an oral morphine equivalent of 120 mg/day without evidence of increasing benefit with increasing dose. Tapering or stopping high-dose opioids needs careful planning and collaboration.

The FPM advise best practice when commencing an opioid should include[13]:

- Explaining that opioids are, in general, poorly effective for long-term pain. For a small proportion of patients, opioids may be successfully used as part of a broader plan, including non-medication treatments and self-management.
- Discussing the degree of pain relief that might be expected and understanding that the aim is not complete pain relief but rather reducing pain sufficiently to engage in self-management.
- Agreeing specific functional goals that might be achieved.
- Discussing the potential harms of opioid treatment (see 'Learning Point Long-term Effects of Opioids').
- Discussing the effect of opioids on driving skills.
- Discussing the circumstances in which opioid therapy will be stopped.
- Discussing arrangements for review.

Evidence Base Pharmacological Strategies

In chronic primary pain, NICE supports the use of antidepressants (amitriptyline, citalopram, duloxetine, fluoxetine, paroxetine, and sertraline), without preference for one class over another.[2] Duloxetine has an evidence base for long-term use. NICE do not recommend paracetamol, benzodiazepines, nonsteroidal anti-inflammatory drugs (NSAIDs) or antiepileptics due to a lack of benefit and potential harm.

There is limited efficacy for the use of topical NSAIDs for chronic musculoskeletal pain. Likewise, for the use of high-concentration capsaicin in postherpetic neuralgia.[14]

Patients may derive benefit from non-opioid medications in some types of chronic secondary pain syndromes, specifically in those with clear neuropathic features. Individualized assessment is key and, if trialling medications, regular review of benefit and adverse effects is important, as is periodic dose tapering to evaluate ongoing need.

Expert Comment

Cannabinoids are broadly defined as constituents of cannabis or synthetic compounds with pharmacological activity on the endocannabinoid system.

Recently published systematic reviews conclude a lack of high-quality evidence for the use of cannabinoids in the treatment of CNCP.

Although there is preclinical data supporting the hypothesis of the use of cannabinoids for pain relief, current uncertainties in the clinical evidence regarding efficacy and safety do not support recommendations for the general use of cannabinoids for relief of chronic pain outside a research setting.

Evidence Base Non-pharmacological Strategies

A Cochrane review verified there is low-quality evidence physical activity and exercise can reduce pain intensity and improve physical functioning, whilst outcomes for psychological function and quality of life were variable.[15] Multiple types of physical interventions were included. Adverse events were few.

Evidence was unable to show benefit for transcutaneous electrical nerve stimulation (TENS).[16]

Although NICE guidelines support consideration of acupuncture based on efficacy in the short but not long term, concerns about cost-effectiveness limit support of this intervention.[2]

Cognitive behavioural therapy (CBT) has moderate-quality evidence of a small benefit for reducing pain and distress, and low-quality evidence for disability.[17] This benefit was seen at both end of treatment, and at 6–12 months. Acceptance and commitment therapy (ACT) is increasingly being used with evidence of being cost-effective, having lasting benefits on pain interference, disability, depression, and quality of life.[6]

Expert Comment

The aims of pain management are to achieve a balance between pain and adverse effects of analgesia, to optimize physical function, and to support self-management.

Closer integration of pain management, oncology and palliative care services can result in more comprehensive pain assessment and a wider range of treatments for patients comprising pharmacological, interventional, rehabilitative, and psychological approaches. Those with less complex pain, but who require more skilful balancing of analgesic medicines, can benefit as well as the clear benefit in complex pain syndromes.

A framework for the provision of pain services for adults in the UK with cancer or life-limiting disease has been published by the FPM.[18]

Clinical Tip Pain Management Programmes

Pain management programmes can be considered for patients with complex pain.[19] They are typically delivered as non-resident, CBT-based, group programmes. The interdisciplinary treatment includes education on pain physiology and psychology, pain self-management, activity management, relaxation, goal setting, and adapting unhelpful beliefs.

Suitable patients are those for whom pain has a significant impact on their lives. Historically this would be in those where previous interventions have failed, but more recently, early, less intensive interventions have shown to be effective.

There is evidence of efficacy, for programmes of at least 25–30 hours, sustained to follow-up at one year. More intensive programmes can achieve greater improvement.

A Final Word from the Expert

Patients with chronic pain frequently present with a complex mixture of medical, psychological, and social factors. Condition specific management alone, offered in 'pursuit of cure', often fails people with chronic pain, leading to unresolved pain and rising distress. Pain management requires a coordinated biopsychosocial approach to support patients effectively. Small incremental positive change is made possible through access to a range of enabling treatments including some specialist treatments. For patients with complex pain, they need specialists with the training and expertise to manage their care holistically.

References

1. Treede R, Rief W, Barke A, et al. Chronic pain as a symptom or a disease: the IASP classification of chronic pain for the international classification of diseases (ICD-11). *Pain* 2019; 160(1): 19–27.
2. National Institute for Health and Care Excellence. Chronic pain (primary and secondary) in over 16s: Assessment of all chronic pain and management of chronic primary pain. NICE Guideline 193. 2017.
3. Ossipov M, Morimura K, Porreca F. Descending pain modulation and chronification of pain. *Curr Opin Support Palliat Care* 2014; 8(2): 143–151.
4. Nicholas MK, Linton SJ, Watson PJ, Main CJ. Early identification and management of psychological risk factors ('yellow flags') in patients with low back pain: a reappraisal. *Phys Ther* 2011; 91(5): 737–753.
5. Chief Medical Officer Annual Report. *Pain: Breaking Through the Barrier*. Crown Copyright; 2008.

6. McCracken L, Yu L, Vowles K. New generation psychological treatments in chronic pain. *BMJ* 2022; 376: e057212–2057212
7. National Institute for Health and Care Excellence. Low back pain and sciatica in over 16s: assessment and management. NICE Guideline 59. 2016.
8. Faculty of Pain Medicine. Opioids aware: Opioids for long term pain. Available at: https://fpm.ac.uk/opioids-aware-clinical-use-opioids/opioids-long-term-pain
9. De Vries F, Bruin M, Lobatto D, et al. Opioids and their endocrine effects: a systematic review and meta-analysis. *J Clin Endocrinol Metab* 2020; 105(4): 1020–1029.
10. Solomon D, Rassen J, Glynn R, Lee J, Levin R, Schneeweiss S. The comparative safety of analgesics in older adults with arthritis. *Arch Intern Med* 2010; 170(22): 1968–1978.
11. Lee M, Silverman S, Hansen H, Patel V, Manchikanti L. A comprehensive review of opioid-induced hyperalgesia. *Pain Physician* 2011; 14: 145–161.
12. Merlin J, Childers J, Arnold R. Chronic pain in the outpatient palliative care clinic. *Am J Hosp Palliat Care* 2012; 30(2): 197–203.
13. Faculty of Pain Medicine. Opioids aware: checklist for prescribers. Available at: https://fpm.ac.uk/opioids-aware-structured-approach-opioid-prescribing/checklist-prescribers
14. Derry S, Wiffen P, Kalso E et al. Topical analgesics for acute and chronic pain in adults—an overview of Cochrane Reviews. *Cochrane Database Syst Rev* 2017; 5: CD008609.
15. Geneen L, Moore R, Clarke C, Martin D, Colvin L, Smith B. Physical activity and exercise for chronic pain in adults: an overview of Cochrane Reviews. *Cochrane Database Syst Rev* 2017; 4: CD011279.
16. Gibson W, Wand B, Meads C, Catley M, O'Connell N. Transcutaneous electrical nerve stimulation (TENS) for chronic pain—an overview of Cochrane Reviews. *Cochrane Database Syst Rev* 2019; 4: CD011890.
17. Williams A, Fisher E, Hearn L, Eccleston C. Psychological therapies for the management of chronic pain (excluding headache) in adults. *Cochrane Database Syst Rev* 2020; 8: CD007407.
18. Royal College of Anaesthetists. Framework for provision of pain services for adults across the UK with cancer or life-limiting disease. 2019. Available at: https://fpm.ac.uk/sites/fpm/files/documents/2019-07/Framework%20for%20pain%20services%20cancer%20and%20life%20limiting%20disease%202019.pdf
19. The British Pain Society. *Guidelines for Pain Management Programmes for Adults: An Evidence-Based Review Prepared On Behalf Of the British Pain Society*. 2013. Available at: https://www.britishpainsociety.org/static/uploads/resources/files/pmp2013_main_FINAL_v6.pdf

SECTION 2

Management of other symptoms in advanced illness

CASE

6 Breathlessness

Natasha Lovell

Expert: Sabrina Bajwah

Case history

Dalian, a 71-year-old retired lorry driver presented to a large teaching hospital with a three day history of increasing shortness of breath. Dalian had been diagnosed with chronic obstructive pulmonary disease (COPD) four years ago and had a past medical history of ischaemic heart disease with reduced left ventricular function on echocardiogram. Prescribed medications on admission included Seretide, Salbutamol, Tiotropium, Carbocisteine, Spironolactone, Furosemide, Aspirin, Bisoprolol, and Atorvastatin. Dalian had no known drug allergies.

Dalian self-identified as of Black Caribbean ethnicity. He lived with his wife, who was his main carer, in a first-floor flat. There was no formal package of care in place. He had a reduced exercise tolerance and was able to mobilize short distances with a stick. He was a current smoker of 15 cigarettes per day and did not drink alcohol. This was his fifth admission to hospital with shortness of breath in the past year.

Observations on arrival to hospital were heart rate; 111 beats per minute, blood pressure 115/65mmHg, respiratory rate 13, and oxygen saturation 92% on air. A CXR showed hyperinflation and emphysematous changes in keeping with COPD but no consolidation. Routine blood tests and an arterial blood gas were within normal parameters. He was diagnosed with a non-infective exacerbation of COPD. Dalian was reviewed by the medical team and expressed concerns about his ongoing breathlessness, which he felt was currently inadequately managed.

Expert Comment

There is a growing body of evidence to suggest that pulse oximeters may be less accurate on patients of colour. A recent study conducted in 2020, at the University of Michigan Hospital compared measures of oxygen saturation by pulse oximetry and arterial blood gas samples from adult inpatients receiving supplemental oxygen.[1] The sample consisted of white patients (n=1,333) and black patients (n=276) and revealed that of the patients who had an SpO_2 reading on pulse oximetry between 92% and 96%, black patients were three times more likely (11.7%) to have an arterial oxygen saturation of less than 88% than white patients (3.6%).[1]

Learning Point

The terminology used to describe breathlessness is evolving and remains inconsistent in the literature. The American Thoracic Society (ATS) definition of 'a subjective experience of breathing discomfort that consists of qualitatively distinct sensations that vary in intensity' is perhaps most commonly referred to.[2] Chronic breathlessness is a common symptom of advanced disease, and often increases as diseases progress. Prevalence is as high as 98% in COPD, 93% in interstitial lung disease (ILD), 88% in chronic heart failure, and 77% in cancer.[3, 4] It is a common cause of acute hospital admission, accounting for up to 20% of ambulance presentations.[5] Breathlessness is a distressing symptom, which commonly occurs alongside other symptoms, impacts social roles and responsibilities, and has significant psychosocial implications.

Clinical Tip

Breathlessness can only be perceived by the person experiencing it and does not necessarily correlate with the level of hypoxia. Systematic review has identified that people with advanced disease living with breathlessness describe concerns across six domains; 1) the physical symptoms of breathlessness and subsequent effect on function; 2) the emotional impact; 3) the spiritual distress experienced; 4) the social impact of breathlessness; 5) concerns relating to aspects of control; and 6) the context of breathlessness (acute episode or chronic).[6] This is shown in the model of total breathlessness (Figure 6.1) and can be used as a practical framework to assess breathlessness in clinical practice.

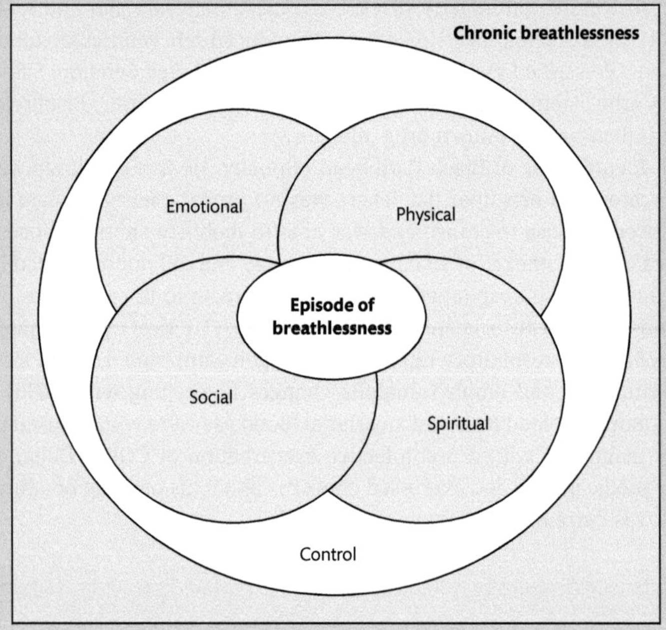

Figure 6.1 Model of total breathlessness.

Dalian spent two days in hospital. Initially, he was noted to be agitated, frequently asking for assistance to leave the ward to smoke. He was reviewed by a respiratory nurse specialist. It was explained to him that, based on his blood gas results, he may be eligible for long-term oxygen therapy at home; however, this would require him to stop smoking. Dalian agreed to speak to the smoking cessation specialist and, when reviewed, expressed motivation to stop smoking. Written information was provided, and a nicotine patch was prescribed. It was explained to Dalian that formal assessment for long-term oxygen therapy could be considered following discharge after a period of stability, and review of his smoking status.

> **Learning Point Long-term Oxygen Therapy and Smoking**
>
> British Thoracic Society guidelines state that patients should not normally have long-term oxygen therapy ordered at the time of an acute exacerbation, and formal assessment should take place after a period of stability of at least eight weeks.[7] Smoking cessation should be discussed, and written education given, and patients should be made aware in writing of the dangers of using home oxygen within the vicinity of any naked flame.

Dalian was reviewed by a physiotherapist and taught breathing exercises and positional techniques to help to manage the symptom of breathlessness. The evidence for pulmonary rehabilitation was discussed and Dalian explained that whilst he had previously been referred, he had been unable to complete the full course due to being admitted to hospital. Dalian agreed to referral to the hospital palliative care team (HPCT) and was reviewed by a clinical nurse specialist on the ward. Dalian explained that when he became breathless, he felt very frightened and worried that he might die. Following a detailed assessment, he was provided with some written information about breathlessness, as well as a hand-held fan which can be helpful in reducing the feeling of breathlessness. It was agreed that on discharge he would be referred to the Fatigue and Breathlessness course based at the local hospice.

> **Evidence Base Non-pharmacological Management of Breathlessness**
>
> Non-pharmacological interventions should take priority initially. The best evidence is for pulmonary rehabilitation, which combines exercise and education, and has been shown to be effective at both relieving breathlessness and enhancing a sense of control for patients with COPD.[8] Holistic services are emerging, designed specifically for those with advanced disease and chronic breathlessness. Treatments are selected based on the needs of individual patients, their families, and carers. Individual studies suggest a positive impact on health outcomes,[9] and systematic review suggests services can reduce distress and improve psychological outcomes of anxiety and depression (Figure 6.2).[10]

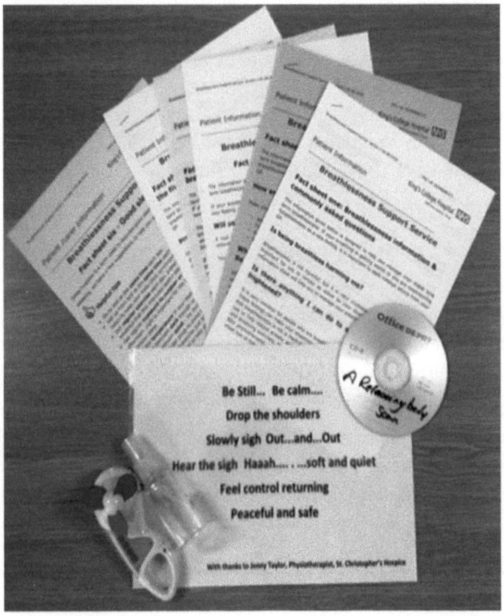

Figure 6.2 Example of resources used in a breathlessness support service.

Dalian asked the medical team whether there were any medications which might help with his breathlessness. It was explained that whilst the best evidence is for non-drug treatments, there are some drug treatments which can be considered in the management of breathlessness. These include ensuring that medications given for the underlying condition are optimized and treating other symptoms where possible. It was explained that oxygen is one kind of medical treatment which was being considered for him. The evidence for lose dose morphine in the management of breathlessness was also explained. Dalian initially expressed some concerns about potential side effects and the risk of addiction but said that he would be willing to consider this if other non-drug measures weren't working. The medical team queried whether a benzodiazepine might be an appropriate treatment for the anxiety relating to Dalian's breathlessness. It was explained that non-pharmacological treatments, for example cognitive behavioural therapy (CBT) would be more appropriate in the first instance.

Evidence Base Pharmacological Management of Breathlessness

The evidence base for pharmacological interventions remains limited, with no evidence of benefit of oxygen compared to room air for relieving breathlessness in the absence of hypoxia in a large randomized controlled trial.[11] Additionally, a Cochrane Review published in 2016 identified eight controlled trials of benzodiazepines and found no evidence of benefit in the absence of breathlessness-related anxiety.[12] The review recommends that benzodiazepines should only be used if other first-line treatments have failed and states a need for well-conducted and adequately powered studies. There is moderate randomized controlled trial evidence from a Cochrane Review to support the use of parental and oral opioids,[13] and a sustained release morphine has recently been licensed for use in chronic breathlessness in Australia. However, optimal dosing, titration, and potential issues arising from long-term use and safety remain to be determined.

Evidence Base Safety of Opioids and Benzodiazepines

Opioids and benzodiazepines are commonly prescribed in the management of breathlessness. However, many clinicians express concerns about possible adverse effects of these drugs including respiratory depression, confusion, falls, and premature death. A population based longitudinal cohort study in Sweden aimed to evaluate the safety of benzodiazepines and opioids in patients with severe COPD.[15] The primary outcome was the effects of benzodiazepines and opioids on rates of admission to hospital and mortality. The study found that any dose of benzodiazepines and higher opioid doses (>30 mg morphine equivalent) were associated with an increase in mortality in the COPD population.

Clinical Tip

Constipation is a common undesirable effect of opioid medications and routine prescribing of a laxative should be considered. Nausea and vomiting are also common but usually transient and will usually improve after five to seven days.

Expert Comment

Benzodiazepines are highly addictive and associated with increased morbidity and mortality in COPD. For patients with a prognosis of months to years, they should only be used for severe anxiety in the very short term (days) whilst starting a longer-term anxiolytic, e.g. mirtazapine. Mild to moderate anxiety should be managed with non-pharmacological measures such as CBT.

For patients at the end of life, benzodiazepines should be used for anxiety and anxiety related breathlessness. COPD patients at the end of life often require both morphine and midazolam in a syringe pump to ensure adequate control of anxiety related breathlessness.

Expert Comment

Most of the evidence for opioids in the management of breathlessness is for morphine and it remains unclear whether there could be a class effect. Interestingly a recently published randomized trial found no benefit of oxycodone when compared to placebo, although results may have been limited by certain aspects of the trial design.[14] There remains a need for well-conducted and adequately powered studies of different classes of opioids.

Future Advances

Neuroimaging studies are beginning to explore complex interactions between neural networks in the brain which may underpin the perception of breathlessness.[16] Studies of induced breathlessness in healthy volunteers confirm activation of the insula, amygdala, and anterior cingulate cortex.[17] Drugs that modify processing and perception of afferent information in the brain, such as antidepressants, may have a role in the treatment of chronic or refractory breathlessness. However, in a large randomized controlled trial, sertraline was shown to have no benefit when compared to placebo.[18] Mirtazapine is a noradrenergic and specific serotonergic antidepressant which may have beneficial effects on breathlessness by inhibiting fear circuits and fear conditioning, and also by causing bronchodilation. Mirtazapine is a potent antagonist of histamine H1, and may also be advantageous for other symptoms such as poor appetite, poor sleep, and anorexia, which are all common in advanced disease and breathlessness.[19]

Prior to discharge with agreement from Dalian the medical team met with his wife. Mrs Agumanu expressed that she was struggling to meet Dalian's increasing care needs. She found episodes of breathlessness very distressing, and felt she had no other options except to phone for an ambulance when this happened. Mrs Agumanu expressed concerns about what might happen in the future but was reluctant to speak to Dalian for fear that she might upset him. A meeting was organized with Dalian and his wife and attended by members of the multidisciplinary team. Dalian acknowledged that they would benefit from some more support at home. He also recognized that he was deteriorating and expressed a wish not to die in hospital. Agreed outcomes from the meeting included organizing a formal care package, and referral to the community palliative care team (CPCT) for ongoing symptom management and to support with advance care planning.

Future Advances

Inducing breathlessness activates areas of the brain relating to fear, and research has shown that viewing images or videos of breathlessness can elicit breathlessness. A live citizen experiment was conducted in collaboration with the Science Gallery, King's College London.[20] The experiment aimed to explore the effect of audio recordings of breathing on self-reported breathlessness.

Participants listened to short audio recordings of breathlessness with the following causes in a random order: exercise, anxiety, chronic lung disease, and approaching the end of life. Participants were asked to identify the cause of breathlessness, and report how breathless they felt (before and after each recording) using a validated 0–10 numerical rating scale. Self-reported breathlessness increased after listening to any of the four recordings and was highest for anxiety.

A Final Word from the Expert

This case is a good example of the distressing nature of breathlessness experienced by many patients. It also demonstrates the significant impact on every part of the patient's life and on those who are close, including friends and family. Ideally, this patient should have had non-pharmacological management of his breathlessness earlier in his disease. This may have reduced some of the earlier anxiety and breathlessness he experienced. It is important to explore the patient's anxiety fully. Many patients are scared about what their increasing breathlessness means and what the future might hold. It is important to address these concerns and maximize the use of cognitive behavioural therapies where possible. If anxiety cannot be managed through non-pharmacological measures, long-term anxiolytics should be used early. When patients become breathless at rest or on minimal exertion, pharmacological therapies such as opioids should be introduced early alongside active treatment of the underlying disease. Multidisciplinary working between respiratory and palliative care teams across primary and secondary care is essential to ensure patients' holistic needs are managed throughout their disease journey.

References

1. Sjoding MW, Dickson RP, Iwashyna TJ, Gay SE, Valley TS. Racial bias in pulse oximetry measurement. *N Engl J Med* 2020; 383(25): 2477–2478.
2. Parshall MB, Schwartzstein RM, Adams L, et al. An official American Thoracic Society statement: update on the mechanisms, assessment, and management of dyspnea. *Am J Respir Crit Care Med* 2012; 185(4): 435–452.
3. Moens K, Higginson IJ, Harding R. Are there differences in the prevalence of palliative care-related problems in people living with advanced cancer and eight non-cancer conditions? A systematic review. *J Pain Symptom Manage* 2014; 48(4): 660–677.
4. Solano JP, Gomes B, Higginson IJ. A comparison of symptom prevalence in far advanced cancer, AIDS, heart disease, chronic obstructive pulmonary disease and renal disease. *J Pain Symptom Manage* 2006; 31(1): 58–69.
5. Hutchinson A, Pickering A, Williams P, Bland JM, Johnson MJ. Breathlessness and presentation to the emergency department: a survey and clinical record review. *BMC Pulm Med* 2017; 17(1): 53.
6. Lovell N, Etkind SN, Bajwah S, Maddocks M, Higginson IJ. Control and context are central for people with advanced illness experiencing breathlessness: a systematic review and thematic synthesis. *J Pain Symptom Manage* 2019; 57(1): 140–155.e2.
7. Hardinge M, Annandale J, Bourne S, et al. British Thoracic Society guidelines for home oxygen use in adults: accredited by NICE. *Thorax* 2015; 70(Suppl 1): i1–i43.
8. McCarthy B, Casey D, Devane D, Murphy K, Murphy E, Lacasse Y. Pulmonary rehabilitation for chronic obstructive pulmonary disease. *Cochrane Database Syst Rev* 2015(2): Cd003793.
9. Higginson IJ, Bausewein C, Reilly CC, et al. An integrated palliative and respiratory care service for patients with advanced disease and refractory breathlessness: a randomised controlled trial. *Lancet Respir Med* 2014; 2(12): 979–987.
10. Brighton LJ, Miller S, Farquhar M, et al. Holistic services for people with advanced disease and chronic breathlessness: a systematic review and meta-analysis. *Thorax* 2019; 74(3): 270–281.
11. Abernethy AP, McDonald CF, Frith PA, et al. Effect of palliative oxygen versus room air in relief of breathlessness in patients with refractory dyspnoea: a double-blind, randomised controlled trial. *Lancet* 2010; 376(9743): 784–793.
12. Simon ST, Higginson IJ, Booth S, Harding R, Weingartner V, Bausewein C. Benzodiazepines for the relief of breathlessness in advanced malignant and non-malignant diseases in adults. *Cochrane Database Syst Rev* 2016; 10: Cd007354.
13. Barnes H, McDonald J, Smallwood N, Manser R. Opioids for the palliation of refractory breathlessness in adults with advanced disease and terminal illness. *Cochrane Database Syst Rev* 2016; 3: Cd011008.
14. Ferreira DH, Louw S, McCloud P, et al. Controlled-release oxycodone vs. placebo in the treatment of chronic breathlessness—a multisite randomized placebo controlled trial. *J Pain Symptom Manage* 2019; 59(3): 581–589.
15. Ekström MP, Bornefalk-Hermansson A, Abernethy AP, Currow DC. Safety of benzodiazepines and opioids in very severe respiratory disease: national prospective study. *BMJ* 2014; 348: g445.
16. Pattinson KT, Johnson MJ. Neuroimaging of central breathlessness mechanisms. *Curr Opin Support Palliat Care* 2014; 8(3): 225–233.
17. Banzett RB, Mulnier HE, Murphy K, Rosen SD, Wise RJ, Adams L. Breathlessness in humans activates insular cortex. *Neuroreport* 2000; 11(10): 2117–2120.
18. Currow DC, Ekstrom M, Louw S, et al. Sertraline in symptomatic chronic breathlessness: a double blind, randomised trial. *Eur Respir J* 2019; 53(1): 1801270.
19. Lovell N, Wilcock A, Bajwah S, et al. Mirtazapine for chronic breathlessness? A review of mechanistic insights and therapeutic potential. *Expert Rev Respir Med* 2019; 13(2): 173–180.
20. Lovell N, Etkind S, Prentice W, Higginson I, Sleeman K. The sound of anxiety: exploring the effect of audio recordings of breathing on self-reported breathlessness. *Eur Respiratory Soc* 2023; 62(1): 2201439.

CASE 7 Nausea, Vomiting, and Hiccups

Holly McGuigan

Expert: Anna Sutherland

Case History

Matthew, a 42-year-old man, was referred to the hospital palliative care team (HPCT) with intractable vomiting and hiccups. Matthew had recently been diagnosed with metastatic small-cell lung cancer and declined life-prolonging treatments. Matthew described early satiety, hiccups, regurgitation, and a sluggish bowel habit. He had noticed food 'getting stuck on the way down'.

Matthew was dehydrated. Abdominal examination was unremarkable, with normal bowel sounds.

The HPCT diagnosed Matthew with gastric stasis and constipation. His Clinical Nurse Specialist (CNS) started a subcutaneous infusion of metoclopramide 30 mg over 24 hours with good effect.

Learning Point Approach to Oral, Pharyngeal, or Mid-oesophageal Causes

The Scottish Palliative Care Guidelines identify this as a separate category, triggered by activation of the vagal and glossopharyngeal nerves.

Symptoms:

- reflux
- retching triggered by coughing
- worse on eating
- triggered by tastes or smells

Reversible causes include:

- oesophagitis
- gastro-oesophageal reflux
- oesophageal candida
- oesophageal stent

Drug management includes anticholinergics or broad spectrum antiemetics, e.g. levomepromazine.[5]

Clinical Tip Serotonin Antagonists

Serotonin antagonists (e.g. ondansetron) are rarely helpful unless there is a raised serotonin level, (e.g. chemotherapy or gastrointestinal radiotherapy) and constipation is a common side-effect.

Expert Comment Serotonin Syndrome

Serotonin syndrome is characterized by a triad of autonomic hyperactivity, neuromuscular hyperactivity, and altered mental status in the presence of serotonergic drugs and the absence of alternative explanations.[2] It may be seen with metoclopramide, levomepromazine, and olanzapine. It is rare clinically at lower antiemetic doses unless a patient is on concurrent high dose antidepressants or antipsychotics.

Clinical Tip General Approach to Hiccups

Common causes include:

- Gastric stasis/distension
- Gastro-oesophageal reflux
- Diaphragmatic irritation
- Side effects of medications (steroids, benzodiazepines, opioids, antidopaminergics)
- Chemical causes such as uraemia[1]
- Causes of aerophagia (breathlessness, anxiety, non-invasive ventilation)
- Structural causes affecting the medulla oblongata

First address potentially reversible causes.

Drugs that reduce gastric distension/gastro-oesophageal reflux include[2]:

- Simeticone
- Prokinetics
- Proton pump inhibitors
- Histamine 2 antagonists

Drugs that centrally suppress hiccups:

- gabapentin or baclofen first line[2]

Evidence Base Hiccup Management

Very Low

A Cochrane review was withdrawn due to a lack of high-quality randomized controlled trial (RCT) evidence.[3]

An independent systematic review advised that 'whenever possible, the treatment of hiccups should be directed at the underlying cause of the condition'.[4]

Haloperidol is widely used for the management of hiccups but there is limited evidence for this.[4]

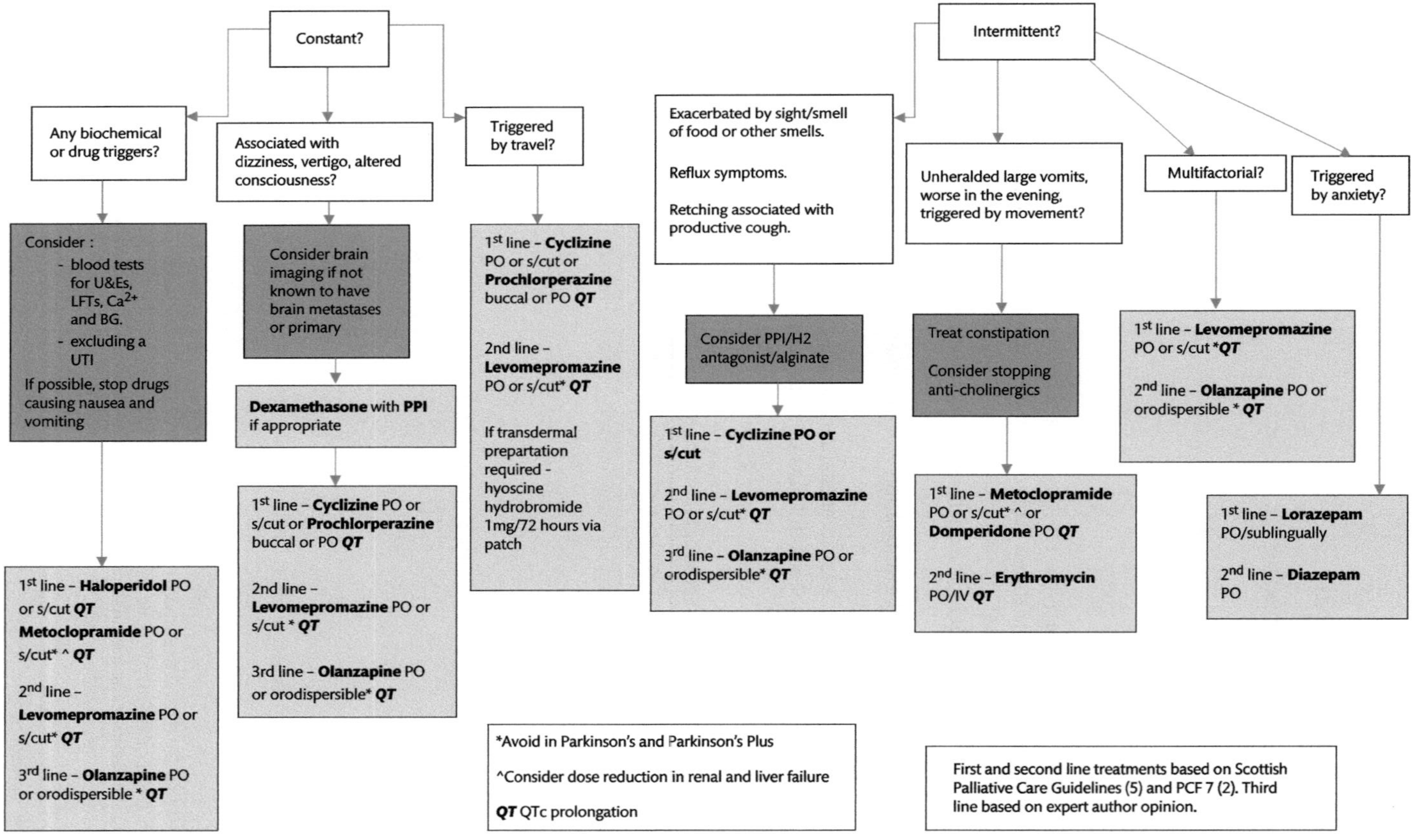

Figure 7.1 Is the nausea and vomiting . . . ?

Clinical Tip Assessing Causes of Nausea and Vomiting

It is essential to establish the pattern of the nausea (Figure 7.1).

History

- Check this is not regurgitation or rotational vertigo
- Assess nausea and vomiting separately
- For each, ask about
  - o triggers, volume, and timing—for example, unheralded vomits at the end of the day suggest gastric stasis
  - o exacerbating and relieving factors, including drugs already tried and response to these
  - o medication that may be contributing
- Ask about and treat associated symptoms, e.g.
  - o colic (might preclude the use of prokinetics)
  - o constipation and confusion (exclude hypercalcaemia)
  - o dehydration (treat uraemia)
  - o postural hypotension

Examination

- For dehydration, infection, or drug toxicity.
- For organomegaly, bowel sounds and ascites. Consider a rectal examination.
- Consider a central nervous system examination, including for papilloedema, if history is suggestive of intracerebral causes or if symptoms are intractable.

Investigations

Blood tests may include:

- urea and electrolytes
- liver function
- calcium
- glucose
- digoxin/aminophylline levels
- phosphate and magnesium

Consider:

- urinalysis for infection
- imaging, including brain, if cause unclear or features suggestive of cerebral metastases[5]

Learning Point Targeting Antiemetics Based On Receptor Theory

Antagonist/Agonist	Receptors					
	AChM	H1	5HT2	D2	5HT3	5HT4
	Ant	Ant	Ant	Ant	Ant	Ag
Metoclopramide ^{QT}				++	+	++
Domperidone ^{QT}				++		
Haloperidol ^{QT}				+++	+	
Cyclizine	++	++				
Ondansetron ^{QT}					+++	
Levomepromazine ^{QT}	++	+++	+++	++	+	
Olanzapine ^{QT}	++	+	++	++	+	+

Expert Comment

Extra-pyramidal Side Effects

Domperidone does not cross the blood-brain barrier and is not associated with extra-pyramidal side effects. Orodispersible tablets are available if imported from Europe.

Antidopaminergic antiemetics which cross the blood-brain barrier risk extra-pyramidal side effects.[5] Haloperidol poses the highest risk.

Prescribing in Parkinson's Disease

- Cyclizine (25 mg initially) and domperidone are widely used first line
- Levomepromazine 2.5 mg subcutaneous or 3 mg oral can be used second line with close monitoring following specialist input.

Clinical Tip Approaches to Specific Causes of Nausea and Vomiting

If subacute or complete bowel obstruction is suspected consider:

- abdominal imaging
- surgical or endoscopic intervention, such as stent if a single transition point is identified, or venting gastrostomy

If oesophageal features such as dysphagia or retching are present, consider:

- barium swallow/OGD

If intractable nausea or features of intracerebral causes:

- Assess for neurological signs and symptoms
- Consider brain imaging

Clinical Tip Review Drug Chart

Consider medications that may contributing to nausea:

- Steroids
- Non-steroidal anti-inflammatory drugs (NSAIDs)
- Antibiotics
- Opioids
- SSRIs
- Digoxin
- Aminophylline
- Creon

Evidence Base The Antiemetic Effect of Corticosteroids

Very Low

The mechanism for the antiemetic effect of corticosteroids is not well understood.[8]

A 2017 Cochrane review concluded that there was insufficient evidence to support or refute the use of dexamethasone to treat nausea and vomiting in advanced cancer.[9]

	Action and Side Effects				
	↓Gut Motiliity and Secretions	Sedation	EPSE	Prokinetic Drugs (Colic)	Lowers seizure threshold
Metoclopramide ^{QT}			Y	Dose related	Y
Domperidone ^{QT}				Dose related	Y
Haloperidol ^{QT}		Y	Y		Y
Cyclizine	Y	Y	*		Y
Ondansetron ^{QT}	Y	Y	Y		Y
Levomepromazine ^{QT}		Y	Y		Y
Olanzapine ^{QT}	Y	Y	Y		Y

Ant - antagonist; Ag - agonist; AChM - anticholinergic/muscarinic; H1 - Histamine 1; 5HT - 5-hydroxytryptamine/serotonin; D2 - Dopamine 2; EPSE - extra-pyramidal side effects; ^{QT} - QT prolongation; AM - allosteric modulator. Based on PCF 7.[2]

*Cyclizine may rarely cause movement disorders, including tremor, dyskinesia, and dystonia.[2]

Other drugs that:

- reduce bowel motility and secretions—prochlorperazine, hyoscine butylbromide, octreotide, cinnarizine
- are prokinetic—erythromycin, stimulant laxatives
- prolong QT—erythromycin, prochlorperazine, mirtazapine

Unfortunately, 36 hours later Matthew developed slurred speech, stiffness, and grimacing. His eyes were in a fixed gaze. He was diagnosed with acute dystonia and started on a short course of oral procyclidine 2.5 mg three times a day.[6] Metoclopramide was stopped and oral domperidone 10 mg three times a day was commenced.

An OesophagoGastroDuodenoscopy (OGD) confirmed extrinsic compression of the oesophagus by mediastinal lymphadenopathy and a stent was inserted. His symptoms resolved and domperidone was discontinued.

A few weeks later Matthew was reviewed at home. He had constant nausea. Bloods revealed a corrected calcium of 3.2 and acute kidney injury (eGFR 55, baseline > 90). He was admitted to hospital and treated with fluids and bisphosphonates.

Matthew's nausea persisted despite a normalized calcium and renal function. It didn't respond to cyclizine 50 mg three times a day. His CNS asked for advice from the palliative care doctor and they started levomepromazine 2.5 mg subcutaneously nocte. Unfortunately, this failed to control the nausea so they discussed the case again. They considered a switch from levomepromazine to olanzapine but decided against this given the high risk of recurrence of dystonia. Instead, they commenced dexamethasone 4 mg with omeprazole 40 mg in addition to cyclizine and levomepromazine. The nausea resolved rapidly.

Expert Comment What Is the Minimum Dose of Levomepromazine for Nausea and Vomiting?

Unknown

Scottish Palliative Care Guidelines suggest a dose of 2.5 mg subcutaneously as a starting PRN dose for nausea and vomiting for all patients.[5] In other areas of the UK 6.25 mg is a standard dose, reflected in the Palliative Care Formulary (PCF) guidance.[2] There is a single RCT comparing levomepromazine 6.25 mg to haloperidol.[7]

The question of 'how low can you go?' to achieve antiemetic effect without sedation is an important research question.

Evidence Base For Each Antiemetic in a Palliative Care Population

Expressed by Oxford Centre for Evidence-Based Medicine (OCEBM) Levels of Evidence

Please note that use of each of these drugs is supported by a large body of empirical practice.

Metoclopramide:

*Evidence Level 1b***[10]

Haloperidol:

*Evidence Level 1b***7

5HT3 Antagonists

Palliative Care Population- *Evidence level 1b***[11]
Chemotherapy-Induced Nausea and Vomiting—*Evidence level 1a** [12]

Levomepromazine:

*Evidence Level 1b***7

Cyclizine

*Evidence Level 5**** 2

Olanzapine:

Palliative Care Population-*Evidence level 1b*** 13
Chemotherapy-Induced Nausea and Vomiting—*Evidence level 1a**[13]

*1a Systematic review of RCTs

**1b Individual RCT

***5 Expert opinion

Expert Comment Olanzapine as an Antiemetic

Olanzapine has a broader spectrum of action than levomepromazine. A Cochrane review found 13 RCTs in chemotherapy and one was in a palliative population. The number needed to treat to fully resolve nausea and vomiting was 5.[13]

We suggest olanzapine third line in many contexts when prokinesis is not need. It is anticholinergic and therefore should be used with caution in patients with paralytic ileus.[6]

Olanzapine is useful:

- in stimulating appetite
- in avoiding a syringe driver
- in concomitant depression or delirium

Dexamethasone was weaned slowly to 2 mg. Matthew developed new dizziness and diplopia. The team suspected brain metastases. An MRI scan revealed a lesion in the posterior fossa. Dexamethasone was increased to 4 mg with good effect.

Expert Comment 2:1 Oral to Subcutaneous Switching Ratio for Cyclizine

Bio-availability of oral cyclizine is 50% suggesting a potential 2:1 oral to subcutaneous conversion. We suggest starting with 75 mg/24 hours but increasing to 150 mg/24 hours if ineffective.[2]

Expert Comment Myasthenia Gravis

In myasthenia gravis, it is important to use non-pharmacological methods, as therapeutic options are extremely limited. All anticholinergic and antipsychotic medications risk worsening muscle weakness.

If initiating antiemetics it is necessary to monitor respiratory rate and oxygen saturations, ideally in an inpatient setting and consider shared decision-making with Neurology, Clinical Pharmacology, and Pharmacy.

Clinical Tip 'Worried Sick'

Anxiety can cause or exacerbate nausea and vomiting. It can present as nausea associated with specific triggers, e.g. medical appointments.

Management:

- CBT referral
- benzodiazepine or an antidepressant

Clinical Tip MI and Angina Risk with Cyclizine and Hyoscine

Hyoscine butylbromide can cause tachycardia, hypotension, and potentially fatal cardiac complications in cardiac disease. It is contraindicated in tachycardia.

It is likely that cyclizine and hyoscine hydrobromide may carry similar risks.

Later, as Matthew approached the end of his life he was no longer able to swallow oral medication. Dexamethasone was converted to a subcutaneous injection of 4 mg (3.3 mg by the base). Cyclizine 75 mg was given subcutaneously via a syringe driver over 24 hours with a daily subcutaneous injection of levomepromazine 5 mg. The medication was effective and controlled his symptoms until death.

Future Advances Alternatives to Subcutaneous Ranitidine

Following withdrawal of ranitidine, alternatives for subcutaneous acid suppression and treatment of gastrointestinal bleeding are unclear. There is growing clinical experience in the subcutaneous administration of proton pump inhibitors such as omeprazole and esomeprazole although the evidence is currently case series.[14, 15]

Future Advances Mirtazapine as an Antiemetic

A 4-week, prospective, open-label study of Mirtazapine in cancer patients found that it reduced nausea (n=28).[19]

Further research is required, although there is a stronger evidence base in chemotherapy-induced nausea and vomiting.

Future Advances Quetiapine as an Antiemetic

Quetiapine withdrawal syndrome causes vomiting. A case report suggests it might have helped a patient's nausea, however more evidence is needed before adopting this in practice.[20]

Clinical Tip Non-pharmacological Management of Nausea and Vomiting

Interventions that may help include:

- Frequent small bland meals
- Peppermint tea/capsules
- Positioning upright
- Not pressurizing the patient to eat
- Encouraging sips of fluid
- Good oral hygiene/saliva replacements
- Acupuncture

A double-blind randomized controlled trial of acupressure was not effective for nausea and vomiting in patients with advanced cancer.[16]

Olfactory distraction using alcohol swabs has been shown to be effective in an emergency care setting[17] and a small case series supports its use in a palliative care population.[18]

Discussion

Matthew presented with intractable nausea and hiccups. His functional gastric stasis was managed with subcutaneous metoclopramide. Later an OGD confirmed an extrinsic compression of his oesophagus, and a stent was inserted. When he developed recurrence of nausea, biochemical causes were identified and treated (hypercalcaemia and uraemia). Towards the end of his life, a centrally mediated nausea was found to have been caused by a brain metastasis.

Nausea and vomiting is one of the most complex symptoms to assess and manage. However, it is vital that it is controlled, not only because nausea is a significant and debilitating symptom, but also because uncontrolled nausea and vomiting can contribute to loss of symptom control for other symptoms due to the loss of the oral route, precipitating acute admissions for parenteral medications and hydration.

A Final Word from the Expert

There remains a relatively low level of evidence for many of the antiemetics we employ. The emphasis therefore needs to be on the identification and treatment (wherever possible) of the cause(s). Whilst the number of interventions available to us is continuing to increase there remains an urgent need for further research, not only into newer options such as olanzapine, mirtazapine, and quetiapine but also into those we consider to be 'routine' management choices. There remains a concerningly low level of evidence to support the use of haloperidol and levomepromazine, in particular.

The pathophysiology of a patient's nausea and vomiting can evolve over time or become multifactorial, as this case demonstrates. The importance of regular reassessment of the patient's symptoms and history cannot be overstated.

References

1. Singh P, Yoon S, Kuo B. Nausea: a review of pathophysiology and therapeutics. *Therap Adv Gastroenterol* 2016; 9(1): 98–112
2. Wilcock A, Howard P, Charlesworth S. *Palliative Care Formulary*, 8th ed. London: Pharmaceutical Press, 2022.
3. Steger M, Schneemann M, Fox M. Systemic review: the pathogenesis and pharmacological treatment of hiccups. *Aliment Pharmacol Ther* 2015; 42: 1037–1050
4. Moretto E, Wee B, Wiffen P, et al. Interventions for treating persistent and intractable hiccups in adults. *Cochrane Database Syst Rev* 2013; 1: CD008768.
5. Scottish Palliative Care Guidelines. Nausea and vomiting. Available at: https://www.palliativecareguidelines.scot.nhs.uk/guidelines/symptom-control/Nausea-and-Vomiting.aspx
6. British National Formulary. Available at: https://bnf.nice.org.uk
7. Hardy J, Skerman H, Philip J. Methotrimeprazine versus haloperidol in palliative care patients with cancer-related nausea: a randomised, double-blind controlled trial. *BMJ Open* 2019; 9(9): e029942.
8. Chu C, Hsing C, Shieh J, et al. The cellular mechanisms of the antiemetic action of dexamethasone and related glucocorticoids against vomiting. *Eur J Pharmacol* 2014; 722: 48–54.
9. Vayne-Bossert P, Haywood A, Good P, et al. Corticosteroids for adult patients with advanced cancer who have nausea and vomiting (not related to chemotherapy, radiotherapy, or surgery). *Cochrane Database Syst Rev* 2017; 7: CD012002.
10. Bruera E, Belzile M, Neumann, C, et al. A double-blind, crossover study of controlled-release metoclopramide and placebo for the chronic nausea and dyspepsia of advanced cancer. *J Pain Symptom Manage* 2000; 19: 427–435.
11. Mystakidou K, Befon S, Liossi C, et al. Comparison of the efficacy and safety of tropisetron, metoclopramide, and chlorpromazine in the treatment of emesis associated with far advanced cancer. *Cancer* 1998; 83(6): 1214–1223.
12. Piechotta V, Adams A, Haque M, et al. Antiemetics for adults for prevention of nausea and vomiting caused by moderately or highly emetogenic chemotherapy: a network meta-analysis. *Cochrane Database Syst Rev* 2021; 11: CD012775.
13. Sutherland A, Naessens K, Plugge E, et al. Olanzapine for the prevention and treatment of cancer-related nausea and vomiting in adults. *Cochrane Database Syst Rev* 2018; 9: CD012555.
14. Agar M, Webster R, Lacey J, et al. The use of subcutaneous omeprazole in the treatment of dyspepsia in palliative care patients. *J Pain Symptom Manage* 2004; 28(6): 529–531.
15. Hindmarsh J, Adelaja M, Abd Latif S, et al. Administering esomeprazole subcutaneously via a syringe driver in the palliative demographic: a case series. *J Clin Pharm Ther* 2021; 47(5): 694–698.
16. Perkins P, Parkinson A, Parker R, et al. Does acupressure help reduce nausea and vomiting in palliative care patients? A double blind randomised controlled trial. *BMJ Support Palliat Care* 2022; 12: 58–63.
17. April M, Oliver J, Davis W, et al. Aromatherapy versus oral ondansetron for antiemetic therapy among adult emergency department patients: a randomized controlled trial. *Ann Emerg Med* 2018; 72(2): 184–193.

18. Corona A, Chin J. Olfactory distraction for management of nausea in palliative care patients. *Am J Hosp Palliat Care* 2022; 39(3): 388–393.
19. Kim S, Shin I, Kim J, et al. Effectiveness of mirtazapine for nausea and insomnia in cancer patients with depression. *Psychiatry Clin Neurosci* 2008; 62: 75–83.
20. Hindmarsh J, Lee M. The use of quetiapine for the management of nausea and vomiting in idiopathic Parkinson's disease. *J Palliat Care* 2022; 37(1): 15–17.

CASE

8 Cancer Cachexia

Lucy Ison

Experts: Barry Laird and Richard Skipworth

Case history

Douglas, a 54-year-old businessman, was seen by his GP with a 3-month history of weight loss, anorexia, and fatigue. Recent medical history involved visits to the GP with symptoms including low mood, fatigue, and loss of appetite.

On further questioning, Douglas described epigastric pain and unintended weight loss of 5 kg (7% body weight) over three months. A trial of omeprazole had no effect on his pain.

Douglas lived at home with his wife and two adult children. He smoked 10 cigarettes a day and had done so for 30 years. He drank a bottle of wine a week. Douglas considered himself fit and active but had noticed a dip in his energy levels recently.

There was no family history of malignancy, inflammatory bowel disease, liver problems, gastrointestinal ulcers, or coeliac disease.

On examination at the GP surgery, Douglas had some mid-epigastric tenderness. He had a soft abdomen with no palpable masses. He was jaundiced.

Douglas was referred for a pancreatic CT scan and blood tests, including tumour markers, liver function tests, and C-reactive protein. CT scan revealed a mass in the head of the pancreas. A fluorodeoxyglucose-positron emission tomography (FDG PET) CT showed no observed local or distant spread. CA19-9 was mildly raised. The hepatopancreaticobiliary multidisciplinary team (HBP MDT) offered Douglas resection of the tumour with sparing of the pylorus and standard lymphadenectomy.

At the time of referral to surgery, he had an Eastern Cooperative Oncology Group Performance Status (ECOG-PS) of zero. Douglas's blood tests revealed an elevated C-reactive protein (CRP), normal albumin (>35 g/L), and thus he had a modified Glasgow Prognostic Score (mGPS) of 1.[1]

Douglas was enrolled in a prehabilitation programme prior to surgery to optimize his functional and nutritional status. He was advised to stop smoking and cut down on his alcohol consumption. He was screened for malnutrition and was found to have moderate malnutrition according to the phenotypic and etiologic criteria as outline by the Global Leadership Initiative on Malnutrition (GLIM) criteria.[2]

Douglas was seen by a dietitian and given advice on nutrient-dense food. He was assessed by a physiotherapist and given specific exercise interventions prior to surgery. He was managed on an Enhanced Recovery for Surgery (ERAS) pathway.[3]

The tumour was resected successfully. Douglas was commenced on pancreatin post-surgery. Once recovered from surgery, he had 6 cycles of chemotherapy (gemcitabine and capecitabine).

Expert Comment

The mGPS has been extensively validated in primary operable and inoperable cancers, in over 150,000 patients and 300 clinical studies. It is the most studied prognostic score in cancer and predicts survival. Work has also shown that this is related to quality of life—the more inflamed, the worse quality of life is likely to be. It can be used as an objective biomarker to guide patient care.

Expert Comment

Prehabilitation and ERAS are component parts of a spectrum of patient optimization and effective peri-operative care, with a view to returning patients to a status of maximal functional recovery, with minimal complications, as soon as possible. It is a responsibility of all multidisciplinary team members, including surgeons, anaesthetists, nursing staff, dieticians, and physiotherapists, but can be encouraged through the institution of formalized pathways, exercise and diet regimens, and dedicated staff.

For one year following chemotherapy, he was well and maintained his postoperative weight. However, over a period of two months, he developed jaundice, and pale, bulky stools. He experienced a further 5% weight loss. A CT scan showed a recurrence of pancreatic cancer with loco-regional recurrence and liver metastases. Re-discussion in the HPB MDT meeting occurred, and he was commenced on chemotherapy (FOLFIRINOX). Due to his ongoing weight loss, he attended a cachexia clinic. He had dietary counselling to ensure adequate protein and calorie intake, physical therapy, and psychological support. Symptoms of nausea and abdominal pain were reviewed.

Expert Comment

Defining cachexia has been the subject of much debate over the last two decades and scientific understanding is still evolving. One of the challenges has been that a true characterization of cachexia has not been done, so it is challenging to understand the trajectory and how symptoms relate to changes in body composition and biological changes. The GLIM criteria[2] are recommended; however, be aware that if a patient has a cancer where cachexia is highly prevalent (e.g. lung or pancreatic cancer) then formal diagnosis using the GLIM criteria may not be applicable at the earliest stages.

Learning Point

The GLIM criteria are now commonly used to assess cachexia.[2]

1. SCREEN FOR THOSE AT RISK FOR MALNUTRITION USING VALIDATED SCREENING TOOL

Malnutrition Universal Screening Tool (MUST)—BMI, unplanned weight loss, acute disease (if patient acutely unwell and likely to have no nutritional intake for 5 days)

Mini Nutritional Assessment Short form (MNA-SF)—questions about food intake, involuntary weight loss, mobility, psychological stress, neuropsychological problems, BMI

Nutritional Risk Screening-2002 (NRS-2002)—BMI, weight loss in last 3 months, reduced intake for last week, in intensive care unit (ICU). If answer yes to these consider—degree of nutritional impairment, severity of disease, and age

↓

2. ASSESS USING PHENOTYPIC AND AETIOLOGIC ASSESSMENT CRITERIA

Phenotypic Criteria:

Weight loss—>5% within past 6 months, or >10% beyond 6 months

Low BMI—<20 if <70 years or <22 if >70 years. (Asia: <18.5 if <70 years or <20 if >70 years)

Reduced muscle mass—Reduced by validated body composition measuring techniques

Aetiologic Criteria

Reduced food intake—< or = to 50% of energy requirements > 1 week or any reduction for >2 weeks or any chronic gastrointestinal (GI) condition that adversely impacts absorption

Disease burden / inflammation

↓

3. DIAGNOSE MALNUTRITION IF MEETS CRITERIA FOR 1 PHENOTYPIC AND 1 AETIOLOGIC CRITERIA

4. ASSESS SEVERITY BASED ON PHENOTYPIC CRITERION

Stage 1 / Moderate: 5–10% weight loss in the last 6 months, 10–20% beyond 6 months, BMI <20 if <70 years or <22 if >70 years, mild to moderate reduced muscle mass.

Stage 2 / Severe: >10% weight loss within the past 6 months or >20% beyond 6 months. BMI <18.5 if <70, <20 if >70. Severe deficit of muscle mass

Learning Point Multimodal Treatment

Increasingly, it has been recognized that cancer cachexia is a multifactorial syndrome, requiring a multimodal approach to management.

Cachexia clinics are run by multidisciplinary teams trained to manage a broad range of issues. Teams may include a registered dietician, physiotherapist, palliative care professional, and a speech and language therapist. The patient is holistically assessed, and family/caregivers are included in the assessment and recommendations. Cachexia clinics have been found to significantly increase patient appetite and to cause weight gain in one-third of patients reviewed.[10]

Evidence Base Pharmacological Agents for Cachexia

There is currently insufficient evidence to strongly endorse any particular pharmacological agent (see Table 8.1).

Table 8.1 Evidence for pharmacological management of cachexia

Weak Evidence to Recommend	
Corticosteroids	Used in the short term for appetite stimulation and weight gain. Most of this gain is in body fat and water not muscle gain.[4]
Progestins e.g. megestrol acetate and medroxyprogesterone acetate	Increase body weight but increases adipose tissue rather than skeletal muscle.[4] Associated with significant side effects including increased risk of venous thromboembolism. Effect on weight gain can take 6-12 weeks.[5]
Supplement long chain N-3 fatty acids /fish oil	Thought to improve body weight and appetite, as well as quality of life.[4]
Metoclopramide	Pro-kinetic agent to stimulate gastric emptying. Can improve nausea, but not appetite.[6]
Olanzapine	Moderate evidence to suggest using olanzapine to reduce nausea and stimulate appetite.[4, 7]
Insufficient Evidence to Recommend	
Branched chain or other amino acids	Insufficient consistent evidence to recommend.[4]
NSAIDs	Reduce the catabolic drive of systemic inflammation and may increase or stabilize body weight.[4]
Cannabinoids	Studies have shown no effect on quality of life or appetite.[4]
Androgenic steroids	Taking androgenic steroids may result in an increase in muscle mass.[4]

Expert Comment

It is the job of everyone in the multidisciplinary team to identify and treat cachexia. Simple advice on diet and exercise can be given by all members of the team, from the consultant to the allied health professional. Be aware that cachexia symptoms may not be volunteered by the patient so enquire about weight loss, appetite, and physical activity as much as possible.

Learning Point Nutrition

In malnourished cancer patients, and those at risk of malnutrition, nutritional intervention is recommended. Energy-rich foods should be increased to meet total energy expenditure (TEE), and protein should be increased to 1–1.5 g/kg/day.[4]

If after these recommendations, nutritional goals are not reached then oral nutritional supplements (ONS) can be used.[4] Vitamins and minerals should be supplied in quantities that are approximately equal to recommended daily amounts unless there are specific deficiencies.[4]

Learning Point Physical Therapy

Exercise is used in cachexia to improve aerobic capacity, muscle strength, and health-related quality of life.[11] Resistance and aerobic exercise in combination may maintain and improve muscle mass.[12] Some evidence suggests that resistance exercise may be more effective at improving muscle strength than aerobic exercise.[12]

Learning Point Cachexia and Frailty

Cachexia is not only seen in cancer but also in many other chronic diseases for example chronic obstructive pulmonary disease, renal failure, heart disease, and diabetes. As with cancer patients, cachexia in these patients can adversely impact quality of life and can lead to increased mortality, and therefore they should be assessed regularly.[14]

Clinical Tip Communication

It is extremely distressing to witness people not eating or losing weight and this can cause tension in the family unit. Patients and family need tailored information on mechanisms of cancer cachexia. Psychosocial interventions can ease distress.[15]

Under Investigation	
Selective androgen receptor modulators (SARM): e.g. enobosarm	One study had initial results that showed enobosarm caused a significant increase in lean body mass and improvement in quality of life. Final results have been released but not been formally published.[8, 9]
Anamorelin	The only licensed medication for cancer cachexia—licensed in Japan. The ROMANA trial showed a significant increase in body weight, but not handgrip strength, from baseline at all time points.[9]

Expert Comment

Cachexia causes a huge amount of stress to patients and their caregivers. It is critical to acknowledge this and also to empower the patient and caregiver to do positive things to address this. These can be simple such as sharing small meals together, going for walks or exercising together, and allowing them to discuss this openly.

Douglas's chemotherapy was stopped due to recurrent hospitalizations to treat neutropenic sepsis. Douglas was referred to the community palliative care team (CPCT). He deteriorated very rapidly, with further weight loss, decline in mobility, fatigue, and increased symptom burden. He was very keen to go to his daughter's wedding, and so was commenced on a trial of dexamethasone 4 mg OD. This increased his appetite and energy levels to a limited degree for a few days, but these effects were short-lived, so steroids were discontinued after a week.

Clinical Tip Corticosteroids

Corticosteroids and progesterones are amongst the only pharmacological agents that have sufficient evidence to recommend their use in cancer cachexia.[4] Steroids however should be used with caution and any benefits carefully balanced against their many side effects. These include susceptibility to infection, peptic ulceration, deterioration of glycaemic control, psychiatric disturbances, muscle weakness, osteoporosis, adrenal suppression, and avascular necrosis.[13] Steroids have the advantage of working within days of commencing the treatment. However, their anticachectic effect may last only for 3-4 weeks. It is recommended therefore that steroids should only be used for a limited period in advanced disease.[4]

Learning Point Nutrition at the End of Life

Nutritional support at the end of life must be goal-orientated and focused on relieving eating and weight loss-related distress, rather than aiming to improve function.[4] A focus should be maintained on managing symptoms, for example pain, depression, and constipation. Referral to a dietician may provide support to patients and relatives, and an opportunity to talk to concerns surrounding nutrition.[7]

Douglas was admitted into the hospice for symptom control. His analgesics and antiemetics were adjusted. Subcutaneous fluids were given after he expressed feelings of distress at being thirsty. He died peacefully at the hospice with his family around him.

Clinical Tip Clinically Assisted Nutrition and Hydration

It is important to explain to patients and carers that hunger is rare at the end of life, but patients can gain comfort from small amounts of their favourite foods. The level of evidence for parenteral nutrition (PN) in advanced cancer is weak, and it has been suggested that PN should be avoided in those with a low performance status. The decision to initiate PN should be an individualized decision and should take into account performance status, metastatic disease, Glasgow Prognostic Score, and crucially the goals of PN. Consideration should be made of the risks and burdens of PN including line sepsis, the need for monitoring electrolytes, and the need to be attached to a line for many hours in a day. Prior to starting PN, discussions should be had on withdrawal of PN at the end of life and which specific criteria may need to be fulfilled for this to be discontinued.[16]

Clinically assisted hydration (CAH) has shown no clear and consistent benefit at the end of life.[17] There is some inconsistent evidence for improvement of agitation.[4] However, studies have shown that CAH is ineffective for dry mouth or thirst and therefore should not be used in this context.[17] The decision to give hydration at the end of life must therefore be individualized. Research in this area is ongoing.[18]

Future Advances

As our understanding of the genesis of cancer cachexia increases, it is likely that pathways targeting the endocannabinoid systems, GDF15, ghrelin, and JAK-STAT may lead to targeted treatments for cachexia. Nevertheless, in the same paradigm that exists in modern cancer therapy, combination treatment is likely to be central with targeted therapies employed on a background of basic nutrition and exercise interventions.

A Final Word from the Expert

Be aware that in patients with cancer, cachexia is more likely to happen than not (and is almost a certainty in some cancers). Therefore, it is imperative that attention is paid to cachexia. Historically, cachexia has been considered an inevitable consequence of cancer and has been viewed with nihilism due to a lack of effective therapies. A step change is needed to recognise and treat cancer cachexia as an integral part of good oncological and palliative care. This case illustrates key principles in these aforementioned factors and provides clinicians with the foundations to identify and effectively treat cancer cachexia.

References

1. McMillan DC. The systemic inflammation-based Glasgow Prognostic Score: a decade of experience in patients with cancer. *Cancer Treat Rev* 2013; 39(5): 534–540.
2. Cederholm T, Jensen GL, Correia MITD, et al. GLIM criteria for the diagnosis of malnutrition—a consensus report from the global clinical nutrition community. *Clin Nutr* 2019; 38(1): 1–9.
3. Melloul E, Lassen K, Roulin D, et al. Guidelines for perioperative care for pancreatoduodenectomy: enhanced recovery after surgery (ERAS) recommendations 2019. *World J Surg* 2020; 44(7): 2056–2084.
4. Muscaritoli M, Arends J, Bachmann P, et al. ESPEN practical guideline: clinical nutrition in cancer. *Clin Nutr* 2021; 40(5): 2898–2913.
5. Yavuzsen T, Davis MP, Walsh D, LeGrand S, Lagman R. Systematic review of the treatment of cancer-associated anorexia and weight loss. *J Clin Oncol* 2005; 23(33): 8500–8511.
6. Bruera E, Belzile M, Neumann C, Harsanyi Z, Babul N, Darke A. A double-blind, crossover study of controlled-release metoclopramide and placebo for the chronic nausea and dyspepsia of advanced cancer. *J Pain Symptom Manage* 2000; 19(6): 427–435.
7. Roeland EJ, Bohlke K, Baracos VE, et al. Management of cancer cachexia: ASCO guideline. *J Clin Oncol* 2020; 38(21): 2438–2453.
8. Dobs AS, Boccia RV, Croot CC, et al. Effects of enobosarm on muscle wasting and physical function in patients with cancer: a double-blind, randomised controlled phase 2 trial. *Lancet Oncol* 2013; 14(4): 335–345.
9. Currow D, Temel JS, Abernethy A, Milanowski J, Friend J, Fearon KC. ROMANA 3: a phase 3 safety extension study of anamorelin in advanced non-small-cell lung cancer (NSCLC) patients with cachexia. *Ann Oncol* 2017; 28(8): 1949–1956.
10. del Fabbro E, Hui D, Dalal S, Dev R, Nooruddin ZI, Bruera E. Clinical outcomes and contributors to weight loss in a cancer cachexia clinic. *J Palliat Med* 2011; 14(9): 1004–1008.
11. Fong DYT, Ho JWC, Hui BPH, et al. Physical activity for cancer survivors: meta-analysis of randomised controlled trials. *BMJ* 2012; 344: e70.
12. Stene GB, Helbostad JL, Balstad TR, Riphagen II, Kaasa S, Oldervoll LM. Effect of physical exercise on muscle mass and strength in cancer patients during treatment—a systematic review. *Crit Rev Oncol Hematol* 2013; 88(3): 573–593.
13. Wilcock A, Howard P, Charlesworth S. *Palliative Care Formulary*, 8th ed. London: Pharmaceutical Press, 2022.
14. Yoshida T, Delafontaine P. Mechanisms of cachexia in chronic disease states. *Am J Med Sci* 2015; 350(4): 250–256.
15. Hopkinson JB, Fenlon DR, Okamoto I, et al. The deliverability, acceptability, and perceived effect of the Macmillan approach to weight loss and eating difficulties: a phase II, cluster-randomized, exploratory trial of a psychosocial intervention for weight- and eating-related distress in people with advanced cancer. *J Pain Symptom Manage* 2010; 40(5): 684–695.
16. Arends J, Strasser F, Gonella S, et al. Cancer cachexia in adult patients: ESMO clinical practice guidelines. *ESMO Open* 2021; 6(3): 100092.
17. Kingdon A, Spathis A, Brodrick R, Clarke G, Kuhn I, Barclay S. What is the impact of clinically assisted hydration in the last days of life? A systematic literature review and narrative synthesis. *BMJ Support Palliat Care* 2021; 11(1): 68.
18. Davies AN, Waghorn M, Webber K, Johnsen S, Mendis J, Boyle J. A cluster randomised feasibility trial of clinically assisted hydration in cancer patients in the last days of life. *Palliat Med* 2018; 32(4): 733–743.

CASE

9 Bowel Obstruction

Sarah Webster and Emily Rea

Expert: Emma Husbands

Case history

Jess, a 53-year-old teacher, attended the clinic with a one-week history of nausea, vomiting, and abdominal distension. She was vomiting small amounts several times a day with some relief of nausea and fullness afterwards, and she was passing liquid yellow stool.

On examination, her abdomen was distended and tense but non-tender with no shifting dullness. Bowel sounds were quiet and infrequent.

Jess had been diagnosed with metastatic uterine carcinosarcoma three months earlier. She initially presented with large-volume ascites secondary to peritoneal disease. She underwent recurrent paracentesis, but her ascites improved once she began chemotherapy.

Learning Point What is Malignant Bowel Obstruction?

A consensus definition of MBO established three diagnostic criteria[1]:

1. Failure to pass stool or flatus
2. Obstruction distal to the ligament of Treitz (at the duodenojejunal flexure)
3. Presence of a primary intra-abdominal cancer or extra-abdominal cancer with peritoneal involvement.

MBO may occur at a single site or multiple sites. Two-thirds of cases involve the small bowel.[1] Data from retrospective studies and post-mortem findings suggest a prevalence in cancer patients of 3–15%, most commonly in patients with gynaecological and gastrointestinal cancers, and those with advanced malignancy.

In MBO, the symptoms relate to bowel distension proximal to the level of obstruction. A cycle of bowel distension, increased gastrointestinal and pancreaticobiliary secretions, and epithelial damage triggering an inflammatory response occurs. Prostaglandins, vasoactive intestinal peptide (VIP) and nociceptive mediators are released. Excess luminal contents can lead to large volume vomiting. The bowel attempts to overcome the obstruction by contracting and this can lead to colicky abdominal pain, bowel ischaemia, perforation, and sepsis.

Learning Point Aetiology

Bowel obstruction may be described as mechanical or functional. It can be partial or complete (see Table 9.1).

Table 9.1 Aetiology of bowel obstruction

MECHANICAL	**Extrinsic compression:** Commonly due to tumour outside the bowel lumen. Other causes include ascites, adhesions, and post-radiation fibrosis.
	Intrinsic compression: Direct disease invasion into the bowel wall e.g. radiation enteropathy.
	Occlusion of the lumen: Caused by intraluminal masses.
FUNCTIONAL	**Peristaltic failure:** Impairment of the mesentery or nerves supplying the bowel e.g. coeliac plexus. This may occur following surgery, with constipating medications e.g. opioids, in electrolyte abnormalities e.g. hypokalaemia, and with diabetes or inflammatory bowel disease.

Learning Point

Diagnosis

A diagnosis of MBO can be made on clinical grounds but would often be confirmed by imaging.

History

The history should include a clear description of bowel habit including flatus, presence of nausea or vomiting, and pain. Remember to ask about medications.

Clinical Tip

When asking about pain try to distinguish between colic (short-lived intense spasms of pain that may occur in waves, often described as sharp, cramping pains) and continuous dull or aching pain which may originate from the tumour.

Clinical symptoms may direct us towards the likely level of obstruction (see Table 9.2).

Table 9.2 Likely clinical symptoms based on level of obstruction

Proximal small bowel	Large volume vomiting that occurs after eating. Vomitus may contain undigested food and can be odourless (a combination of swallowed saliva and gastric secretions) or may be bile-stained. Colic may be minimal - tending to be associated with vomiting. Stool distal to the obstruction may still be passed but with diminishing frequency/volume.
Distal small bowel	Nausea and vomiting are often less severe. Vomitus may be mixture of bile-stained and faeculent. Abdominal distension may occur. Colic tends to be severe. Constipation and diarrhoea can precede complete obstruction.
Large bowel	Nausea and vomiting are a later feature, usually in small amounts. Vomitus will likely be faeculent. Abdominal distension is prominent. Colic is usually less severe. Alternating constipation and diarrhoea may precede complete obstruction.

Examination

Examination may reveal abdominal distension and less commonly, visible distended loops of bowel. Tumour mass, ascites, and faecal masses may be palpable. Rectal examination may reveal hard faeces or if the rectal ampulla is empty and distended this suggests stool higher in the colon.

Investigations

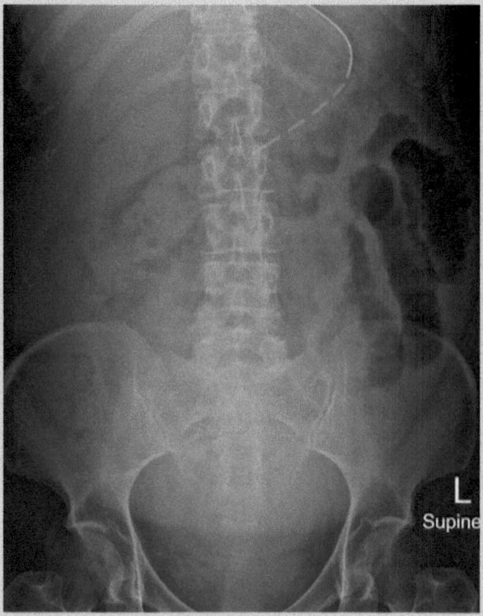

Figure 9.1 AXR demonstrating left-sided dilated small bowel loops. Note the presence of nasogastric tube (NG tube) and faecal loading in the ascending colon.

Clinical Tip

Plain AXR may demonstrate faecal loading and dilated loops of bowel or significantly distended stomach (Figure 9.1). Other findings may include air-fluid levels proximal to the site of obstruction with a paucity or absence of intraluminal gas distal to the point of obstruction. Functional obstruction will show a uniform gaseous distension of the stomach, bowel, or rectum. Although perforation in MBO is unusual, presence of free air may be seen on AXR. The presence of tumour encasing the bowel may render AXR unremarkable, even if obstruction is present.

Expert Comment

Investigations should only be undertaken if they will influence management. In suspected MBO, it can be useful to confirm the diagnosis, as this may impact prognosis and thus advance care planning.

Bloods should be taken to assess hydration and exclude other causes for MBO e.g. hypokalaemia, hypercalcaemia, or hypothyroidism. AXR can establish a diagnosis of small bowel obstruction (up to 70% accuracy) but provides limited information on the cause and is unlikely to show multilevel obstruction.

CT scans (see Figure 9.2) can identify transition points and associated mass effect and may be helpful to guide options for stenting or surgery. Gastrograffin contrast is preferred due to its hyperosmolar composition and it has been shown to improve chance of resolution of the obstruction.[2] Barium has been shown to increase the risk of exacerbating the obstruction.

Jess was diagnosed with functional bowel obstruction. Hospital or hospice admission were discussed but Jess wished to remain at home with input from the community palliative care team (CPCT).

As Jess's history suggested a partial rather than complete obstruction, initial management focused on 'acceleration' of the bowel, alongside reducing inflammation and

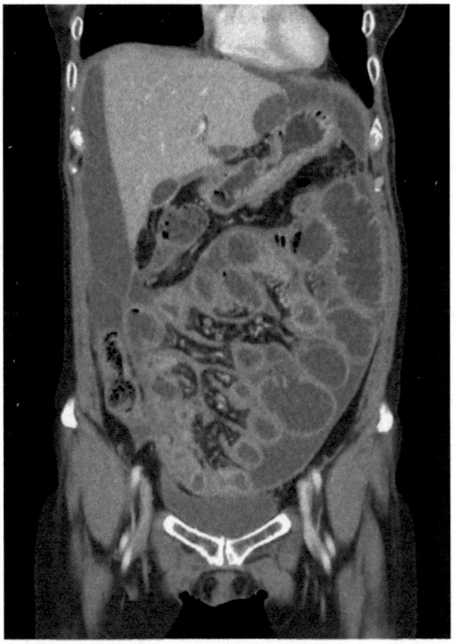

Figure 9.2 CT abdomen/pelvis showing multilevel obstruction and small volume ascites.

gastric secretions. A decision was made to trial medications orally in the first instance in line with Jess's wishes:

- Metoclopramide 10 mg TDS orally
- Dexamethasone 8 mg OD orally
- Lansoprazole orodispersible 30 mg OD orally, later titrated to 30 mg BD

Clinical Tip

The approach to MBO management can be likened to traffic control. When MBO occurs, there will be a build-up of 'traffic' (gastric contents). Management should focus on reducing the build-up with decompression, redirecting fluid through a nasogastric (NG) tube if appropriate, and reducing fluid production with a proton pump inhibitor (PPI)/Histamine-2 antagonist (H2A).

Always assess for a 'road block' (tumour/complete stricture) and consider if it can be removed (i.e. whether surgical management is appropriate).

If there is no obvious 'road block', consider whether the pace of 'traffic' can be increased by 'acceleration' (i.e. use of prokinetics). If there is a 'bottle neck', accelerating may exacerbate symptoms and 'shifting to neutral' may be preferable (i.e. discontinuing prokinetics). You may need to 'put the brakes on' (i.e. use an antisecretory and/or antispasmodic medication) because a transport lorry cannot get through a standard car lane.

Be prepared to react and change 'direction' or 'speed' accordingly.

None of these approaches reduce the chance of resolution of MBO.

Expert Comment

Whilst an approach of maintaining prokinesis is often appropriate in the absence of colic and with no signs of complete obstruction, increasing 'painless' vomiting may represent mechanical colic and so increased vomiting is a red flag to consider shifting away from prokinesis. If there are significant adhesions, colic can sometimes also be experienced as back pain and again this may suggest a need to stop prokinesis.

The presence and severity of colic or symptoms above is likely to be the main guide to stopping prokinesis but location of care may also influence the approach – particular caution should be used in the community where frequent monitoring and review of symptoms is more challenging.

Evidence Base

A Cochrane systematic review reported that fewer patients developed constipation when using transdermal fentanyl compared to oral morphine.[10] However, there is no evidence to support switching opioids in the presence of MBO.

Expert Comment

Passage of liquid stool can sometimes make it seem MBO is resolving but may represent liquefaction of stool in the lower bowel.

Evidence Base

The evidence for the use of steroids is poor but a Cochrane review concluded they may relieve symptoms and the risk of adverse events is very low.[6] They remain a mainstay of MBO treatment in clinical practice exerting anti-inflammatory, antiemetic, and analgesic effects.

Clinical Tip

Always consider side effects of steroids, such as hunger, which can become distressing.

Forty-eight hours later Jess represented to the hospital Emergency Department with vomiting. The diagnosis remained partial bowel obstruction and in the absence of colic, the 'acceleration' approach was continued, but medications were given parenterally:

- continuous subcutaneous infusion (CSCI) with morphine sulphate 5 mg and metoclopramide 30 mg over 24 hours
- dexamethasone 8 mg subcutaneously OD

Jess declined hospital admission, so an urgent CT scan was requested as an outpatient.

The following day, Jess developed severe colic with continued vomiting, reflux, and belching. She continued to pass liquid yellow stool. Management shifted into creating a 'neutral bowel'.

- Metoclopramide was stopped
- CSCI haloperidol 2.5 mg over 24 hours was started for nausea

Learning Point Management

As MBO usually occurs in patients with advanced disease, management should be guided by the patient's goals of care and functional status. When MBO presents with no further oncological treatment possible, prognosis is likely measured in weeks.

- Early surgical intervention may enable patients to continue treatment for their underlying malignancy but morbidity, mortality, and rates of recurrence of MBO are high. Careful patient selection is necessary. Patients with a single transition point and a good performance status are more likely to have a successful outcome.[3]

Future Advances

There are no consensus core reported outcome measures for MBO and at the time of writing, a multicentre study was underway to try and reach a consensus.[4] Use consistent approaches such as volume of NG output, frequency of vomiting, or pain to assess response to medication.

Intervention may involve bowel resection, metal stent insertion, or venting gastrostomy, depending on the site of the obstruction, local services, and patient fitness.[5]

Principles of medical management include:

- Rest bowel by minimizing oral intake. Give medications parenterally where possible or convert to suspension/dispersible preparations if necessary. Ensure regular mouth care.
- Decompress the bowel. This may involve inserting a nasogastric tube or using a venting gastrostomy.
- Give dexamethasone (6–16 mg, depending on local guidelines). This is usually given parenterally, but this will depend on the setting.
- Reduce intraluminal secretions. H2As and PPIs reduce gastric secretions.[7] Ranitidine, the H2A with the largest evidence base, is no longer available. Other H2As, e.g. famotidine and nizatidine are not available parentally in the UK. Whilst orodispersible PPIs can be tried, parenteral formulations of omeprazole and esomeprazole can be administered subcutaneously.[8,9]
- Give analgesia as required. Opioids remain the mainstay of pain management despite constipating side effects. If severe colic, anticholinergics such as hyoscine

butylbromide can be used, but with caution due to the slowing effects on the gastrointestinal (GI) tract.

- Consider hydration including correction of electrolyte imbalance if appropriate.
- Manage nausea and vomiting. Choice of antiemetic should be guided by the status of obstruction and presence of colic:
  - **Partial obstruction with NO colic: '*Acceleration*'**
    - Trial of parenteral metoclopramide, monitoring closely for colic.[11]
    - If metoclopramide isn't tolerated or is ineffective, erythromycin can be used intravenously (IV) or as an oral suspension.[12]
  - **Partial obstruction WITH colic or complete obstruction: '*Neutral*'**
    - First line—haloperidol.[11]
    - Second line—olanzapine.[11]

    Ondansetron and granisetron may be of benefit. Cyclizine is commonly used in clinical practice but there is no conclusive evidence around its role in MBO.[11]
  - **Partial obstruction WITH severe colic or complete obstruction: '*Apply brakes*'**
    - Antisecretory agents—anticholinergics and somatostatin analogues. Hyoscine butylbromide is the most commonly used anticholinergic. Hyoscine hydrobromide may be more useful for profound nausea as it crosses the blood brain barrier.
    - Octreotide, a somatostatin analogue, causes splanchnic vasoconstriction and inhibits production of VIP resulting in reduced intestinal and pancreatic secretions, decreased gastric emptying, and slowing of smooth muscle contractions. Due to its cost, octreotide should be used judiciously, ensuring regular review. One placebo controlled RCT demonstrated no statistically significant reduction in days free of nausea, vomiting, or pain when octreotide was added alongside bowel rest, dexamethasone, ranitidine, and PRN hyoscine buytylbromide.[13] If there is no clinical improvement (i.e. reduced volume of NG tube output/no. of vomits) after 5–7 days, octreotide should be discontinued.

> **Expert Comment**
>
> Long-acting intramuscular forms of octreotide are available but due to cost and duration of effect, should not be offered until response and the appropriate dose have been established.

Several days later, Jess was admitted to hospital with persistent vomiting, abdominal distension, and constipation. A CT scan showed multilevel obstruction with multiple transition points.

A NG tube was inserted and fluids were administered intravenously. Dexamethasone was increased to 8 mg SC BD. No surgical options were appropriate due to the multilevel nature of obstruction.

Despite the NG tube Jess continued to vomit large volumes. Octreotide 300 micrograms over 24 hours via syringe pump was started. This was titrated to 800 micrograms over 24 hours. This significantly improved her symptoms enabling her to attend her wedding reception, temporarily without the NG tube, which had long been a priority.

Advance care planning discussions took place and Jess chose to return home. IV fluids were stopped and subcutaneous fluids were offered at home in discussion with Jess' GP, community nursing team, and CPCT. Jess stayed at home for a month before being admitted to her local hospice for end of life care.

Learning Point Ongoing Management

The approach to management depends on resolution of MBO and any interventions that have been trialled. Establishing the patient's priorities will guide care. A preference to avoid hospital admission may require accepting limitations in management. As recurrence of MBO is common it is important to consider and plan for future episodes.

- If MBO resolves, care should continue to focus on maintaining 'acceleration' and avoiding build-up of 'traffic'. A low fibre/residue diet is recommended, and laxatives should be considered.
- For people who remain in complete obstruction, care should be focused on comfort, using parenteral medication and fluids to alleviate symptoms. Patients may accept episodes of vomiting in preference to having a nasogastric tube or in order to continue oral intake.

Nutrition and Hydration

Parenteral fluids may provide symptom control in patients with MBO who deteriorate due to dehydration, rather than as a consequence of their disease. Parenteral nutrition is occasionally used to support patients with MBO with ongoing disease modifying treatments which may reverse the MBO, or to bridge a patient to interventions such as surgery or stenting. There is no evidence to suggest improved survival or quality of life with the use of clinically assisted nutrition and hydration in the setting of irreversible MBO from end-stage disease.[14] Clinically assisted nutrition and hydration may influence options such as place of care and limit the patient's freedom in the final phase of their illness.

Future Advances

Establishing wider access to parenteral fluids across all care settings should optimize the ability to support management of MBO in non-acute settings. Current provision of hydration in community settings is inconsistent across the UK.

A Final Word from the Expert

The pattern of fluctuation seen in this case is typical of MBO. Awareness of the potential for rapid progression from partial to complete bowel obstruction (and indeed resolution of obstruction), is vital in adjusting treatment.

The use of medical approaches will form standard care, but surgical intervention should always be considered. A focus on parenteral administration where possible, and suspension or orodispersible formulations is encouraged to give greater assurance of absorption.

Understanding an individual's priorities helps to guide care and the interventions offered will be influenced by this. Care should be tailored where possible, including for very specific events such as removal of NG tube for Jess's wedding reception in this case. Monitoring of outcomes should be agreed with the patient given a lack of consensus patient reported outcome measures. Close multidisciplinary team (MDT) working will ensure that care can be managed in the most appropriate setting and any changes in clinical condition coordinated both in and out-of-hours.

References

1. Tuca A, Guell E, Martinez-Losada E, Codorniu N. Malignant bowel obstruction in advanced cancer patients: epidemiology, management, and factors influencing spontaneous resolution. *Cancer Manag Res* 2012; 4: 159–169.
2. Branco BC, Barmparas G, Schnüriger B, et al. Systematic review and meta-analysis of the diagnostic and therapeutic role of water-soluble contrast agent in adhesive small bowel obstruction. *Br J Surg* 2010; 97(4): 470–478.

3. Cousins SE, Tempest E, Feuer DJ. Surgery for the resolution of symptoms in malignant bowel obstruction in advanced gynaecological and gastrointestinal cancer. Cochrane Database Syst Rev 2016; 1: CD002764.
4. Baddeley E, Bravington A, Johnson M, et al. Development of a core outcome set to use in the research and assessment of malignant bowel obstruction: protocol for the RAMBO study. *BMJ Open* 2020; 10(6): e039154.
5. van Hooft JE, van Halsema EE, Vanbiervliet G, et al. European Society of Gastrointestinal Endoscopy. Self-expandable metal stents for obstructing colonic and extracolonic cancer: European Society of Gastrointestinal Endoscopy (ESGE) Clinical Guideline. *Endoscopy* 2014; 46(11): 990–1053.
6. Feuer DJ, Broadley KE. Corticosteroids for the resolution of malignant bowel obstruction in advanced gynaecological and gastrointestinal cancer. *Cochrane Database Syst Rev* 2000; 2000(2): CD001219.
7. Clark K, Lam L, Currow D. Reducing gastric secretions—a role for histamine 2 antagonists or proton pump inhibitors in malignant bowel obstruction?. *Support Care Cancer* 2009; 17: 1463.
8. Wilcock A, Howard P, Charlesworth S. *Palliative Care Formulary*, 8th ed. London: Pharmaceutical Press, 2022.
9. Woodman M, Curtin J, Howard P. Esomeprazole for subcutaneous infusion: compatibility with other alkaline medications. *BMJ Support Palliat Care* 2022. spcare-2022-003936.
10. Hadley G, Derry S, Moore R, Wiffen P. Transdermal fentanyl for cancer pain. *Cochrane Database Syst Rev* 2013; 10: CD010270.
11. Davis M, Hui D, Davies A, et al. Medical management of malignant bowel obstruction in patients with advanced cancer: 2021 MASCC guideline update. *Support Care Cancer* 2021; 29(12): 8089–8096.
12. Rea E, Husbands E. Erythromycin: prophylaxis against recurrent small bowel obstruction. *BMJ Support Palliat Care* 2017; 7(3): 261–263.
13. Currow DC, Quinn S, Agar M, et al. Double-blind, placebo-controlled randomized trial of octreotide in malignant bowel obstruction. *J Pain Symptom Manage* 2015; 49: 814–821.
14. Sowerbutts A, Lal S, Sremanakova J, Clamp A, et al. Home parenteral nutrition for people with inoperable malignant bowel obstruction. *Cochrane Database Syst Rev* 2018; 8: CD012812.

CASE 10 Pruritis

Rose O'Duffy

Expert: Maggie Presswood

Case history

Bill, a 75-year-old man, presented to the acute medical unit at a tertiary hospital with jaundice and general deterioration. On acute medical clerking, Bill also reported severe, generalized itch.

> **Expert Comment**
>
> Itch is rarely the first reported symptom by patients and is sometimes not volunteered unless an explicit enquiry is made by the clinician. This can be due to patient perception that little can be done to alleviate the symptom. It is good practice in a thorough review of symptoms to ask about the presence of itch in all patients with palliative care needs.

Bill had been diagnosed with colorectal cancer five months previously after he started experiencing unexpected weight loss and rectal bleeding. Bone and liver metastases were present at the time of diagnosis. He had ischaemic heart disease, congestive cardiac failure, and hypertension. He lived with his wife who was in good health. He was generally frail, remaining in bed for more than 50% of the day and needed carers twice a day. Taking this into consideration, there was a multidisciplinary team (MDT) discussion of his case and the possible treatment options. This meeting concluded that there would be limited benefit from chemotherapy or radiotherapy, and no role for surgery. After discussion with his oncologist and his family, Bill decided not to have any oncological treatment and to focus on his quality of life.

Following diagnosis, Bill managed well for several weeks but subsequently developed abdominal pain. Morphine sulphate immediate release (IR) was very effective for the pain, so his GP commenced regular morphine sulphate modified release (MR) at a starting dose of 5 mg BD. The dose was gradually titrated over a period of weeks up to 20 mg BD according to the severity of the pain and the amount of breakthrough pain relief required.

Bill developed marked jaundice and pruritis, so presented to his local A + E department. Bill's itch was generalized. He had tried his wife's E45 cream, and although this helped a bit, his itch appeared to be worsening and it was stopping him from sleeping. On admission to the acute medical unit he was markedly icteric. His Liver Function Tests (LFTs) demonstrated Bilirubin 132 umol/L, Alkaline Phosphatase (ALP) 535 U/L, Alanine Transaminase (ALT) 174 U/L, Albumin 19 g/L. His serum-corrected calcium was normal and eGFR was 55 ml/min. There were no signs or symptoms of opioid toxicity and his pain was well controlled, so no changes were made to his opioid regimen at this stage. CT Thorax/Abdomen/Pelvis (CT TAP) demonstrated new liver metastases, including a lesion obstructing the common bile duct, as well as progression of his known lung and bone metastases. After discussion with the interventional radiology team, it was thought that the obstructing lesion in the bile duct would be amenable to a stent. This was placed via Endoscopic Retrograde CholangioPancreatography (ERCP) and within 72 hours his LFTs began to normalize and his itch drastically improved. Bill returned home, back to the care of his GP, with some advice about simple measures to take if his itch returned, i.e. keeping his fingernails short.

Eight weeks later, Bill's itch returned and he again became jaundiced. He did not want to return to hospital for further investigation (including possible repeat ERCP), so his GP started chlorphenamine in the community. This did not help, and just made him drowsy, so his GP made a referral to community palliative care team (CPCT) for support with symptom management.

The CPCT decided to switch him from morphine sulphate to oxycodone with a dose reduction in view of ongoing itch and drowsiness. There was no myoclonus, hallucinations, or respiratory depression. Opioid rotation would not be standard practice given his deranged LFTs, but this was a reasonable step to take here (see the section on opioid-induced itch for a fuller explanation of the rationale).

After 48 hours, his itch had improved only slightly. The team concluded that the likeliest cause of ongoing generalized itch was due to cholestasis (due to progression of hepatic metastases), and he agreed to trial sertraline 25 mg OD for this. He continued to clinically decline over the next week, however, and taking oral medications became increasingly difficult. After a discussion with Bill and his wife, it became clear that his preferred place of care and death was home. He became drowsy and nauseated, and a Continuous Subcutaneous Infusion (CSCI) was commenced to manage his nausea and pain as he was no longer able to take oral medications. He did not show signs of agitation, suggesting itch was no longer bothering him, and so the decision was made to monitor and use PRN medication as needed. He died peacefully at home.

Expert Comment

Opioid-induced itch—troublesome, ongoing pruritus—only occurs in approximately 1% of patients taking systemic opioids.[1] However, mild pruritis occurs in up to 10% of patients. See later in the text for a suggested strategy to manage this.

Learning Point

Itch, or pruritus, has been defined as 'an unpleasant cutaneous sensation that provokes the desire to scratch'.[2] This response helps to distinguish it from pain; when we feel pain the impulse is to withdraw—in itch the impulse is the opposite.[3] It can be debilitating for those who suffer from it, cause significant psychosocial morbidity, and is often challenging to treat.[4]

Scratching an Itch

Scratching has been demonstrated to attenuate the transmission of itch via the spinothalamic tract, and scratching appears to deactivate areas of the brain that associate itch with an unpleasant feeling.[5,6]

Meanwhile, scratching in the presence of itch appears to activate areas of the brain, i.e. the putamen, which is particularly associated with the anticipation of pleasure.[5]

Sensitization

Like pain, people can also become sensitized to itch if repeatedly exposed to itchy stimuli. They can develop[7]:

- Allokinesis, wherein non-itchy stimuli are interpreted as itchy
- Hyperkinesis, wherein mildly itchy stimuli are amplified and interpreted as severely itchy

This sensitization occurs both peripherally and centrally.[7]

Evidence Base

What Happens Peripherally

Unmyelinated C-fibres convey the sensation of itch from the skin to the central nervous system. There are multiple possible pruritogens, including neuropeptides, cytokines, and amines.[8] Some of these have been demonstrated to have their own specific neuronal pathway, e.g. histamine. Schmelz et al.[9] demonstrated a histamine-specific itch pathway mediated by about 5% of the C-fibres present in the skin.[2]

95% of C-fibres with the potential to convey itch are therefore unaffected by histamine. In the literature, this pathway is often demonstrated using cowhage spicules, which transmit itch via histamine-independent polymodal C-fibres.[6]

What Happens Centrally

The itch impulse is transmitted along the C fibre to the dorsal root ganglion in the spinal cord, immediately crosses over to the contralateral spinothalamic tract, and ascends to multiple nuclei in the thalamus. Multiple areas of the brain are activated, including those involved with emotion, attention, and motor planning. There are also notable similarities with the areas activated by pain.[3]

Clinical Tip General Approach

A thorough history and examination can help determine the likeliest cause(s) of the itch, facilitating a logical treatment strategy (see Figure 10.1). Information about recent travel, recent medication changes, or associated symptoms can be particularly useful.

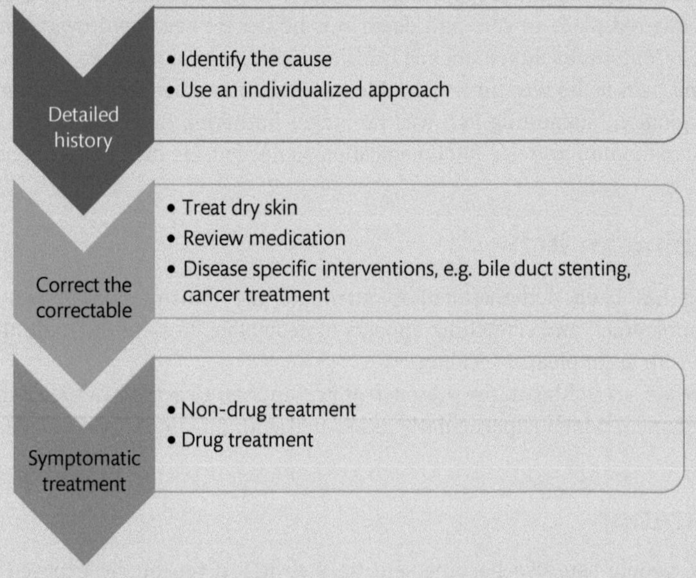

Detailed history
• Identify the cause
• Use an individualized approach
Correct the correctable
• Treat dry skin
• Review medication
• Disease specific interventions, e.g. bile duct stenting, cancer treatment
Symptomatic treatment
• Non-drug treatment
• Drug treatment

Figure 10.1 A guide to approaching itch.

Non-drug Treatment

Some simple measures can be taken to reduce the impact of itch[2]:

1. Keeping cool, i.e. light clothing
2. Keeping fingernails short
3. Avoid drying out skin, i.e. substituting emollients for soap

Expert Comment

Drug-induced pruritus: In a study of 200 patients with cutaneous drug reactions, 12.5% had pruritus without a rash.[10] Ensure a detailed history of all medication changes or additions within the few months preceding the onset of itch. Ask about the use of over-the-counter (OTC) medications, herbal remedies, and recreational drugs. There are many proposed mechanisms for drug-induced pruritus but many are idiopathic. Some of the commonest offending medications in patients with palliative care needs are: opioids, allopurinol, amiodarone, diuretics, ACE inhibitors, statins, NSAIDs, and antibiotics. The benefit/risk ratio of stopping a suspect medication needs to be considered on a case-by-case basis. Allergic reactions to drugs involve the release of histamine and response to H1 antihistamines, and stopping the offending drug.

Complementary therapies can be useful as well as psychological therapies to help break the itch-scratch cycle.[2, 8]

Common Causes of Pruritus in Palliative Care and Management

Dry Skin

Even where there is a possible endogenous cause of itch, treating dry skin may avoid the need for systemic or disease-specific treatment.

Suggestion for treatment:

- The best emollient is the greasiest one the patient is willing to use regularly. The emollient needs to be reapplied throughout the day.[8]

Topical Antipruritics

- Capsaicin cream 0.025–0.075% has been used successfully for localized areas of uraemic pruritus, although the burning sensation can be intolerable and it is not suitable for use for generalized pruritis. Capsaicin initially causes hypersensitivity, followed by a long period of desensitization as substance P stores are depleted.[11]
- Levomenthol or 1–2% menthol in aqueous cream—menthol activates a transient receptor potential (TRP) channel called TPRM8, which is thought to inhibit pruritogenic signals within the dorsal horn of the spinal cord.[12]

Cholestatic Itch

Cholestatic itch is likely due to endogenous release of opioids from the liver. Opioid antagonists have been shown to reduce scratching in patients with cholestatic itch, and have also induced withdrawal-like effects in patients who were not receiving exogenous opioids.[2]

There are several treatment options available:

- Sertraline: based on the findings of a small study (n = 12) that suggested an improvement in symptoms.[13]
- Rifampicin: Kremer et al suggested in their 2012 paper that rifampicin reduces the expression of autotaxin, a lysophospholipase that is produced by hepatic cells. Raised plasma levels of autotaxin were shown correlate with itch severity.[14]
- Danazol (synthetic hormone): based on a 1952 case study,[8] and is thought to be effective as a result of the directly toxic effect of 17α-alkyl androgens on hepatocytes, thereby preventing the liver from producing the enkephalins that contribute to itch.[2]
- Opioid antagonists: there is a risk of analgesic reversal. It has been suggested that an opioid antagonist that does not cross the blood brain barrier, like methylnaltrexone may be of use,[13] as it preserves the analgesic effect of the opioid, whilst reversing its peripheral side effects.

Opioid-induced Itch

There are two types of opioid-induced itch:

1. Histamine-related. This occurs in around 1% of cases.[2, 8]
2. Non-histamine-related. This is centrally mediated, and appears related to interactions with other neurotransmitters, especially serotonin.[2, 8]

Expert Comment

Emollients, creams, lotions, and ointments contain oils, which can catch fire. When emollient products come into contact with dressings, clothing, bed linen, or hair, there is a danger that a naked flame or cigarette smoking could cause these to catch fire. To reduce the fire risk, patients using skincare products are advised to be very careful near naked flames to reduce the risk of clothing, hair, or bedding catching fire.

Expert Comment

Some specialist guidelines recommend colestyramine first line for cholestatic pruritus in incomplete biliary obstruction. Because it sequesters bile salts inside the gastrointestinal tract it is ineffective in complete biliary obstruction. Unfortunately, many patients find they cannot tolerate colestyramine. It is unpalatable and can cause nausea, vomiting, and diarrhoea.[8]

Expert Comment

Despite the fact that many causes of itch are histamine-independent, a short trial of antihistamine may be indicated. This is because the onset of action will be relatively quick in comparison to other systemic therapies. Sedating first generation antihistamines can be of benefit particularly if itch is worse at night.

Some common approaches to opioid-induced itch include:

- Antihistamine.
- Opioid switch, e.g. morphine to oxycodone. The effect of an opioid rotation is thought to be mediated by an imbalance in the opioid receptor sub-types (see Future Advances). Morphine has a very high affinity for mu receptors, whilst oxycodone has a much lower affinity for mu receptors, and therefore balances kappa and mu more effectively, whilst also maintaining analgesia.[15]
- As mentioned earlier, serotonin may mediate opioid-induced pruritus. Therefore a 5-HT3 receptor antagonist like ondansetron may be helpful. It is particularly useful for itch caused by spinal morphine.[2,8,16]

Uraemic Itch

Uraemic itch is thought to be multifactorial, and likely due to a number of pruritogens accumulating in the skin including substance P, vitamin A, and histamine.[2,8,16]

Dry skin is also common in patients with renal failure. There are more mast cells in the dermis in this cohort of patients, possibly because of secondary hyperparathyroidism, possibly because of scratching.[2,16]

For localized uraemic itch, possible treatments include:

- Capsaicin cream (to deplete substance P)[11]
- UVB phototherapy (to deplete vitamin A)[16]

For systemic uraemic itch, treatments include:

- Gabapentin/pregabalin: thought to work by hindering the transmission of the pruritic signal in the central nervous system[13]
- Naltrexone

> **Future Advances**
>
> An interesting observation in patients with uraemic itch is that the kappa (κ) and Mu(μ) opioid receptors become imbalanced. While μ receptors are itch-inducing, κ receptors are itch-suppressing. In chronic itch, there is a proliferation of μ receptors, thereby promoting itch. Nalfurafine, a κ agonist, has shown promise in randomized controlled trials, although is not yet licensed in the UK.[8, 13]

Other Important Causes of Itch

Haematological Disease

- Itch is experienced by around 30% of people with Hodgkin's lymphoma, and may precede the diagnosis[16]
- Generally the best treatment is treatment of the cancer itself,[16] but other treatment options include:
  - Prednisolone: mechanism unknown[2]
  - Cimetidine: suggesting the possibility that itching in Hodgkin's lymphoma is mediated by H_2 receptors[16]
  - Carbamazepine: an incidental benefit found when treating patients for trigeminal neuralgia in a 2008 case study[17]

Paraneoplastic Disease

The approach to itch in paraneoplastic disease is the same step-wise approach as mentioned above. However paroxetine in particular can be helpful,[8] likely related either to its inhibition of the CYP2D6 hepatic enzyme or the modulating effect of increased serotonin on central opioid receptors[18]

The following suggestions are less frequently used, and tend to be reserved for itch that has proved resistant to other treatments:

- Thalidomide: thought to work via its anti-inflammatory effects[19]
- Midazolam: used in a case study by Prieto et al., and used successfully at low doses to treat refractory cholestatic itch with minimal sedation[20]
- Lidocaine via CSCI: used successfully in itch secondary to cutaneous T-cell lymphoma[8]

A Final Word from the Expert

Intractable itch can impact on quality of life in a manner akin to chronic pain and is deserving of the same degree of attention. The pathogenesis of itch can be complex, with multiple pruritogens and a complex interplay between skin cells and sensory nerve afferents relaying the itch signals to the brain. Multiple higher centres produce the sensation of itch and govern the response. The symptoms of pruritus, like pain, can initiate both peripheral and central sensitization. Only a small proportion of itch pathways are mediated by histamine. Itch can either be the presenting symptom or, more commonly, can present alongside other symptoms in patients with palliative care needs. A thorough symptom review should therefore involve direct enquiry regarding the presence of itch. Investigation into the likeliest causes of itch should then guide treatment. Simple measures such as ensuring good skin hydration and minimizing the 'scratch-itch' cycle can help. A short trial of antihistamine may be appropriate with recourse to other medication with specific rationale if this is ineffective.

There has been extraordinary progress recently in the understanding of the pathophysiology of pruritus. The onus is on palliative care to adopt new evidence-based strategies to tackle this distressing symptom as they become clear.

References

1. Kam PC, Tan KH. Pruritus--itching for a cause and relief? *Anaesthesia* 1996; 51(12): 1133–1138.
2. Twycross R, Greaves MW, Handwerker H, et al. Itch: scratching more than the surface. *QJM* 2003; 96(1): 7–26.
3. Lavery MJ, Kinney MO, Mochizuki H, Craig J, Yosipovitch G. Pruritus: an overview. What drives people to scratch an itch? *Ulster Med J* 2016; 85(3): 164–q73.
4. van Os-Medendorp H, Eland-de Kok PC, Grypdonck M, Bruijnzeel-Koomen CA, Ros WJ. Prevalence and predictors of psychosocial morbidity in patients with chronic pruritic skin diseases. *J Eur Acad Dermatol Venereol* 2006; 20(7): 810–817.
5. Bin Saif GA, Papoiu AD, Banari L, et al. The pleasurability of scratching an itch: a psychophysical and topographical assessment. *Br J Dermatol* 2012; 166(5): 981–985.
6. Davidson S, Zhang X, Yoon CH, Khasabov SG, Simone DA, Giesler GJ, Jr. The itch-producing agents histamine and cowhage activate separate populations of primate spinothalamic tract neurons. *J Neurosci* 2007; 27(37): 10007–10014.
7. Ikoma A. Updated neurophysiology of itch. *Biol Pharm Bull* 2013; 36(8): 1235–1240.
8. Wilcock A, Howard P, Charlesworth S. *Palliative Care Formulary*, 7th ed. London: Pharmaceutical Press, 2020.
9. Schmelz M, Schmidt R, Bickel A, Handwerker HO, Torebjork HE. Specific C-receptors for itch in human skin. *J Neurosci* 1997; 17(20): 8003–8008.
10. Raksha MP, Marfatia YS. Clinical study of cutaneous drug eruptions in 200 patients. *Indian J Dermatol Venereol Leprol* 2008; 74(1): 80.

11. Papoiu AD, Yosipovitch G. Topical capsaicin. The fire of a 'hot' medicine is reignited. *Expert Opin Pharmacother* 2010; 11(8): 1359–1371.
12. Liu B, Jordt SE. Cooling the itch via TRPM8. *J Invest Dermatol* 2018; 138(6): 1254–1256.
13. Siemens W, Xander C, Meerpohl JJ, et al. Pharmacological interventions for pruritus in adult palliative care patients. *Cochrane Database Syst Rev* 2016; 11: CD008320.
14. Kremer AE, van Dijk R, Leckie P, et al. Serum autotaxin is increased in pruritus of cholestasis, but not of other origin, and responds to therapeutic interventions. *Hepatology* 2012; 56(4): 1391–400.
15. Tarcatu D, Tamasdan C, Moryl N, Obbens E. Are we still scratching the surface? A case of intractable pruritus following systemic opioid analgesia. *J Opioid Manag* 2007; 3(3): 167–170.
16. Krajnik M, Zylicz Z. Understanding pruritus in systemic disease. *J Pain Symptom Manage* 2001; 21(2): 151–168.
17. Korfitis C, Trafalis DT. Carbamazepine can be effective in alleviating tormenting pruritus in patients with hematologic malignancy. *J Pain Symptom Manage* 2008; 35(6): 571–572.
18. Zylicz Z, Krajnik M, Sorge AA, Costantini M. Paroxetine in the treatment of severe non-dermatological pruritus: a randomized, controlled trial. *J Pain Symptom Manage* 2003; 26(6): 1105–1112.
19. Hercz D, Jiang SH, Webster AC. Interventions for itch in people with advanced chronic kidney disease. *Cochrane Database Syst Rev* 2020; 12: CD011393.
20. Prieto LN. The use of midazolam to treat itching in a terminally ill patient with biliary obstruction. *J Pain Symptom Manage* 2004; 28(6): 531–532.

CASE 11 Mouth Care

Grace Rowley

Expert: Philip Lodge

Case history

Karen, a 59-year-old teacher, presented with an ulcerated swelling in her oral cavity. She had no significant past medical history, never smoked, and drank four units of alcohol per week. A biopsy showed a severe dysplastic lesion of her lower alveolus. Localized rim resection and sentinel node biopsy were performed, followed by wide local excision and neck dissection. The tumour was staged as a T4 squamous cell carcinoma.

Prior to postoperative radiotherapy, a review was carried out by community dentistry and the ear, nose, and throat (ENT) specialist nurse who counselled Karen on the importance of regular oral assessment and management of oral complications.

Clinical Tip Mouth Assessment

Oral examination involves general observation of the patient, including nutritional status. Use of an assessment tool such as the Oral Health Assessment Tool (OHAT) may be helpful. It systematically works through examination of the mouth, lips, tongue, gums, buccal tissues, saliva, natural teeth, dentures, oral cleanliness, and enquires about dental pain.[1]

Clinical Tip Basic Oral Care

Basic oral care maintains cleanliness, reduces infection, promotes comfort, and can contribute to reducing adverse outcomes in oral mucositis.[2] It includes regular oral care carried out by the patient or caregiver. Prior to oncological treatment, it is important to educate the patient on the importance of oral care and provide them with the means to carry it out. Dental assessment and care before, during and after treatment is essential. Bland oral rinses such as saline or sodium bicarbonate may be helpful in maintaining hygiene and comfort.[3]

Clinical Tip Dental Review

Before commencing treatment, a dental review is advised where the patient is assessed and any necessary dental work carried out. Patients need regular dental reviews as they are prone to caries and periodontitis due to xerostomia, reduced oral hygiene, and radiotherapy. Restorative dental input, good oral hygiene, and the use of topical sodium fluoride are important. Dental pain affects nutrition and quality of life.[4]

Postoperative radiotherapy, 60 Gy in 30 fractions, was delivered over 6 weeks. During this, Karen developed erythema and ulceration of the oral cavity causing pain and difficulty eating. Karen had severe oral mucositis (grade 3). She could not tolerate solids and a nasogastric (NG) tube was sited to ensure adequate nutrition. Pain was initially managed with oral morphine then switched to a continuous subcutaneous morphine infusion

Expert Comment

Low-level laser therapy for mucositis is not widely available. It has been approved by NICE.

due to challenge of taking oral medications. She was prescribed Caphasol© QDS to protect the oral mucosa. Karen struggled with thick secretions for which a saline nebulizer was prescribed. She received photobiomodulation (PBM) therapy twice weekly during radiotherapy. Karen's symptom management was supported by the hospital palliative care team (HPCT). Importantly, the continuous subcutaneous infusion (CSCI) morphine dose was gradually weaned and stopped as her mucositis symptoms improved, in order to prevent opioid toxicity developing. During and following radiotherapy, she had a dry mouth requiring artificial saliva, this persisted for several months.

Learning Point Photobiomodulation (PBM)

Low-level laser therapy induces a PBM which can accelerate healing by decreasing inflammation. The mechanism is not fully understood but is thought to increase the mitochondrial and cell membrane photoreceptor adenosine triphosphate (ATP) synthesis.[5] Intraoral treatment for chemotherapy or radiotherapy-induced mucositis uses a probe in the mouth and may be used for the duration of the oncological treatment. Key outcomes include improved quality of life, reduction in oral mucositis, and reduction in pain. It has also been shown to improve nutrition and reduce the need for clinically assisted nutrition.[6]

Clinical Tip Addressing Nutritional Needs

Patients undergoing buccal radiotherapy, with palliative or curative intent, are at significant risk of malnutrition. Early review and intervention by a dietician is essential. The risks of malnutrition include increased infections, delayed healing, muscle weakness, reduced response to cancer treatments and increased mortality.[7] Enteral feeding may need to be considered. This is also important to ensure reliable administration of medications. Taste disorders are common in patients undergoing chemotherapy or radiotherapy and can be affected by other factors, including medication, mucosal lesions, and renal dysfunction with reduction in appetite and quality of life. It is important that patients are prepared for these adverse effects and are supported to optimize nutritional intake.[8]

Learning Point Grading of Mucositis

There are a variety of mucositis scales which are used to rate the overall status of the mouth including symptoms, signs, and functional disturbance. Many are based on the scale developed by the World Health Organization (WHO) (Table 11.1).[9] Regular assessment is important to highlight any changes and for the formulation of a management plan.

Table 11.1 World Health Organization oral mucositis scale/common toxicity criteria

Grade 0 (none)	None
Grade 1 (mild)	Oral soreness, erythema
Grade 2 (moderate)	Oral erythema, ulcers, solid diet tolerated
Grade 3 (severe)	Oral ulcers, liquid diet only
Grade 4 (life-threatening)	Oral alimentation impossible

Learning Point Mucositis

Oral mucositis is characterized by erythema, ulceration, and pain. In a neutropenic patient, it can predispose to sepsis. It affects quality of life, nutritional state, and can lead to hospitalization.[10] Mucositis may interrupt treatment and can affect the gastrointestinal tract causing nausea, vomiting, diarrhoea, cramping, and anal pain.[3]

The pathogenesis of oral mucositis is complex. Initial injury to the cells occurs via direct DNA damage resulting from chemotherapy or radiotherapy or indirectly by the generation of reactive oxygen species. This leads to enzyme and transcription factor activation which upregulates genes coding for inflammatory cytokines. This causes tissue damage with ulceration and bacterial infiltration, causing a cycle of inflammation. Healing is spontaneous dependent on extracellular matrix signals and the reestablishment of the mucosal barrier.[10]

Mucositis can affect up to 80% of patients undergoing radiotherapy[10] and it may persist for several weeks after treatment has been completed. [11] In those undergoing chemotherapy, the duration of mucositis is typically up to two weeks.[10]

Evidence Base Management of Mucositis

Prevention and treatment of oral mucositis varies between centres. Education on basic oral care is important, including the use of saline and sodium bicarbonate rinses and regular teeth brushing.[3, 10] It is important to empower patients to report any oral changes. Cryotherapy can be used in prevention. It causes superficial vasoconstriction, which reduces the cytotoxic drug delivery to oral tissues therefore reducing mucosal damage.[3] There is evidence for the use of intraoral photobiomodulation therapy.[3] Keratinocyte growth factor-1 has evidence of benefit in reducing the severity and duration of mucositis in patients undergoing chemotherapy for haematological malignancies.[3, 10] Benzydamine has anti-inflammatory, antimicrobial, and cytoprotectant properties which can be used in prevention and treatment.[3, 10] Oral glutamine has been suggested for the prevention of mucositis patients undergoing treatment for head and neck cancer.[3] Honey has also been suggested for preventative management.[3] Topical morphine 0.2% mouthwash can be used for the treatment of pain.[3] There are several topical agents used to moisten and protect the oral cavity through different mechanisms. A calcium phosphate solution can be used to moisten, lubricate, and repair the mucosa.[11]

Evidence Base Analgesia

Mucositis causes pain due to tissue damage involving sloughing of the epithelium, mucosal inflammation, and ulceration leading to sensitization of pain receptors and an increase in inflammatory and pain mediators.[12] Basic oral hygiene is important in all aspects of mouth care, including pain. Topical agents can be helpful. Benzydamine mouthwash, a non-steroidal anti-inflammatory medication, has evidence of effect along with 0.2% morphine mouthwash.[3] Systemic analgesics may be required. Patient-controlled analgesia (PCA) morphine has been recommended for patients undergoing haematopoetic stem cell transplant with mucositis, for other causes following current general acute pain guidelines is recommended.[12] The use of ice chips or cryotherapy can provide temporary relief with some cytotoxic agents.[3]

Karen's disease went into remission. Eighteen months later, she developed a non-healing ulcer and recurrent infections due to osteomyelitis of her anterior mandible requiring antibiotic treatment. She developed a thick coating on her tongue, which added to the difficulties she was experiencing with oral discomfort and altered taste. She was treated for oral candida infection with a seven-day course of 100 mg fluconazole OD.

Expert Comment

The pain from severe mucositis cannot be underestimated and, as noted, there is a place for parenteral opioids. Outside the acute hospital setting, a subcutaneous continuous infusion via a syringe driver is a reasonable alternative to PCA opioid and is included in many local guidelines.

Learning Point Oral Candidiasis

Oral candidiasis is an opportunistic infection which can be a mark of systemic disease such as diabetes. It is caused by the overgrowth or infection of a yeast-like fungus called candida. *Candida albicans* is the most common species colonizing the oral cavity. Other species include *Candida glabrata* and *Candida tropicalis.*[13] Overgrowth of candida causes local discomfort, altered taste,

Expert Comment

Management of oral candidiasis includes assiduous oral hygiene with particular attention paid to cleaning dentures. Managing a QDS schedule of nystatin suspension as an oral rinse is often a challenge and a pragmatic approach with the use of fluconazole first line may be necessary.

Expert Comment

Osteonecrosis of the jaw associated with bisphosphonate and denosumab therapy in patients with metastatic bone disease has an incidence of 1-2%. The morbidity associated with the condition is significant with uncertainty regarding optimal management. Lowering the risk by optimizing oral and dental care is therefore essential.

dysphagia, and even extended inpatient hospital admissions. In immunocompromised patients, it can pose a serious risk of systemic infection.[14] Overgrowth happens as a consequence of the interplay between host, micro-organism, and environmental factors. Host factors include immunosuppression, poor performance status, renal failure, diabetes, and medications including broad-spectrum antibiotics and corticosteroids. Poorly fitting dentures, poor oral hygiene, smoking, and alcohol can all be contributing factors.[14]

Basic oral hygiene and topical antifungals are often adequate for an uncomplicated oral candidiasis.[13] Dentures require thorough regular cleaning.

Moderate to severe infections, oesophageal candidiasis, or infections in immunocompromised patients may require systemic therapy such as fluconazole.[15] Culture and sensitivity testing should be done to guide treatment if initial therapy is unsuccessful.[13]

Azole antifungals inhibit cytochrome P450 enzymes, particularly CYP3A4. It is important to review concurrent medications as antifungals may increase plasma drug concentrations. If prescribed alongside a strong CYP3A4 inducer, the plasma concentrations of the antifungal may reduce.[15]

Learning Point Osteonecrosis of the Jaw

Osteonecrosis of the jaw can result from bisphosphonates and denusomab therapy. Osteonecrosis is defined as the presence of necrotic bone for greater than 8 weeks in patients using bisphosphonates or similar medication. Inhibition of osteoclast function and bone remodelling can lead to bone collapse. It may present with an oral fistula. Pain is often associated with infection but may also be neuropathic. Management involves long term systemic antibiotics, analgesia and, occasionally, surgery is required in advanced disease.[16] Osteoradionecrosis can be induced by radiation causing ischaemic necrosis of the mandible in the absence of a local primary tumour necrosis, disease recurrence, or metastatic spread. Management ranges from conservative measures to systemic antibiotics and, occasionally, surgical debridement. Hyperbaric oxygen has also been used.[16]

CT and biopsy showed disease recurrence leading to further surgery with excision of the mandibular bone. Further radiotherapy was not an option. A repeat CT three months post-surgery unfortunately demonstrated extensive disease progression. Karen was referred to the community palliative care team (CPCT) for ongoing symptom management, psychological support, and advanced care planning.

Learning Point Xerostomia

Saliva has several functions. Mucin glycoproteins help lubricate food and protect the oral cavity. Amylase aids the digestion of starches and lingual lipase digestion of fats. Saliva contains lysozymes with antibacterial properties. Xerostomia causes difficulties with chewing, speaking, swallowing, and taste. It increases the risk of infection, dental caries, and oral candidiasis. It is also a distressing symptom for patients.[17] The commonest cause is drugs, particularly those with anticholinergic effects. Sjogren's syndrome can also cause xerostomia. Radiotherapy can affect the salivary glands causing fibrosis, with fine vasculature, and parenchymal degeneration reducing the flow and composition of saliva. There may be resolution over several months however, it can persist.[9]

Evidence Base Management of Xerostomia

Basic oral care, regular sips of water and ice can be helpful general measures. Review of medication is important, however it can be difficult to discontinue drugs that are important for symptom management. Salivary substitutes can be used, which require regular application. Oxygenated glycerol trimester (OGT) saliva substitute has been found to be more effective than water-based electrolyte sprays. Chewing gum can increase saliva production.[18] Salivary stimulants improve the flow of saliva by acting as an agonist at muscarinic cholinergic receptors.[17] Pilocarpine is licenced for use in radiotherapy-induced xerostomia and Sjogren's syndrome, although side effects may limit its use.

Clinical Tip End of Life Mouth Care

Mouth care continues to be of utmost importance as death approaches. Patients are often unable to carry out basic care themselves, so this needs to be carried out by healthcare professionals and family. Each patient needs individualized care, and clarity as to who is responsible for care is important.[19] Mouth care needs to be included in care plans. Any non-essential medication that may be contributing to oral symptoms should be reviewed. The mouth can be moisturized with sprays, sponges, and lip lubricants.

Expert Comment

Xerostomia is under-estimated as a cause of distress and the conscientious use of OGT oral moisturizer is key before considering muscarinic drug therapy in the most severely affected patients.

Future Advances

The use of PBM is a growing field with multiple ongoing studies. Recent guidance recognizes the use for both treatment and prevention of oral mucositis.[3] As research advances are made, it is likely that there will be changes to indications and protocols and practice may extend to paediatric patients.[3]

Discussion

Oral health is easily overlooked in palliative care even though it directly impacts overall quality of life.[19] Patients can lose the ability to communicate their oral health needs or to carry out oral care. Oral problems can predispose patients to malnutrition due to reduced oral intake. Oral conditions can affect psychological well-being with impaired communication and social isolation. This can lead to depression and in turn poor oral hygiene.[20] The proactive management of oral conditions is an essential component of holistic care.

A Final Word from the Expert

We have presented a case where the interventions applied have been those included in national or international guidance with an established evidence base and we have avoided those with either poor- or low-quality evidence for use.

Advice regarding good oral hygiene and rigorous dental assessment have been emphasized as a fundamental need for patients prior to embarking on therapies with a high risk of mucositis and where osteonecrosis is a potential complication. The need for education and regular support for patients through their treatment is vital.

The use of PBM and Keratinocyte growth factor-1 are not widespread, therefore the mainstays of treatment remain simple symptom control measures as described.

References

1. NICE. The Oral Health Assessment Tool. National Institute for Clinical Excellence. 2009. Available at: https://www.nice.org.uk/guidance/ng48/resources/oral-health-assessment-tool-pdf-2543183533
2. McGuire DB, Fulton JS, Park J, et al. Systematic review of basic oral care for the management of oral mucositis in cancer patients. *Support Care Cancer* 2013; 21(11): 3165–3177.
3. Elad S, Cheng KKF, Lalla RV, et al. MASCC/ISOO clinical practice guidelines for the management of mucositis secondary to cancer therapy. *Cancer* 2020; 126(19): 4423–4431.
4. Mulk BS, Chintamaneni RL, Prabhat MPV, Gummadapu S, Salvadhi SS. Palliative dental care: a boon for debilitating. *J Clin Diagnostic Res* 2014; 8(6): 1–6.

5. Dompe C, Moncrieff L, Matys J, et al. Photobiomodulation—underlying mechanism and clinical applications. *J Clin Med* 2020; 9(6): 1–17.
6. NICE. Low-level laser therapy for preventing or treating oral mucositis caused by radiotherapy or chemotherapy. 2018; pp. 4–7. Available at: https://www.nice.org.uk/guidance/ipg615
7. Talwar B, Donnelly R, Skelly R, Donaldson M. Nutritional management in head and neck cancer: United Kingdom National Multidisciplinary Guidelines. *J Laryngol Otol* 2016; 130(S2): S32–S40.
8. Murtaza B, Hichami A, Khan AS, Ghiringhelli F, Khan NA. Alteration in taste perception in cancer: causes and strategies of treatment. *Front Physiol* 2017; 8(MAR): 1–10.
9. Sen S, Priyadarshini S, Sahoo P, Dutta A, Singh A, Kumar U. Palliative oral care in patients undergoing radiotherapy: integrated review. *J Fam Med Prim Care* 2020; 9: 5127–5131.
10. Georgiou M, Patapatiou G, Domoxoudis S, Pistevou-Gompaki K. Oral mucositis: Understanding the pathology and management. *Hippokratia* 2012; 16(3): 215–216.
11. Kiprian D, Jarzabski A, Kawecki A. Evaluation of efficacy of Caphosol in prevention and alleviation of acute side effects in patients treated with radiotherapy for head and neck cancers. *Wspolczesna Onkol* 2016; 20(5): 389–393.
12. Lalla RV, Bowen J, Barasch A, et al. MASCC/ISO clinical practice guidelines for the management of mucositis secondary to cancer therapy. *Cancer* 2014; 120(10): 1453–1461.
13. Akpan, M. Oral candidiasis. *Postgr Med J* 2002; 78: 455–459.
14. Coronado-Castellote L, Jiménez-Soriano Y. Clinical and microbiological diagnosis of oral candidiasis. *J Clin Exp Dent* 2013; 5(5): 279–286.
15. Wilcock A, Howard P, Charlesworth S. *Palliative Care Formulary*, 7th ed. London: Pharmaceutical Press, 2020, pp. 501–504.
16. Smith HS, Pilitsis JG. *The Art and Science of Palliative Medicine: Supportive and Palliative Care in Dentistry and Oral Medicine*, 1st ed. Hong Kong: AME, 2014, pp. 385–406.
17. Fleming M, Craigs CL, Bennett MI. Palliative care assessment of dry mouth: what matters most to patients with advanced disease?. *Support Care Cancer* 2020; 28(3): 1121–1129.
18. Furness S, Bryan G, Mcmillan R, Birchenough S, Worthington HV. Interventions for the management of dry mouth: non-pharmacological interventions. *Cochrane Database Syst Rev* 2013; 2013(9): CD009603.
19. Gustafsson A, Skogsberg J, Rejnö Å. Oral health plays second fiddle in palliative care: an interview study with registered nurses in home healthcare. *BMC Palliat Care* 2021; 20(1): 1–11.
20. Venkatasalu MR, Murang ZR, Ramasamy DTR, Dhaliwal JS. Oral health problems among palliative and terminally ill patients: an integrated systematic review. *BMC Oral Health* 2020; 20(1): 1–12.

CASE

12 Constipation

Anna Bradley

Expert: Jason Boland

Case History

Alice, an 82-year-old retired teacher, was admitted to a hospice. She had a diagnosis of advanced lung adenocarcinoma with bone metastases and was too frail for systemic oncological treatment. Her past medical history included osteoporosis and hypothyroidism. She had no known drug allergies.

Her GP had commenced regular morphine for management of her cancer pain four weeks earlier and had titrated the dose until her pain was well controlled. She began complaining of mild, generalized abdominal pain, early satiety, nausea, and bloating three days prior to admission. She had last opened her bowels five days previously; she would have normally opened them daily.

Her regular medications were: morphine sulphate modified release (MR) 40 mg PO BD; morphine sulphate immediate release (IR) 10 mg PO PRN (using 1–2 daily); paracetamol 1 g PO QDS; levothyroxine 125 micrograms OD; alendronic acid 70 mg once weekly; adcal D3 1 tablet BD. She was prescribed lactulose when initiating morphine treatment, but Alice discontinued it due to excessive flatulence.

Learning Point Diagnosing Constipation

Some tools for diagnosing constipation exist but the gold standard is clinician assessment.[4] The sensation of constipation is subjective[1] and tools should be patient-reported.

The Rome IV Criteria[5] for diagnosing functional constipation have been found to be highly specific (94.5%) but have a low sensitivity (33.9%) when compared to assessment by an experienced clinician.[6] Its role in clinical practice is therefore unclear as not everyone with constipation will meet the diagnostic criteria.

Other constipation assessment scales have been validated. They have a role in research and training, but it is recommended that they are not used in routine clinical practice.[7]

Clinical Tip Assessment of Constipation

All patients with advanced cancer should be regularly assessed for constipation.[3] A detailed history is essential and should include[7,8]:

- Comparison of current bowel habit to normal pattern
- Frequency and consistency of bowel movements
- The presence of pain, straining, tenesmus, or blood/mucus in stool
- Exploration of possible cause(s)
- Previous management and its effectiveness

The Bristol Stool Chart[9] can be used to assess stool consistency.

Associated symptoms include flatulence, colicky abdominal pain, abdominal distension, anorexia, nausea and vomiting, halitosis, and overflow diarrhoea. Constipation should be considered if the person has urinary frequency or retention, and if they are agitated or confused (if elderly or have impaired brain function).[8]

Learning Point Definition of Constipation and Prevalence

Definition: 'The slow movement of faeces through the large intestine, resulting in infrequent bowel movements and the passage of dry, hard stool'.[1]

Constipation is very common in advanced cancer patients and is known to have a negative impact on their quality of life.[2] Prevalence is estimated to be between 32–87%. This variation is attributed to different populations and different diagnostic methods used between studies.[3]

Examination should include abdominal and digital rectal examination (DRE) unless there is a contraindication.

Further investigations are not required routinely for most patients. Investigations that may be considered in the event of severe or suddenly occurring symptoms might include[1]:

- Blood tests: corrected calcium levels, urea and electrolytes, and thyroid function tests.
- Imaging: AXR or CT of the abdomen and pelvis (to exclude bowel obstruction or another pathology).

Expert Comment

Diagnosing constipation is the crucial step for its management. It must be considered and included as part of symptom review. Questions include whether bowel habit has changed, the presence of overflow diarrhoea or other new gastrointestinal symptoms, which interventions, if any, the patient has tried, and the impact upon the patient's life. If faecal impaction in the rectum is suspected, especially with overflow diarrhoea, then a DRE will help guide treatment.

Learning Point Pathogenesis of Constipation

The pathogenesis of constipation in patients with advanced cancer is due to prolonged gut transit time caused by a combination of[10]:

- Changes in gut fluid handling
- Impaired intestinal motility

This may be due to factors arising directly from the cancer, from its treatment or for other associated reasons.

On further assessment, Alice reported that her last bowel motion had the consistency of small, hard lumps (type 1 on Bristol Stool Chart). She had to strain and experienced tenesmus afterward. She was passing wind daily. Over the two weeks prior to admission, Alice had been feeling generally weaker and less mobile. Going to the bathroom had been an effort and a commode was ordered to have by her bedside. She was drinking several cups of tea daily but nausea and fullness had made it difficult to eat more than a few mouthfuls. On examination, her abdomen was soft and non-tender, with sluggish bowel sounds. A DRE revealed hard stool in her rectum. Based on the assessment, the medical team diagnosed Alice as being severely constipated. It was decided to perform some routine blood tests to check calcium levels, potassium, and thyroid function but imaging was not felt to be necessary at this point, given suspicion of bowel obstruction was low.

Expert Comment

Once diagnosed as being present, assessing the cause of constipation is critical, as if a cause is found and reversible this might resolve the constipation. Multiple aetiologies may be found. The appropriateness of investigation and management of cause must also be individually assessed.

Learning Point Causes of Constipation in Palliative Care Patients

The cause of constipation in palliative care patients is usually multifactorial. Table 12.1 gives a summary of common causes.[1, 8]

Table 12.1 Common causes of constipation

Environmental	Lack of privacy Unfamiliar toileting arrangements Needing assistance with personal care Poor positioning (use of bedpan being particularly challenging)
Dietary	Dehydration Poor food intake (especially low fibre)
Medication	Opioids, anticholinergics, antidepressants, diuretics, anti-emetics (e.g. 5-HT_3 receptor antagonists), iron, neuroleptics, antacids, cytotoxics (e.g. vinca alkaloids)
Metabolic	Hypercalcaemia, hypothyroidism, hypokalaemia
Neuromuscular	Myopathy
Neurological	Metastatic spinal cord compression, spinal tumours, autonomic dysfunction
Structural	Abdominal or pelvic tumours, radiation fibrosis, painful anorectal conditions
Other	Inactivity, depression, sedation, global weakness, pain

Source: Data from Larkin, P.J. et al (2018). Diagnosis, assessment and management of constipation in advanced cancer: ESMO Clinical Practice Guidelines. *Ann Oncol*.1;29(Suppl 4):iv111-iv125. DOI: 10.1093/annonc/mdy148 and National Institute for Health and Care Excellence (NICE) (2021). Clinical Knowledge Summary. *Palliative care - constipation*. https://cks.nice.org.uk/topics/palliative-care-constipation/.

Clinical Tip Non-pharmacological Management of Constipation

Environmental factors should be addressed. For example, patients should be given privacy to defaecate and be facilitated to adopt the optimal toilet position (i.e. semi-squatting, knees above hips, leaning slightly forward) with a foot stool.[4]

Lifestyle factors such as increasing fluid and fibre intake and increasing physical activity may help but may not be feasible in palliative care patients.

Learning Point Classification of Commonly Used Laxatives

Table 12.2 shows the classification of commonly used laxatives.[11]

Table 12.2 Classification of common laxatives

Class of laxative	Mode of action	Examples of laxatives	Common side effects
Faecal softeners			
Surface-Wetting agents	Lower surface tension, allowing water and fats to penetrate hard faeces.	Docusate sodium Poloxamer 188 (in co-danthramer)	Liquid form unpalatable.
Osmotic laxatives	Water is retained in the gut lumen, causing an increase in faecal volume (and subsequent increased peristalsis).	Lactulose Macrogols Magnesium hydroxide suspension Magnesium sulphate	Bloating, intestinal colic, flatulence. Magnesium and sulphate salts can lead to hypermagnesaemia in renal impairment.
Stimulant laxatives	Act on the submucosal and myenteric plexus in the large bowel, leading to improved intestinal motility. Increase water secretion into the bowel, which softens stool.	Bisacodyl Dantron Senna Sodium picosulfate	Intestinal colic Dantron: discoloration of urine, prolonged skin contact in incontinence can cause a dantron burn. Potentially carcinogenic - therefore prescribing limited to terminally ill.
Lubricants	Coat the surface of the stool making it slippery and easier to pass.	Liquid paraffin Arachis oil	Anal seepage Absorption can cause a foreign body granulomatous reaction. Avoid in peanut allergy.
Bulk-forming agents (fibre)	Increase stool bulk through water-binding and increasing bacterial cell mass. This causes intestinal distension and so stimulates peristalsis.	Ispaghula husk Methylcellulose Sterculia	Limited role in palliative care due to need to maintain fluid intake.

Adapted with permission from Pharmaceutical Press. Table 1 Commonly Used Laxatives, Chapter: Constipation. Wilcock A, Howard P, Charlesworth S. *Palliative Care Formulary*. 7th ed. Pharmaceutical Press; 2020.

Evidence Base Laxatives in Palliative Care

Systematic reviews have concluded that there is no evidence that any laxative is more effective than others in the palliative care population.[12, 13] Guidelines are therefore largely based on consensus best practice and expert opinion.[11]

Expert Comment

Laxatives remain the mainstay of pharmacological management of constipation. There is limited research data for many laxatives. In general, laxatives soften stool or stimulate the bowel. Laxative choice depends on if the stool is hard and/or decreased bowel frequency. Often both are an issue. Choice also depends on tolerability, what the patient has tried before and the effect/side effects of this. Reassessment every day or two is important to guide decision making regarding whether the laxative dose should be titrated, whether an additional laxative should be tried or whether the laxative should be changed.

Clinical Tip Laxative Choice

It has been recommended by some that macrogol laxatives should be the first-line treatment for constipation for patients with advanced cancer.[4]

Others suggest that the first-line laxative should be a stimulant laxative, with addition of an osmotic or surface-wetting laxative if colic is a problem.[8]

If patients do not respond to optimal dosing of first-line conventional laxatives, the patient should be reassessed and there should be consideration of adding or switching to another conventional laxative from a different class.[4] More specialist medications exist, such as linaclotide, lubiprostone, and prucalopride. These should generally only be prescribed by experienced clinicians.[4]

Expert Comment

Rectal interventions should be considered if the patient has faecal impaction, especially with overflow diarrhoea. If detected on DRE, then the hard stool can be fragmented and suppositories can be administered at the same time. Enemas might also be needed.

Alice's blood tests revealed normal calcium levels, normal potassium levels, and normal thyroid function. She was initially commenced on oral macrogol, 2 sachets BD, and received rectal glycerine suppositories as hard stool was found on DRE. She was also prescribed metoclopramide 10 mg TDS for nausea. She was assisted to the bathroom by nursing staff, provided with a footstool, and given privacy. These interventions had some success and she passed type 2 stool after suppositories. Over the following week, she opened her bowels only every 2–3 days with straining and difficulty. A stimulant was therefore added (senna 15 mg BD).

Learning Point Opioid-induced Constipation (OIC)

The use of opioids is the commonest cause of constipation in cancer patients.

The effect of opioids on the bowel is primarily due to the activation of enteric mu-opioid receptors found throughout the gastrointestinal (GI) tract.[14] The pathogenesis of OIC is demonstrated in Figure 12.1.

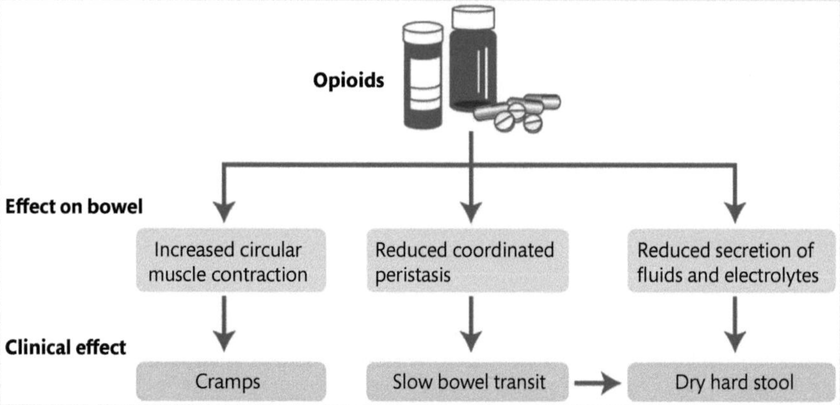

Figure 12.1 Pathogenesis of Opioid-induced Constipation.
Reproduced from *Pharmacological therapies for opioid induced constipation in adults with cancer*, Boland JW, Boland EG, 358:j3313, 2017 with permission from BMJ Publishing Group.

OIC can be defined as: 'A change, when initiating opioid therapy, from baseline bowel habits and defecation pattern that is characterized by any of the following:

a) reduced bowel frequency
b) development or worsening of straining
c) a sense of incomplete evacuation
d) the patients' perception of distress related to bowel habits'[14]

The gold standard for diagnosing OIC is clinical assessment.[4] It can also be evaluated using outcome measures such as the Bowel Frequency Index (BFI).[15]

Expert Comment

OIC is a very common cause of constipation in the presence of opioid use. It can be a dose limiting side effect, even causing people to stop their opioids. Opioids affect the whole gastrointestinal tract, so other symptoms are often present.

Learning Point **Management of Opioid-induced Constipation**

Anyone prescribed opioids should receive prophylactic laxatives,[8] a stimulant is generally recommended.[11]

For someone with OIC it is important to consider if the opioid can be stopped or switched to a less-constipating alternative. Studies have shown that those prescribed transdermal buprenorphine, oral tramadol, or transdermal fentanyl were less likely to be constipated than those taking oral morphine.[4,16] Despite a pooled data analysis[16] showing OIC is associated with increasing opioid dosage, a recent observational study did not show such an association.[4] Further controlled studies evaluating this effect over the longer term are needed.

Peripherally acting mu-opioid receptor antagonists (PAMORAs) reverse the effects of opioids on the gastrointestinal tract without reversing the central analgesic effects. Systematic reviews have found them to be safe and effective in treating OIC.[13, 16, 17] National Institute for Health and Care Excellence (NICE) guidelines recommend that they are considered if traditional laxative therapy is ineffective.[18]

Conventional laxatives may be stopped when the PAMORA is introduced in order to assess its efficacy[19] but OIC alone is rarely the only cause of constipation in a palliative care patient, therefore other laxatives may need to be co-prescribed.

Clinical Tip **Available Peripherally Acting mu-opioid Receptor Antagonists**

Naldemedine: Oral tablet, usually prescribed once daily. There is evidence that naldemedine improves bowel function in cancer patients with OIC but there is an increased risk of adverse events, most commonly diarrhoea.[16]

Naloxegol: Oral tablet, usually prescribed once daily. It has been approved by NICE for use in OIC when a patient has not responded to conventional laxatives.[18]

Methylnaltrexone: Subcutaneous injection only licensed in the UK (oral preparations available elsewhere). Weight-based dose, usually given once every other day, or according to individual response with most patients opening their bowels within 90 minutes of administration.[1]

Prolonged release oxycodone-naloxone: Oral tablet prescribed twice daily. Oral naloxone has little systemic availability due to extensive first-pass metabolism and therefore has limited effect on the central action of oxycodone.[19] Evidence suggests that it is effective in improving OIC compared to oxycodone alone.[20]

Expert Comment

There are a range of targeted therapies for OIC. These reverse the peripheral effects of opioids, including constipation and bowel dysfunction, without affecting analgesia. Naldemedine and naloxegol are the main oral PAMORAs available. Be familiar with the option(s) available for you to use. Subcutaneous methylnaltrexone is useful when patients cannot swallow. PAMORAs can be very effective, especially if opioids are the main cause for constipation. They can be so effective, that diarrhoea might result as the constipating effect of opioids is antagonized.

Future Advances

Further high-quality studies to manage constipation in palliative care patients are needed. Evidence of effectiveness of PAMORAs for OIC is largely limited to studies in non-cancer patients using opioids, although studies in cancer patients are in progress.[19]

Alice's symptoms of incomplete evacuation and straining persisted. It was suspected that her constipation may have been partly related to OIC. She was prescribed naldemedine 200 micrograms OD alongside her conventional laxatives resulting in Alice opening her bowels every 1–2 days. She was discharged home with support after a two-week hospice admission.

A Final Word from the Expert

This case exemplifies the important points of diagnosing and managing a patient with constipation. Constipation is very common in palliative care, often underdiagnosed, and ineffectively managed. It is important to consider the symptom, enquire about it, and assess thoroughly. Understand the impact on the patient, possible causes, and reversible factors. There are a range of laxatives with limited evidence, but which can be helpful in practice. For opioid-induced bowel dysfunction, which causes constipation and a range of gastrointestinal symptoms, there are several PAMORAs, with evidence of effectiveness. These should be considered in patients with OIC.

References

1. Larkin PJ, Cherny NI, la Carpia D, et al. Diagnosis, assessment and management of constipation in advanced cancer: ESMO Clinical Practice Guidelines. *Ann Oncol* 2018; 29: iv111–125.
2. van den Beuken-van Everdingen MHJ, de Rijke JM, Kessels AG, Schouten HC, van Kleef M, Patijn J. Quality of life and non-pain symptoms in patients with cancer. *J Pain Symptom Manage* 2009; 38(2): 216–233.
3. Davies A, Leach C, Caponero R, et al. MASCC recommendations on the management of constipation in patients with advanced cancer. *Support Care Cancer* 2020; 28: 23–33.
4. Davies A, Leach C, Butler C, et al. Opioid-induced constipation in patients with cancer: a 'real-world', multicentre, observational study of diagnostic criteria and clinical features. *Pain* 2021; 162(1): 309–318.
5. Drossman D. Functional gastrointestinal disorders: history, pathophysiology, clinical features and Rome IV. *Gastroenterology* 2016; 150(6): 1262–1279.
6. Palsson OS, Whitehead WE, van Tilburg MAL, et al. Development and validation of the Rome IV diagnostic questionnaire for adults. *Gastroenterology* 2016; 150(6): 1481–1491.
7. Larkin PJ, Sykes NP, Centeno C, et al. The management of constipation in palliative care: clinical practice recommendations. *Palliat Med* 2008; 22(7): 796–807.
8. National Institute for Health and Care Excellence (NICE). Clinical knowledge summary: palliative care—constipation. 2021. Available at: https://cks.nice.org.uk/topics/palliative-care-constipation/management/
9. Lewis SJ, Heaton KW. Stool form scale as a useful guide to intestinal transit time. *Scand J Gastroenterol* 1997; 32(9): 920–924.
10. Sykes NP. The pathogenesis of constipation. *J Support Oncol* 2006; 4(5): 213–218.
11. Wilcock A, Howard P, Charlesworth S. *Palliative Care Formulary*, 7th ed. London: Pharmaceutical Press; 2020.
12. Candy B, Jones L, Larkin PJ, Vickerstaff V, Tookman A, Stone P. Laxatives for the management of constipation in people receiving palliative care. *Cochrane Database Syst Rev* 2015; 2015: CD003448.
13. Ahmedzai SH, Boland J. Constipation in people prescribed opioids. *BMJ Clin Evid* 2010; 2010: 2407.
14. Camilleri M, Drossman DA, Becker G, Webster LR, Davies AN, Mawe GM. Emerging treatments in neurogastroenterology: a multidisciplinary working group consensus statement on opioid-induced constipation. *Neurogastroenterol Motil* 2014; 26: 1386–1395.
15. Star A, Boland JW. Updates in palliative care—recent advancements in the pharmacological management of symptoms. *Clin Med (Lond)* 2018; 18(1): 11–16.
16. Candy B, Jones L, Vickerstaff V, Larkin PJ, Stone P. Mu-opioid antagonists for opioid-induced bowel dysfunction in people with cancer and people receiving palliative care. *Cochrane Database Syst Rev* 2018; 6: CD006332.
17. Nee J, Zakari M, Sugarman MA, et al. Efficacy of treatments for opioid-induced constipation: systematic review and meta-analysis. *Clin Gastroenterol Hepatol* 2018; 16: 1569–1584.e2.
18. National Institute for Health and Care Excellence (NICE). Naloxegol for treating opioid-induced constipation. 2015. Available at: https://www.nice.org.uk/guidance/ta345
19. Boland JW, Boland EG. Pharmacological therapies for opioid induced constipation in adults with cancer. *BMJ* 2017; 358: j3313.
20. Morlion BJ, Mueller-Lissner SA, Vellucci R, et al. Oral prolonged-release oxycodone/naloxone for managing pain and opioid-induced constipation: a review of the evidence. *Pain Practice* 2018; 18: 647–665.

CASE 13 Diarrhoea

Robert McConnell

Experts: Michael Connolly and Leona Butterly

Case history

Dorothy, a 70-year-old woman, was admitted to hospital and hospice three times over a period of eight months, for symptom control of severe diarrhoea. A rectal carcinoma was diagnosed six years previously, stage T2N0R0, and surgically treated, resulting in anterior resection. There was no evidence of residual disease found; therefore, her team did not offer systemic anticancer treatment. Stoma reversal to preserve bowel continuity was offered two years later as Dorothy's health remained good. Following the stoma reversal, Dorothy had intermittent diarrhoea, but it was easily self-managed with loperamide.

Five years following the original diagnosis, Dorothy presented with left leg swelling and a deep vein thrombosis (DVT) was diagnosed. A CT scan showed a large soft tissue mass on the left side of her pelvis. A CT-guided biopsy demonstrated a recurrence of the rectal adenocarcinoma. The multidisciplinary team (MDT) deemed the recurrent tumour inoperable. Dorothy was referred for an oncology opinion and consideration of palliative chemotherapy.

Initial treatment consisted of FOLFIRI (folinic acid, fluorouracil, and irinotecan) chemotherapy and cetuximab, however, the disease progressed on this treatment. Treatment switched to second-line therapy FOLFOX (folinic acid, fluorouracil, and oxaliplatin). Radiotherapy was used to manage pain arising from the growing pelvic mass. Following four cycles of FOLFOX scan results showed a reduction in the size of the pelvic mass. However, diarrhoea increased to 5–6 times daily. The oncology team discontinued the 5FU (fluorouracil) from the chemotherapy regime to see if the diarrhoea would improve. Despite stopping it, diarrhoea worsened to grade three (Table 13.1). Dorothy had her first hospital admission with an acute kidney injury (AKI) secondary to dehydration due to diarrhoea. Her renal function improved with fluid resuscitation, but her performance status deteriorated to 2–3. Given Dorothy's deteriorating performance status and the results of a mid-treatment CT scan, showing disease progression with new metastatic liver disease, the oncology team stopped the chemotherapy. Together with Dorothy, the MDT ruled out further anticancer treatment.

Despite stopping chemotherapy, diarrhoea had a significant impact on Dorothy's quality of life (QOL). Dorothy had a second hospital admission with AKI and hyperkalaemia. Stool cultures were negative, so the team commenced loperamide 4 mg QDS and transferred Dorothy to the hospice for symptom control. Diarrhoea remained a significant problem, with 6–7 episodes in 24 hours, including nocturnal symptoms. With increasing fatigue and worsening functional status, she started experiencing faecal incontinence, which was significantly distressing. Her diarrhoea did not improve, the palliative care team prescribed codeine 30 mg QDS but this offered little benefit. The team increased the loperamide to 32 mg in 24 hrs and trialled an orodispersible formulation to improve absorption.

Expert Comment Clinical Presentation

O' Reilly et al. (2020)[1] suggest that the clinical presentation of gastrointestinal (GI) side effects for patients during cancer treatment can include abdominal pain, diarrhoea, rectal bleeding, bloating, and weight loss. They suggest choice of investigations be guided by the patient's symptoms. In cases of abdominal pain or systemic toxicity, CT or MRI should be performed to rule out acute intra-abdominal pathology, i.e. abscess or perforation, which may need emergency intervention.[1]

> **Evidence Base Fluorouracil and Dihydropyridmidine Dehydrogenase DPD**
>
> Dihydropyridmidine dehydrogenase (DPD) is the rate-limiting enzyme in the metabolism of fluorouracil (5FU) and is encoded by the *DPYD* gene. Between 2-8% of people have a partial DPYD deficiency[2] and therefore have reduced metabolism of 5FU, putting them at greater risk of toxicities and side effects, including severe diarrhoea. Those with a deficiency should have a dose reduction to reduce adverse effects. Therapeutic drug monitoring should be undertaken to ensure patients are not underdosed.[3-7]

Table 13.1 Common toxicology criteria–diarrhoea[4]

National Cancer Institute Common Toxicology Criteria (CTC) for diarrhoea				
0	1	2	3	4
No Diarrhoea	Increase of <4 stools daily over baseline. Mild increase in ostomy output compared to baseline	Increase of 4-6 stools daily over baseline. IV Fluids indicated <24hrs. Moderate increase in ostomy output compared to baseline, not interfering with ADL	Increase of ≥7 stools daily over baseline. Incontinence. IV fluids ≥24hrs. Hospitalization. Severe increase in ostomy output compared to baseline, interfering with ADL	Life-threatening consequences (e.g.: Haemodynamic collapse)

Reproduced from National Cancer Institute (2017). *Common Terminology Criteria for Adverse Events (CTC) Version 5.* US Department of Health and Human Services. https://ctep.cancer.gov/protocoldevelopment/electronic_applications/docs/ctcae_v5_quick_reference_5x7.pdf.

> **Clinical Tip Loperamide**
>
> Loperamide hydrochloride is often the first medication used in diarrhoea management. In severe diarrhoea and high output stoma, using orodispersible formulations can be beneficial as absorption is quicker, which is important where fast bowel transit times exist. Loperamide works by binding the μ-opioid receptor of the bowel, slowing gut transit time. It does not cross the blood brain barrier or cause central side effects such as sedation.
>
> Case studies have shown the benefit of using higher off-licence doses.[8] The maximum recommended dose in palliative care is up to 32 mg in 24 hrs due to increased risk of side effects, including paralytic ileus.[9-11]

Following the increased dose of loperamide, the frequency of diarrhoea reduced to 3–4 episodes in 24 hours with no nocturnal symptoms. The surgical team suggested a repeat stoma formation with a de-functioning loop colostomy to manage the diarrhoea and incontinence; however, Dorothy decided against this and did not want any further surgical interventions.

Diarrhoea remained problematic since stoma reversal but escalated during chemotherapy. Between the reversal of her stoma and the diagnosis of cancer recurrence, Dorothy also underwent a cholecystectomy for gallstones. Bile acid malabsorption (BAM) is a side effect of this type of surgery, so the medical team prescribed a trial of cholestyramine 4 g OD on discharge home.

> **Learning Point Bile Acid Malabsorption**
>
> BAM is a common cause of diarrhoea.[12] Bile acids are secreted in the liver and reabsorbed in the terminal ilium and play a role in fat absorption. In BAM, there is a failure of the enterohepatic circulation of bile acids due to terminal ilium resection in cancer surgery, cholecystectomy, pancreatitis, pancreatic surgery, or radiotherapy colitis.
>
> In the colon, the presence of bile acids results in increased fluid and mucus secretion and a reduction in bowel transit time, both of which lead to diarrhoea.
>
> A nuclear medicine scan (Selenium-Homo-Taurocholic Acid Test (SeHCAT)) is diagnostic. However, this can take time to arrange due to limited availability of this type of scan. In patients with advanced disease, a trial of treatment and assessment of response may be preferable.
>
> Treatment
>
> - Cholestyramine: A powder mixed with water at an initial dose of 4 g daily titrated to a maximum of 12–24 g/24 hours. This is often poorly tolerated due to taste and GI discomfort.
> - Colesevelam: A tablet which is off-licence for the treatment of BAM. Often better tolerated than cholestyramine. The dose used is 3.75 g in 1–2 divided daily doses.

One month later Dorothy had a final hospice admission due to escalating diarrhoea and an AKI that resulted in mild opioid toxicity.[15] Management included intravenous fluids and an opioid switch with dose reduction. An antisecretory drug was added to the other antidiarrhoeal treatment. Octreotide 250 microgram/24 hrs was commenced and delivered by continuous subcutaneous infusion. It was titrated to 1,000 microgram/24 hrs with some symptom improvement. Stool consistency thickened and frequency reduced, however, Dorothy's overall condition continued to deteriorate. She became unable to take oral medications, including loperamide. The symptoms of diarrhoea were unchanged despite stopping the loperamide. Dorothy deteriorated further and died in the hospice.

Learning Point Octreotide

Octreotide is a synthetic somatostatin analogue commonly used in hormone-secreting tumours. Octreotide's effect on the GI tract is to reduce motility, reduce small bowel and pancreatic secretions, and increase water and electrolyte reabsorption. It is through this mechanism that octreotide is useful in the management of diarrhoea and/or high stoma output.

Octreotide is used at a starting dose of 250–500 microgram/24 hrs up to a maximum of 1,500 microgram/24 hrs.[14]

Smaller doses can be given as BD subcutaneous injections if there is a preference to avoid a syringe pump.

Discussion

Diarrhoea is a troublesome symptom that can have a significant impact on QOL for patients with advanced disease and short prognosis. Successful management of diarrhoea can improve QOL and reduce the frequency of hospital admissions.

In patients with advanced disease, there can be multiple causes for diarrhoea. It is important to try to establish the cause/s and target therapy. In Dorothy's case, possible causes include chemotherapy, radiotherapy-induced colitis, medications, constipation causing overflow diarrhoea, BAM, infections, and small bowel bacterial overgrowth. Other causes may include immunotherapy-induced colitis, short bowel syndrome,[11] pancreatic insufficiency, presence of malignancy in the bowel and pre-existing conditions such as inflammatory bowel disease.

The management of diarrhoea is dependent on the cause. Before using antisecretory or antimotility agents it is important to exclude constipation with overflow diarrhoea and infection, as the use of medications may lead to complications, including bowel obstruction and toxic megacolon.

Expert Comment Excluding Constipation

The ESMO clinical practice guidelines[5] state that there is a lack of information surrounding the incidence of diarrhoea in elderly patients. The guidelines suggest diarrhoea occurs less frequently than constipation, with a prevalence of less than 10% among patients with cancer who are admitted to the hospital or to a hospice.[5] The ESMO suggest faecal impaction or partial bowel obstruction can manifest as alternating constipation and diarrhoea, therefore, accurate assessment is essential to exclude other causes.[4]

The ESMO has published guidelines on assessment, examination, and investigation of chemotherapy-related diarrhoea.[5] The guidelines propose an algorithm for management that separates those with complicated and uncomplicated diarrhoea (the latter includes features of fluid depletion, fever, and vomiting). Patients with uncomplicated diarrhoea require a more intensive treatment approach which includes daily evaluation of serum electrolytes and urine output, stool evaluation, use of loperamide, and consideration of octreotide and antibiotics.

Expert Comment Bile Acid Malabsorption

Lyutakov et al. (2019)[13] suggest that BAM is frequently unrecognized as a cause of chronic diarrhoea, because there is a lack of guidance around diagnostic testing and the mechanisms that centre on the unnecessary build-up of bile acids.[13] SeHCAT, although limited to selected centres can be used to determine what type of BAM is causing diarrhoea. However, patients are subject to testing taking place over two days and are exposed to radiation during the scan.[13, 14]

Clinical Tip Medications Commonly Causing Diarrhoea

Medications are a common cause of diarrhoea. When investigating the cause of diarrhoea, a medication history is essential. These medications include but are not limited to: antibiotics, laxatives, antacids, proton pump inhibitors, non-steroidal anti-inflammatories, iron supplements, magnesium supplements, and metformin.

Clinical Tip Drug Absorption

Diarrhoea and fast gut transit time can affect the absorption of drugs through the GI tract. Patient's with significant diarrhoea may require alternative routes of medication administration such as buccal, parenteral routes, or use of alternative formulations such as immediate release liquid and dispersible medications.

A Final Word from the Expert

This case demonstrates the complexities associated with managing diarrhoea in patients with advanced disease. A multidisciplinary approach is essential, including input from oncology, palliative care and radiology. It is essential that the highest standard of care and symptom management is provided for patients whose quality of life is already impacted in the face of an incurable disease.

References

1. O'Reilly M, Mellotte G, Ryan B, O'Connor A. Gastrointestinal side effects of cancer treatments. *Ther Adv Chronic Dis* 2020; 11: 1–7.
2. Amstutz U, Henricks LM, Offer SM, et al. Clinical Pharmacogenetics Implementation Consortium (CPIC) Guideline for dihydropyrimidine dehydrogenase genotype and fluoropyrimidine dosing: 2017 update. *Clin Pharmacol Ther* 2018; 103(2): 210–216.
3. Wörmann B, Bokemeyer C, Burmeister T, et al. Dihydropyrimidine dehydrogenase testing prior to treatment with 5-Fluorouracil, capecitabine, and tegafur: a consensus paper. *Oncol Res Treat* 2020; 43(11): 628–636.
4. Common Terminology Criteria for Adverse Events (CTC) Version 5; National Cancer Institute; 27 November 2017. Available at: https://ctep.cancer.gov/protocoldevelopment/electronic_applications/docs/ctcae_v5_quick_reference_5x7.pdf
5. Bossi P, Antonuxxo A, Cherny NI, et al. Diarrhoea in adult cancer patients: ESMO Clinical Practice Guidelines. *Ann Oncol* 2018; 29(Suppl 4): iv126–iv142.
6. Andreyev J, Ross P, Donnellan C, et al. Guidance on the management of diarrhoea during cancer chemotherapy. *Lancet Oncol* 2014; 15(10): e447–e460.
7. De-Jian M, Zeng-Jun L, Xi-Yan W, Xian-Jun Z, Yan-Lai S. Octreotide treatment of cancer chemotherapy-induced diarrhoea: a meta-analysis of randomized controlled trials. *Transl Cancer Res* 2019; 8(6); 2284–2294.
8. Mackowski A, Chen H-K, Levitt M. Successful management of chronic high-output ileostomy with high dose loperamide. *Case Reports* 2015; 2015(apr22 1): bcr2015209411-bcr2015209411.
9. Regnard C, Twycross R, Mihalyo M, Wilcock A. Loperamide. *J Pain Symptom Manage* 2011; 42(2): 319–323.
10. Lexicomp (n.d). Loperamide: Drug information. UpToDate. Available at: https://www.uptodate.com/contents/loperamide-drug-information?search = loperamide&source = panel_search_result&selectedTitle = 1 ~ 115&usage_type = panel&kp_tab = drug_general&display_rank = 1#F50991639
11. Nightingale J. Guidelines for management of patients with a short bowel. *Gut* 2006; 55(suppl_4): iv1–12.
12. Wilcox C, Turner J, Green J. Systematic review: the management of chronic diarrhoea due to bile acid malabsorption. *Aliment Pharmacol Ther* 2014; 39(9): 923–939.
13. Lyutakov I, Ursini F, Penchev P, Caio G, Corroccio A, Volta, De Giorgio R. Methods for diagnosing bile acid malabsorption: a systematic review. *BMC Gastroenterol* 2019; 19(158): 185.
14. Wilcock A, Howard P, Charlesworth S (eds.). *Palliative Care Formulary*, 7th ed. London: Pharmaceutical Press, 2020.
15. Haanen JBAG, Carbonnel F, Robert C, et al. Management of toxicities from immunotherapy: ESMO Clinical Practice Guidelines for diagnosis, treatment and follow-up. *Ann Oncol* 2017; 28: iv119–42.

SECTION 3

Management of the dying patient

CASE

14 Uncertainty and Prognostication

Simon Noah Etkind

Expert: Paddy Stone

Case history

Evelyn was referred to palliative care following multiple hospitalizations. Aged 82, she had multiple myeloma with secondary amyloidosis and congestive cardiac failure. She also had chronic obstructive pulmonary disease (COPD) and chronic renal impairment. She was receiving oral chemotherapy for her multiple myeloma. She was under the care of haematology, cardiology, respiratory, renal, and palliative care teams.

She gave up driving six months ago and was increasingly reliant on support with daily activities. She lived with her daughter, who assisted with washing and dressing. She was mobile indoors with a walking frame. Her Clinical Frailty Score was 6, representing 'moderate frailty'.

She had four emergency department attendances in the last six months relating to exacerbations of COPD and decompensated heart failure, and her main symptom is breathlessness. She was reluctant to return to hospital, but uncertain how she would manage at home if she became breathless or developed a chest infection. The last time she was discharged, she was told, 'There's nothing we could do for you if you came back to hospital' and this has left her feeling distressed. She was worried about the burden on her daughter and is considering moving to a care home.

Learning Point Uncertainty in Advanced Illness

Uncertainty can be defined as the subjective perception of ignorance, i.e. 'known unknowns'.[1] It is frequently experienced by patients with advanced illness, their carers, and health professionals.[2] Though not necessarily harmful, uncertainty is often interpreted as a threat and can cause considerable distress.[3] Some uncertainties are due to a lack of information and can be resolved by information provision, but uncertainty is often irreducible, and can only be ameliorated, not eliminated. Uncertainty can be considered in terms of *how* things are uncertain (are they complex, unpredictable or ambiguous); *what* is uncertain (does uncertainty relate to the illness, treatment, care processes, the future illness course, or a combination of issues); and *who* is uncertain (does uncertainty lie with the patient, their informal carers, or with health professionals).[1, 4]

Clinical Tip Approaches to Uncertainty

It is first important to understand what uncertainties are experienced and how people respond to uncertainty. Some respond by information seeking, whereas others actively avoid uncertainty, focusing on those things about which they can be certain. A third group accept uncertainty, attempting to integrate it into their daily lives. This latter group may report that they 'live day-to-day' and disengage from future care planning. Health professional approaches to uncertainty should take account of patients' responses. Patients who are engaged, wish for information, and are focused on the future, may benefit from more detailed discussion of future possibilities than those who are disengaged. Tailored communication is key to closing 'uncertainty gaps' and supporting the development of a shared plan for care.[2, 5]

Learning Point Uncertainty in Multimorbidity

Multimorbidity, defined in palliative care as the coexistence of multiple life-limiting illnesses, provides additional challenges in decision-making and prognostication because each additional illness represents another layer of complexity. Multimorbidity is common and increasing: projections suggest that nearly half of people will die with >1 life-limiting illness by 2040.[6] For Evelyn, the unpredictable illness course and fragmented care related to multimorbidity, with involvement of multiple specialist teams, may precipitate uncertainties about her current and future care.

Expert Comment

It should be remembered that illness trajectories relate to the average properties of large groups and are not particularly helpful at predicting individual survival. There is, for example, a huge variation in the prognoses of cancer patients even though, in general, cancer patients follow a similar trajectory. Illness trajectories may be helpful for thinking about service needs or provision but are less useful for individual prognostication.

Expert Comment

Uncertainty is often a reason why clinicians avoid prognostic conversations. Current guidelines emphasize the importance of stating prognostic uncertainty, but this is not the same as abrogating responsibility for making any effort to prognosticate likely survival.[13] Describing prognosis in broad terms such as 'days', 'weeks', 'months', or 'years' may be a useful way of providing helpful prognostic information without being spuriously (in)accurate.

Evidence Base Illness Trajectories

Functional trajectories in life-limiting illnesses have been extensively studied at a group level. Lunney, Lynn, and Adamson retrospectively measured functional status prior to death, identifying four distinct trajectories of terminal decline.[7] These are: *sudden death*, where function is normal until death; *cancer*, characterized by a long period of good function and rapid decline in the final months; *organ failure*, characterized by intermittent illness exacerbations causing temporary dips in function on the background of gradual decline; and *frailty/dementia* with fluctuant low-level function for a long period prior to death. Subsequent research has explored trajectories of psychological, social, and spiritual function, identifying that even where physical function remains good, other domains may be impacted earlier in the illness course.[8]

Learning Point Prognosis and Palliative Care Referral

Models of palliative care should flexibly accommodate people throughout unpredictable illness trajectories. Whilst prognosis remains relevant when identifying patients suitable for specialist palliative care referral, it is seldom the only consideration. Prognosis-based approaches such as the 'surprise question', 'Would you be surprised if this person died within the next year?' can be useful for identifying people who might benefit from a palliative care approach. However, the optimum point at which to refer to specialist palliative care remains uncertain. Tools such as the Supportive and Palliative Care Indicators Tool (SPICT) can help to identify those with palliative care needs without undue focus on prognosis.[9]

Expert Comment How Accurate is the Surprise Question?

Although the overall accuracy of the Surprise Question is quite good, this mostly reflects the fact that when clinicians 'would be surprised if a patient were to die within the next year?', they seldom do. Conversely, the positive predictive value of the Surprise Question for identifying patients who will die within the next year is low. In White's metanalysis, doctors indicated that they would not be surprised if 218 patients died, but only 71 (33%) of those patients did so within the predicted timeframe.[10]

Evidence Base Factors Associated with Poor Prognosis in Older Adults

Numerous factors may indicate poor prognosis; sometimes a combination of factors is most telling. Using routinely collected data, Kelley et al. identified that the combination of a severe medical condition, functional impairment, and recent hospitalization conferred a 28% chance of dying within one year.[11] At older ages, hospitalization alone is associated with high one-year mortality; in one study, 42% of those aged over 85 years died within a year of hospital admission.[12] Hospitalization in an older person may therefore be sufficient reason to trigger discussions about future care planning.

Future Advances Addressing Uncertainty

We don't yet know how best to approach uncertainty in advanced illness. Training clinicians to deal with uncertainty is essential, and future work should focus on how best to identify, address, and communicate uncertainty.

Subsequently Evelyn became less well and decided she would not wish to return to hospital under any circumstances. She ceased chemotherapy and asked for her care to focus on comfort. She had spoken to her family and decided that she would remain at home for end of life care. Her care needs were increasing and her daughter was finding it increasingly difficult to balance her job with caring for her mother. During a discussion with the palliative care nurse she expressed these concerns and asked how long her mother might have left to live.

Learning Point Estimating Prognosis in Advanced Cancer

Prognostic estimates in advanced cancer can be informed by survival data from common tumours, alongside evidence from clinical trials. Based on these data, it is possible to estimate how much a given treatment may extend life, or possible life expectancy without treatment, in patients with a similar clinical picture. But in isolation, these data cannot be used to predict survival for an individual. For those receiving newer anticancer treatments such as immunotherapy, where response to treatment can exceptionally be far greater than the average, predicting prognosis is particularly challenging. Even for those not receiving anticancer treatment, prognosis is not necessarily obvious. For example, if multimorbidity is present, prognosis may be driven by comorbidities rather than cancer.

Expert Comment Prognostic Tools in Advanced Cancer

Broad characteristics such as cancer diagnosis, performance status, and disease stage can give a general indication of prognosis. This can be refined using factors such as low serum albumin or raised C-reactive protein, or indeed the simple combination of these two variables in the form of the Glasgow Prognostic Score.[14] However, to predict individual survival, it is necessary to use individualized risk prediction models, such as the Palliative Prognostic Index (PPI), the Prognosis in Palliative Care Study (PiPS) predictor models or the Palliative Prognostic Score (PaP).[15] These scores statistically combine individual prognostic factors, and general markers of disease severity, to make an individualized prediction about length of survival. The best individualized risk prediction models are as good as (but not consistently better than) expert clinical judgement. Prognosis often becomes clearer at the very end of life, and in one recent study when doctors predicted that patients had less than one week to live, the Positive Predictive Value [PPV] of this estimate was 77%.[16]

Clinical Tip Markers of the Last Days of Life

In the absence of reversibility and in the context of an advanced progressive illness, the combination of becoming bedbound, minimal oral intake, and reduced consciousness level are often indicative of imminent death.[17] Other signs of impending death include poor performance status, agitation/sedation, dysphagia of liquids, and respiration with mandibular movement.[18] No single sign reliably predicts imminent death and it is important to pay attention to the recent illness trajectory and the recent rate of change. A rapid recent decline, particularly in the context of advanced cancer, usually indicates a shorter prognosis.

Clinical Tip Communicating Prognosis

Patients usually wish for an honest assessment of their prognosis, but health professionals can be reluctant to provide this, and may withhold information. Such avoidance can lead to harm, by preventing adequate preparation for the end of life. Clinicians should provide a prognosis when asked. However, given inherent uncertainty, it is important to communicate this information with care and compassion.[13] A confidently given specific prognosis that turns out to be inaccurate can do more harm than a vaguer prognosis accompanied by an explanation about the range of uncertainty. Before providing a prognosis, it is good practice to ensure the patient feels ready to hear prognostic information, and that they have family members with them if that is their preference. It is important to ascertain their current understanding and how much information they wish to know. Prognostication should be contextualized in terms of recent illness trajectory, and a prognosis should usually be given in broad periods of time (e.g. days/weeks/months). Information from prognostic conversations should be recorded in the clinical record and communicated to other health professionals.

Evidence Base Accuracy of Prognostic Estimates

Subjective clinical predictions of survival are often inaccurate. In one study, clinicians' prognoses for patients at time of referral to hospice care were only accurate (within 33% of actual survival) in 20% of cases, and survival was overestimated on average by a factor of 5.3.[19, 20] A systematic review of 42 studies in palliative care settings identified that prognoses ranged from an underestimate of 86 days to an overestimate of 93 days.[21] Some clinicians buck this trend, demonstrating high accuracy in prognostication, especially when death is imminent. In a vignette study of 'expert' clinicians, White et al. found that those who accurately predicted whether a patient would die within 72 hours relied on particular clinical features to make their judgement: Cheyne-Stokes breathing, agitation, or sedation, decline in condition, peripheral cyanosis, palliative performance status, noisy respiratory secretions.[21]

Expert Comment What is Meaningful Accuracy?

The idea that clinician predictions are inaccurate and over-optimistic may be somewhat of a simplification. It depends on what one means by 'accurate'. For example, if a clinician predicts a patient will die within one week, and they die after two weeks, this represents a >33% error in accuracy. Nonetheless, the clinician and the family may regard this prognosis to have been 'accurate enough' to allow them to make appropriate preparations for impending death. If suitable allowances are made for the level of accuracy that is clinically important, then clinicians' predictions (at least about imminent death) are reasonably good.

Evidence Base The Prognosis in Palliative Care Study Predictor Models

The PiPS predictor models are good examples of individualized tools that support prognostication in advanced cancer. There are two versions of PiPS (A and B) which use clinical data such as diagnosis and presence of metastatic disease, physiological parameters such as heart rate, and (for PiPS-B only) results from blood tests, to predict survival in terms of 'months', (>8 weeks), 'weeks' (2–8 weeks), or 'days' (<2 weeks), accompanied by individualized risk predictions about the probability of surviving to each timepoint. In validation studies, the accuracy of PiPS-B was comparable to expert clinician estimates.[21, 22]

Future Advances

Although some prognostic tools (e.g. PaP and PiPS-B) have similar accuracy to that of expert clinicians for people with advanced cancer, no tool has yet demonstrated consistent superiority to expert clinician estimates.[23] Few individualized survival prediction models have been developed or validated for people with advanced non-malignant diseases. Future work should investigate non-cancer illnesses, seeking both to determine prognosis and to optimize communication of uncertainty in this population.

Discussion

This case illustrates challenges relating to clinical uncertainty: multimorbidity and frailty make for a *complex* clinical picture; the nature of COPD and heart failure means that the future illness course is *unpredictable*; and there is *ambiguity* about the benefits of future hospital care. Such uncertainties can be distressing for patients and difficult for clinicians, forming a barrier to future care planning. A key challenge is to support the person to live day-to-day, whilst also enabling them to express preferences so that they achieve the end of life care that they wish for. Addressing uncertainty is essential to achieve this but requires good rapport and a rounded knowledge of the individual, best gained through relational continuity over multiple consultations.

Subsequently, the dying trajectory becomes more apparent. At this stage, the challenge is to give sufficient information about the likely prognosis without making spuriously accurate predictions liable to be incorrect.

A Final Word from the Expert

Although it is important to strive to improve prognostic accuracy through the development and validation of algorithms and improved clinical training, ultimately the most important aspects of prognostication are compassionate communication and the ability to deal with uncertainty. This requires excellent communication skills, empathy, gentle exploration of what is known, explanation of the bounds of uncertainty and honest answering of questions.

References

1. Han PK, Klein WM, Arora NK. Varieties of uncertainty in health care a conceptual taxonomy. *Med Decis Making* 2011; 31(6): 828–838.
2. Etkind SN, Bristowe K, Bailey K, et al. How does uncertainty shape patient experience in advanced illness? A secondary analysis of qualitative data. *Palliat Med* 2016; 31(2): 171–180.
3. Mishel MH. Uncertainty in illness. *Image J Nurs Sch* 1988; 20(4): 225–232.
4. Etkind SN, Li J, Louca J, et al. Total uncertainty: a systematic review and thematic synthesis of experiences of uncertainty in advanced multimorbidity. *Age Ageing* 2022; 51(8): afac188.
5. Etkind SN, Koffman J. Approaches to managing uncertainty in people with life-limiting conditions: role of communication and palliative care. *Postgrad Med J* 2016; 92(1089): 412–417.
6. Finucane AM, Bone AE, Etkind S, et al. How many people will need palliative care in Scotland by 2040? A mixed-method study of projected palliative care need and recommendations for service delivery. *BMJ Open* 2021; 11(2): e041317.
7. Lunney JR, Lynn J, Foley DJ, et al. Patterns of functional decline at the end of life. *JAMA* 2003; 289(18): 2387–2392.
8. Lloyd A, Kendall M, Starr JM, et al. Physical, social, psychological and existential trajectories of loss and adaptation towards the end of life for older people living with frailty: a serial interview study. *BMC Geriatr* 2016; 16(1): 1–15.
9. Highet G, Crawford D, Murray SA, Boyd K. Development and evaluation of the supportive and palliative care indicators tool (SPICT): a mixed-methods study. *BMJ Support Palliat Care* 2014; 4(3): 285–290.
10. White N, Kupeli N, Vickerstaff V, et al. How accurate is the 'Surprise Question' at identifying patients at the end of life? A systematic review and meta-analysis. *BMC Med* 2017; 15(1): 139.
11. Kelley AS, Covinsky KE, Gorges RJ, et al. Identifying older adults with serious illness: a critical step toward improving the value of health care. *Health Serv Res* 2016; 52(1): 113–131.
12. Moore E, Munoz-Arroyo R, Schofield L, et al. Death within 1 year among emergency medical admissions to Scottish hospitals: incident cohort study. *BMJ Open* 2018; 8(6): e021432.
13. Clayton JM, Hancock KM, Butow PN, et al. Clinical practice guidelines for communicating prognosis and end-of-life issues with adults in the advanced stages of a life-limiting illness, and their caregivers. *Med J Aust* 2007; 186(S12): S77–s105.
14. McMillan DC. The systemic inflammation-based Glasgow Prognostic Score: a decade of experience inpatients with cancer. *Cancer Treat Rev* 2013; 39(5): 534–540.
15. Chu C, White N, Stone P. Prognostication in palliative care. *Clin Med (Lond)* 2019; 19(4): 306–310.
16. Stone P, Chu C, Todd C, et al. The accuracy of clinician predictions of survival in the prognosis in palliative care study II (PiPS2): a prospective observational study. *PLoS ONE* 2022; 17(4) e0267050.
17. National Institute for Health and Care Excellence (NICE). Quality standard 144: Care of dying adults in the last days of life. 2017. Available at: https://www.nice.org.uk/guidance/qs144
18. Hui D, Dos Santos R, Chisholm G, et al. Bedside clinical signs associated with impending death in patients with advanced cancer: preliminary findings of a prospective, longitudinal cohort study. *Cancer* 2015; 121(6): 960–967.
19. Christakis NA, Lamont EB. Extent and determinants of error in doctors' prognoses in terminally ill patients: prospective cohort study. *BMJ* 2000; 320(7233): 469–472.
20. White N, Reid F, Harris A, et al. A systematic review of predictions of survival in palliative care: how accurate are clinicians and who are the experts? *PLoS ONE* 2016; 11(8): e0161407.
21. White N, Harries P, Harris AJL, et al. How do palliative care doctors recognise imminently dying patients? A judgement analysis. *BMJ Open* 2018; 8(11): e024996.
22. Stone PC, Kalpakidou A, Todd C, et al. The prognosis in palliative care study II (PiPS2): a prospective observational validation study of a prognostic tool with an embedded qualitative evaluation. *PLoS ONE* 2021; 16(4): e0249297.
23. Stone P, Vickerstaff V, Kalpakidou A, et al. Prognostic tools or clinical predictions: which are better in palliative care? *PLoS ONE* 2021; 16(4): e0249763.

CASE

15 De-escalation from Intensive Therapy Unit

Sarah Longwell

Expert: Lucy Wyld

Case history

Sandra, a 58-year-old teaching assistant, presented to the Oncology Assessment Unit with a 3-day history of breathlessness. She had a background of metastatic, triple-negative breast cancer diagnosed 11 years ago and had completed a sixth cycle of third-line palliative chemotherapy, Capecitabine 10 days ago. She lived with her husband, Steve and had three children aged 18, 22, and 24. Her previous courses of chemotherapy had been complicated by neutropenic sepsis and worsening liver function tests.

She looked unwell and was breathless at rest. Her initial observations were: oxygen saturation 82% (on air), respiratory rate 26, heart rate 127, blood pressure 101/74 mmHg, temperature 37.9°C. On examination, she had bilateral crepitations on auscultation of the chest and mild right upper quadrant tenderness on palpation of the abdomen. Blood tests confirmed neutropenia, 0.3×10^9 per litre and worsening liver function tests. Her renal function and serum calcium were within normal range. She was commenced on intravenous fluids and Piperacillin-Tazobactam. Samples of blood, urine, and sputum were sent for microscopy, culture, and sensitivities.

The Oncology team referred her to the critical care outreach team regarding increasing oxygen requirements and hypotension and not responding to fluid resuscitation. She was reviewed by the Intensive Care and Oncology consultants. After discussion with Sandra and her family, a decision was made for admission to intensive care for inotropic and non-invasive respiratory support. Sandra was clear that if, despite the above measures, her condition were to deteriorate she would not wish to be intubated. Instead, she would wish the focus of her care to be on comfort and time with her family. These ACP discussions were clearly documented in the medical notes.

Expert Comment

Timely and sensitive communication is key to ensure decisions regarding escalation of care are consistent with a patient's wishes or made in their best interests. Prognostication is an important part of informed decision-making and communicating the likely effectiveness of ITU interventions. There are several prognostic tools used within ITU, for example, the Acute Physiology and Chronic Health Evaluation, which predict risk of mortality based mainly on acute physiology measures collected at ITU admission.[1] However, although these tools have a role at a service and population level, predictions for individual patients can be inaccurate. When there is uncertainty surrounding a patient's prognosis, it is important that this is communicated to the patient and their family. In this case, this uncertainty was discussed prior to escalation to ITU to enable the patient to make an informed decision. As in this case, involvement of relevant specialities such as Respiratory Medicine, Medical Oncology, and Intensive Care will be helpful to inform the decision-making process.

Learning Point Family Meetings

A key part of caring for patients in the ITU is ensuring effective communication with family members, who are often required to help inform the decision-making process for patients who lack capacity. Early meetings with family to specifically discuss goals of care and prognosis in patients can reduce ITU length of stay and disagreements over care decisions.[2] This should ideally be within the first 3 days of ITU admission. Some patients may have already documented their wishes as part of advance care planning (ACP) processes. In the absence of this, it is important that the treating teams engage fully in early conversations with family to discuss the benefits and risks of available treatment options. One potential barrier to early communication about prognosis is clinical uncertainty about the expected outcome. However, studies show that families understand this uncertainty and still value discussions relating to prognosis.[3]

Expert Comment

In the ITU, patients' decision-making capacity is often compromised due to critical illness. Legislation guiding decision-making varies internationally. In England and Wales, the Mental Capacity Act sets out the statutory framework for decision-making for patients who lack capacity.[4] When a person lacks capacity to make a particular decision at the time it needs to be made, all decisions must be in the person's best interests. The person must be placed at the heart of the decision-making process and supported to be involved in the decision-making process as far as possible. Legally, families cannot give consent to, or refuse treatment on the patient's behalf unless they have been formally appointed as a Lasting Power of Attorney for Health and Welfare, however families and carers do have a crucial role in providing information about the patient as part of a best interests assessment. It is good practice to convene a formal best interests decision meeting to form part of the process of sharing information. On occasion, this may involve an Independent Mental Capacity Advocate (IMCA), where there is no other party that may be consulted regarding the patient's wishes or best interests. A record of this meeting should be kept in the medical records alongside decisions around goals of care and escalation.

Sandra was transferred to ITU and commenced on non-invasive ventilation (NIV) with 50% oxygen, inotropes, and nasogastric (NG) feeding were also started. A staging computerized tomography (CT) scan showed bilateral consolidation consistent with pneumonia, further progressive liver metastases and new lesions within the thoracic spine—concerning for metastatic disease. There was no evidence of spinal cord compromise in the limited study. In view of the CT changes consistent with bilateral pneumonia (see Figure 15.1) a respiratory opinion was sought and bronchoalveolar samples were sent, which confirmed Influenza A pneumonia.

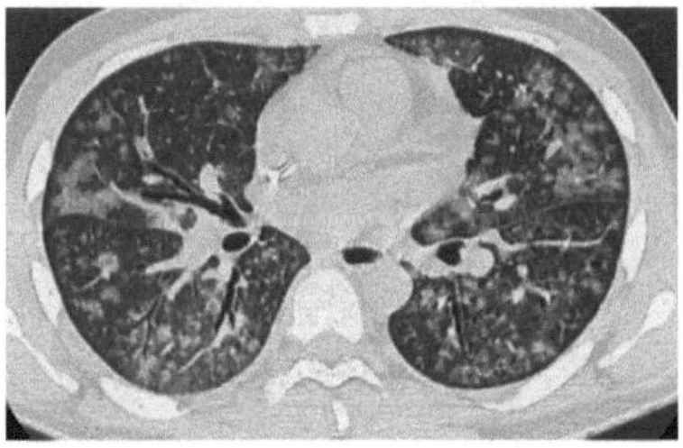

Figure 15.1 CT scan bilateral pneumonia.

Despite treatment, Sandra continued to deteriorate, with worsening hypoxia, breathlessness, and fatigue. The ITU team made a referral to the HPCT for symptom management advice and support for Sandra and her family. On the seventh day of her admission to ITU, she became drowsy, confused, and agitated. She was no longer tolerating her NIV mask and was repeatedly trying to remove her NG tube. Sandra's family were asked to attend to discuss her care going forwards and to inform a best-interests decision-making process, recognizing that she currently did not have the capacity to make decisions about her care. All specialties involved were consulted alongside her family, and all agreed that the burdens of continuing treatment outweighed the benefits and that the focus of her care should be comfort and supporting time with her family. The process of removing NIV support was discussed with her family.

Expert Comment

Treating teams and patients may reach a stage where a decision is made that the burdens of continuing NIV outweigh the benefits.[5] It is important to consider practical aspects of how to best support the patient, their family, and the multidisciplinary team in managing this process of withdrawal. Consideration should be given to the timing of withdrawal which in general should be planned during normal working hours when all necessary staff are available to support. If a patient is dependent upon high levels of oxygen, it is likely they will die soon after NIV is withdrawn; however, it is important to explain to all involved that in some cases it may be longer, lasting hours or days. It is important to anticipate and effectively manage symptoms of breathlessness or distress. For some patients highly dependent upon NIV and already on opioids, benzodiazepines, or other sedatives, a significant increase in doses may be required to control symptoms, with potentially sedating side effects. In general, symptom control should be optimized prior to withdrawal. This may require a continuous infusion of medication, regular review, and adjustments to ensure comfort is key.

Learning Point Symptom Management

Patients in ITU environments may be receiving a diverse range of treatments, including inotropes, respiratory support, and renal replacement therapy. When a multidisciplinary decision has been made to focus on comfort, it is important that all treatments and interventions are reviewed and discussed with patient and family members. This is an opportunity to discuss the benefits and burdens of all interventions, from artificial nutrition and hydration, to blood pressure monitoring and suctioning, ensuring there is a clear plan in place which is sensitively communicated to all and documented.

Clinical Tip Medication Review

On the ITU, almost all patients will have intravenous (IV) access, and so the IV route will usually be the initial route of administration for medication. Where patients are already receiving sedatives (propofol, ketamine, or midazolam), doses and routes will need review in collaboration with the ITU team. It is important to consider de-prescribing all therapies that may not be contributing to the patient's comfort. Specific consideration should be given to antiseizure medications, anti-Parkinson medications, and insulin which will often be continued. It is essential for all patients to have anticipatory medications prescribed and regularly reviewed. If it is expected that a patient may be transferred from the ITU to a ward environment, planning of symptom management, anticipatory prescribing, including conversion of medications to subcutaneous route and a comprehensive handover are key.

Expert Comment

Clinically Assisted Nutrition and Hydration (CANH) refers to all forms of tube-feeding (e.g. via nasogastric tube, percutaneous endoscopic gastrostomy (PEG) or parenteral nutrition). It does not cover oral feeding, by cup, spoon, or any other method for delivering food or nutritional supplements into the patient's mouth. CANH is considered a form of medical treatment and should only be provided when it is in the patient's best interests. The UK General Medical Council have published guidelines in line with current legislation stipulating that health professionals are not required to offer treatments which they consider to be of no clinical benefit.[6]

When reviewing any decision related to CANH, it is always important to adopt an individualized approach. In this case the patient is expected to die imminently and therefore, in line with guidance from several national bodies, it will usually not be appropriate to continue CANH.[7] However, it is important that this decision be kept under review, fully documented, and the reasons why CAHN is not recommended sensitively explained to the family. Other interventions that can be overlooked, but which are vital in maximizing comfort include regular assessment of pressure areas and good mouthcare.

Learning Point Facilitating End of Life Care in Intensive Therapy Unit

Death on the ITU is common, ranging between 15–20% in the UK,[8] internationally there are varying statistics based on country and reason for ITU admission, however, one large audit found a mortality of 16.2%.[9] Therefore, it is vital to ensure that compassionate end of life care is provided. Fundamental considerations include hygiene care, symptom management, and reviewing medical treatments, including those specific to the ITU. Family and, where possible, the patient should be involved in these decisions.

It is important to consider the environment. Most people when asked would choose to die at home and the ITU setting is far away from this. Removing unnecessary medical equipment, interruptions from staff, and noises such as alarms can help. Allowing families to bring in personal items such as bedding, photos, and music can bring comfort. Family should be supported to spend time with their loved one, provision of free parking, and accessible accommodation should be offered where possible. The risk of complicated grief is higher in families of patients who die on ITU, bereavement care should be considered and specialist support may be required.[9]

Evidence Base Spirituality

Admission to the ITU can be an incredibly stressful experience for patients and families; emotional and spiritual support play an important role. Evidence shows that addressing the spiritual needs of a patient improves their health outcomes and quality of life. Conversely, spiritual distress displayed by patients and relatives can increase the burden of illness.

Providing spiritual care in the ITU has challenges, particularly when patients are unable to communicate due to their illness or treatment.[10] Novel approaches have been used such as a spiritual care communication card in patients who were unable to speak but could point to pictures or words. Spiritual support is part of the holistic care that intensive care professionals provide, however, there are often varying levels of confidence. The role of hospital chaplains has evolved and they can be a useful support for the patient, families, and healthcare team.

The team discussed potentially transferring Sandra to a local hospice however it was unclear how long she would live following the withdrawal of NIV, and therefore her family decided that they would prefer for her to stay in hospital. A syringe driver was started for symptom control containing 20 mg morphine sulphate and 20 mg of midazolam and her NG tube was removed for comfort. Her family including her three children were present when her NIV was removed 6 hours later. Her breathing pattern altered shortly after, and she was felt to be in the last hours of her life; therefore, she remained on the unit and died the following morning with her family present.

Expert Comment

As part of discussions about patient preferences and previous wishes, it may be appropriate to sensitively explore the option of organ or tissue donation. The timing of these discussions will vary for each patient, guided by the goals of care. Often this conversation is broached, with the support of the Specialist Nurse for Organ Donation (SN-OD), when the withdrawal of life-sustaining treatment is being considered. If this is something that families would like to explore and the patient appears to be a potential organ donor, a SN-OD will attend to carry out an in-depth assessment and access the Organ Donor Register to establish if the patient had made a decision in advance about organ donation.

Future Advances Palliative Care in Intensive Therapy Unit

Currently, there are two recognized models of palliative care in the ITU setting. The consultative model is based on the involvement of hospital specialist palliative care teams following referral. The integrative model promotes palliative care being incorporated into intensive care teams' daily practice; however, frequently there is a crossover between each model. Over the last decade, closer integration of palliative care and ITU services has led to more patients being transferred directly from the ITU to hospices for end of life care.[11] This involves careful planning and collaborative working from the ITU, HPCT, and hospice teams.

Traditional ITU outcome measures focus on reducing mortality and length of stay. Specialist palliative care teams frequently use patient-reported outcome measures as part of their day-to-day assessment and management of symptoms.[12, 13] More work is needed to develop and implement evidence-based patient and family-centred outcome measures in the ITU.

Discussion

In summary, this is a complex case of a patient with progressive metastatic disease who has had complications throughout her chemotherapy with repeated episodes of neutropenic sepsis. She has been admitted to hospital with further disease progression and bilateral pneumonia requiring NIV. The key learning points are to ensure early discussions between the treating teams, patients, and their relatives surrounding the goals of care. Palliative care teams can help support these conversations and also symptom management. Compassionate end of life care is multifaceted and the ITU environment can pose a challenge to this. However, with individualized patient care and good communication, it can be achieved.

A Final Word from the Expert

High-quality end of life care is a core part of critical care medicine. This case outlines some of the common challenges encountered in ITU, from prognostication in the face of clinical uncertainty to complex decision-making. In most cases, patients in ITU die after life-sustaining treatments are withdrawn, and this case highlights the importance of early and regular communication with all involved to ensure a patient-centred approach to decision-making. Multidisciplinary working across specialities and the involvement of Chaplaincy and bereavement support services are essential in supporting patients and their families.

Timely referral to Palliative Care can be helpful for patients in ITU who often have a high symptom burden, the management of which may be complicated by multiorgan failure. Alongside symptom control advice, the Palliative Care Team may also provide support in complex ethical or legal decision-making processes or complex discharges to other care settings.

References

1. Thompson JP, Bouch DC. Severity scoring systems in the critically ill. *Cont Educ Anaesth Crit Care Pain* 2008; 8: 181–185.
2. Lilly CM, De Meo DL, Sonna LA, et al. An intensive communication intervention for the critically ill. *Am J Med* 2000; 109: 469–475.
3. Evans LR, Boyd EA, Malvar G, et al. Surrogate decision-makers' perspectives on discussing prognosis in the face of uncertainty. *Am J Respir Crit Care Med* 2009; 179(1): 48–53.
4. Department of Health. *Mental Capacity Act*. 2005. Available at: https://www.legislation.gov.uk/ukpga/2005/9/contents
5. Faull C, Oliver D. Withdrawal of ventilation at the request of a patient with motor neurone disease: guidance for professionals. *BMJ Support Palliat Care* 2016; 6: 144–146.
6. General Medical Council. *Treatment and Care Towards the End of Life: Good Practice In Decision Making*. 2022. Available at: https://www.gmc-uk.org/ethical-guidance/ethical-guidance-for-doctors/treatment-and-care-towards-the-end-of-life#: ~ :text = It%20reminds%20you%20that%20decisions,updated%20on%2015%20March%202022
7. Royal College of Physicians, British Medical Association. *Clinically Assisted Nutrition and Hydration (CANH) and Adults Who Lack Capacity to Consent: Guidance for Decision Making in England and Wales*. 2018. Available at: https://www.bma.org.uk/media/1161/bma-clinically-assisted-nutrition-hydration-canh-full-guidance.pdf
8. Intensive Care National Audit & Research Centre (ICNARC). *Report 1. deaths in adult, general critical care units in England and Wales, 1 January 2007 to 31 December 2009*. 2011.
9. Vincent JL, Marshall JC, Namendys-Silva SA, et al. Assessment of the worldwide burden of critical illness: the intensive care over nations (ICON) audit. *Lancet Respir Med* 2014; 2(5): 380–386.
10. Kentish-Barnes, N, Chaize M, Seegers V, et al. Complicated grief after death of a relative in the intensive care unit. *Eur Respir J* 2015; 45(5): 1341–1352.
11. Willemse S, Smeets W, van Leeuwen E, *et al*. Spiritual care in the intensive care unit: An integrative literature research. *J Crit Care* 2020; 57: 55–78.
12. Grundy A, Ewart V, Wakefield D. From an intensive care unit (ICU) to a hospice; a case study highlighting the need for tailored staff education in response to the increasingly complex case-mix in specialist palliative care. *BMJ Support Palliat Care* 2020; 10: 16–17.
13. Bausewein C, Le Grice C, Simon ST, et al. The use of two common palliative outcome measures in clinical care and research: A systematic review of POS and STAS. *Palliat Med* 2011; 25: 304–313.

CASE

16 Community Patient Transferred into Emergency Department/Acute Medical Unit

Alice Copley

Expert: Sarah Yardley

Case history

George, a 71-year-old retired warehouse operative, presented to the emergency department (ED) from a nursing home. An ambulance was called due to worsening dyspnoea and productive cough on a background of reduced oral intake and general deterioration over the last three weeks.

There were pre-existing diagnoses of severe chronic obstructive pulmonary disease, peripheral vascular disease, and right lung squamous cell carcinoma, diagnosed two years ago. He was a current smoker and had a 45-pack-year smoking history. His carcinoma had been treated with palliative radiotherapy (30Gy in six fractions). Five months prior, a restaging CT scan confirmed recurrence and a decision for best supportive care was made. He was discharged from oncology follow-up with a recommendation he was placed on a primary care register for palliative care.

Assessment the previous day by his general practitioner concluded that George might be approaching the end of his life, but paramedics found him unaware of his limited prognosis with no anticipatory medicines available. Clinically, he had a respiratory rate (RR) of 28 breaths per minute and oxygen saturations of 76% on room air, so was brought to the ED.

Clinical Tip Rapid Assessment in the Emergency Department (ED)/Acute Medical Unit (AMU)

The ED and AMU frequently care for patients with advanced end-stage disease and acute life-threatening illness.[1] It is crucial that ED and AMU healthcare professionals can quickly assess the palliative care needs of their patients, recognize those nearing the end of life and deliver personalized care.[2]

Key components:

- Assessing symptoms
- Individual's concerns and expectations
- Understanding of illness and prognosis
- Preferences for emergency care and treatment, including resuscitation
- Collateral history: discussion with family, carers, ambulance service
- Values, well-being, spirituality
- Care needs
- Advance care planning: readmission, preferred place of care and death

Expert Comment What Does Best Supportive Care Mean?

Associations of the word 'palliative' with the very end of life have led to 'best supportive care' being used to describe the management of physical and psychological symptoms alongside the treatment of side-effects from disease-modifying treatment. Collaboration of palliative care clinicians with oncology has allowed services to positively frame supportive care for the whole person and emphasizes that this should be an integral part of treatment and care at any point of serious illness. In oncology, 'Enhanced Supportive Care' services provide concurrent care from diagnosis, through anticancer treatment to rehabilitation, post-treatment care, and survivorship as well as in the last phase of life.

The broader term supportive care is now being adopted elsewhere, and the approach is seen in other specialities such as post-intensive care rehabilitation services.

Expert Comment Communication Challenges in Advance Care Planning

Advance care planning (ACP) is essential for high quality patient care in the last phase of life. The creation of electronic patient records accessible to all care providers is an important aspect of this work as it improves timely access to information on which to base care. However, the quality of advance care plans varies greatly and this can significantly impact on the confidence of care home staff, paramedics, and other healthcare professionals to act on planning at the point of need. It remains the case that ACP is not always completed despite it being appropriate and is not always accessible, but also that even when these two issues are addressed ACP is not always followed. Underlying themes include lack of knowledge, confidence, competence of those faced with implementing the plans, but also uncertainty about the trustworthiness of interpreting and applying the documentation in the situation faced. Causes of uncertainty include when plans have not been reviewed for a long time, lack of understanding about mental capacity and/or what constitutes a valid ACP, and concerns about potential medicolegal consequences leading to escalation of interventions or transfer to an acute hospital to demonstrate all 'life-saving' treatment had been offered.[3]

Expert Comment Why Are People in the Last Phase of Life Transferred from Care Homes to Hospital by Ambulance? What Constitutes Appropriate Admission/Complexity?

Serious incidents in the provision of palliative care when someone is in a care home are likely to be under-reported but professional fear of complaints and failure to recognize dying are recognized as drivers for acute hospital admissions at the end of life.[4] Acute hospital staff and specialist palliative care teams must recognize that what seems appropriate and logical in an acute hospital environment can appear very differently in any community setting without easy access to investigations or rapid help from other professionals.[5] While the configuration of palliative care services is changing, there is much to be done if 'potentially avoidable' hospital admissions are to be reduced. Clinical and organizational factors within the healthcare system mean care home staff are commonly exposed to a lack of support from other agencies, including GPs and out-of-hours support, lack of access to training and variable access to appropriate medications.[6] While it would be ideal to avoid admissions, it is important to consider each case individually and create a plan with the care home to address concerns and avoid repeat occurrence.

Four weeks prior, following an admission with community-acquired pneumonia under the respiratory team, he had been discharged to the nursing home rather than his previous address. During this admission, a do not attempt cardio-pulmonary resuscitation (DNACPR) decision was made and shared with the GP and nursing home. George required assistance with washing and dressing due to shortness of breath and used a mobility scooter around the nursing home.

George's usual medications included inhaled salbutamol 2.5 mg nebules as required, oral morphine sulfate modified-release 10 mg twice daily, oral morphine sulfate immediate-release 2.5–5 mg as required and Trelegy Ellipta® inhaler once daily.

On examination, he was alert, orientated, and able to speak in short sentences. His blood pressure (BP) was 110/67 mmHg, heart rate 90 beats per minute, oxygen

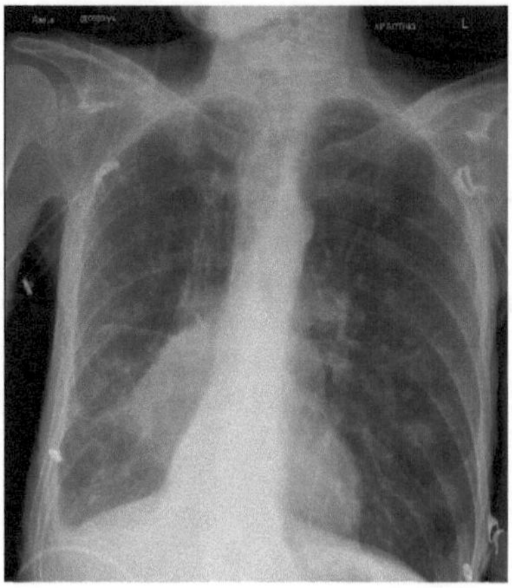

Figure 16.1 Chest X-ray showing chronic changes and right mid-zone atelectasis

saturations 88% on two litres/minute oxygen via nasal cannula, and he was apyrexial. He was cachexic and had finger clubbing. Chest auscultation revealed right mid-zone crepitations and scattered wheeze. He had normal heart sounds, was clinically euvolaemic, and his calves were soft and non-tender.

Blood tests showed elevated inflammatory markers (white cell count 12 × 10^9/L, C-reactive protein 78 milligrams/L), normocytic anaemia (haemoglobin 88 g/dL) and normal renal and liver function. A chest X-ray showed chronic changes and right mid-zone atelectasis (Figure 16.1). An arterial blood gas showed type 1 respiratory failure, and point-of-care testing for COVID-19 was negative.

Expert Comment How Should We Assess When to Investigate and What Action If Any Should Be Taken Based on Abnormal Investigations?

It is a truism that if you don't want to know the answer to a question you should not ask it, yet both professionals and patients can (perhaps inadvertently) get drawn into the biomedical approach of healthcare systems and focus on 'what the numbers say' or what the scans show rather than taking a step back to consider the whole situation. Key questions that should always be asked in palliative care are:

1. Is something potentially reversible happening? If so, what are the possible options for attempting to reverse it? What difference will these options make at the current stage of illness, and what are the burdens?
2. What does the patient understand about their overall situation? What are their preferences about what can be offered in different places of care and where they want to be cared for?
3. Are further investigations needed to provide good clinical care that will achieve the agreed goals established by considering questions 1. and 2.?
4. Do the agreed goals mean that abnormal results of investigations already undertaken need to be acted on in any way?

George was referred to the medical team and commenced oxygen therapy and treatment for community-acquired pneumonia. He was given oral immediate-release morphine sulfate 2.5 mg which alleviated his dyspnoea. Upon further discussion, this gentleman disclosed concerns that he was starting to die. His priority was enjoying the remainder of life (smoking cigarettes and using his electric wheelchair to socialize with other people). His preferred place of care and death was the nursing home. He did not wish to be in hospital even if this choice might reduce the length of his life. He accepted oral antibiotics to treat his pneumonia and was keen to see the palliative care team. The risks and benefits of home oxygen therapy, including fire risk, were discussed and a decision was made not to provide home oxygen as he wished to continue smoking.

Learning Point Capacity to Refuse Interventions

Adults with mental capacity have the right to refuse any medical treatment, even if doing so puts their life at risk. It is important to explain options to patients in a non-judgemental and impartial way to support shared decision-making. Capacity should be assessed following the legal framework in the relevant country. Patients with capacity can draw up documents to refuse specific interventions when they no longer have capacity, as part of an advance decision to refuse treatment.[7]

Evidence Base Oxygen Therapy for Breathlessness in Palliative Care

Long-term oxygen therapy (LTOT) is usually a treatment for hypoxaemia rather than dyspnoea in respiratory disease (e.g. COPD, pulmonary fibrosis, sleep-related hypoventilation) and is usually managed by respiratory specialists. There is some evidence for the use of oxygen therapy for dyspnoea in the hypoxic dying patient with non-malignant disease. However, in malignant disease, there is little evidence that oxygen therapy is beneficial, with occasional exceptions (e.g. the severely anaemic patient who is no longer being transfused)—oxygen use should be personalized according to the assessment of clinical benefit in each individual and balanced with adverse effects including oxygen toxicity, lung atelectasis, drying of the airways, and fire risk, as in the clinical case.[8]

Learning Point Discharging the Dying Patient With Oxygen Therapy

The use of oxygen in the palliative phase of illness should only be considered if the patient has symptomatic breathlessness refractory to other measures and is hypoxic (Figure 16.2). Oxygen is a treatment for hypoxaemia and not effective for breathlessness without hypoxia, nor is it indicated in palliation if the patient is hypoxic but not breathless. Oxygen can be supplied via a concentrator or cylinders, based on the patient's individual needs. It is important to consider the steps below to ensure oxygen is indicated, that safety and practicalities are considered and the need for oxygen is regularly reviewed.

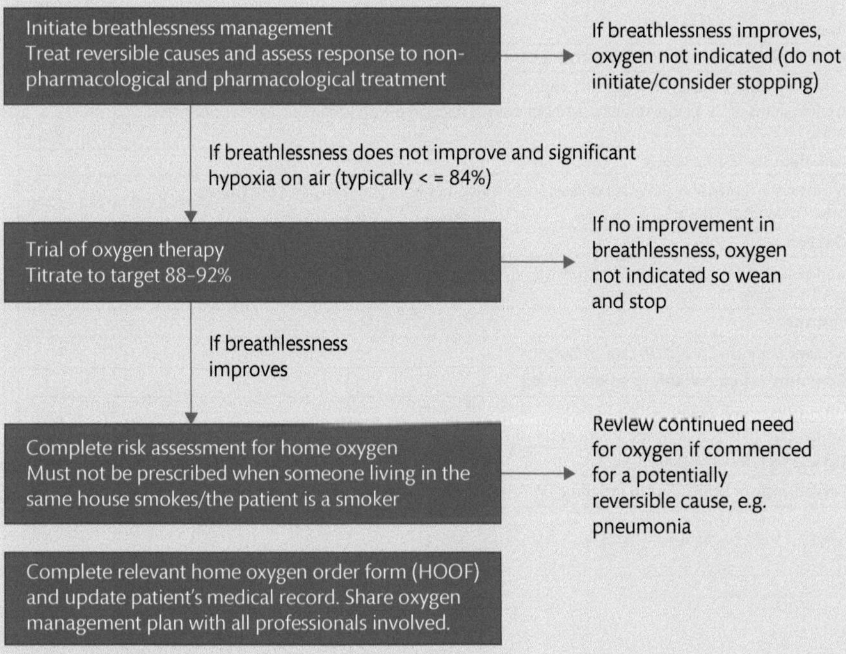

Figure 16.2 Oxygen flowchart.

Source: data from North Central London Integrated Care System *Use of oxygen in the palliative phase of illness and Long-term Respiratory Disease*.

George was discharged the same day with a supply of anticipatory medicines, oral antibiotics, and steroids. He was referred to the community palliative care team and a Recommended Summary Plan for Emergency Care and Treatment (ReSPECT) was completed to make his wishes accessible to all professionals in the future (see Case 18, 'Coordination and Transfer of Care'). He died comfortably three weeks later in the nursing home without being readmitted to hospital.

Clinical Tip Rapid Discharge Pathways from the Emergency Department to Home

Rapid discharge pathways from the ED exist to facilitate rapid transfer to the usual place of residence (home, residential home, or nursing home) for end of life care (Figure 16.3). The following steps act as a guide to ensure safe and effective discharge.

Are the following statement true?	Tick when complete
Rapidly deteriorating condition and may be entering the terminal phase	
The dying patient has expressed wish to transfer to usual place of residence	
Limitations, availability of services involved in rapid discharge discussed with patient and carer	
Safeguarding issues considered	
The patient has capacity to make this decision, or a best interest decision has been reached	
Senior clinician has discussed with the person and family/carer	
Significant change in condition, goals of care including DNACPR, prognosis, treatment escalation, and preferences for hospital readmission	
Person's wishes and preferences (e.g. preferred place of care and death)	
Record recommendations on ReSPECT form	
Own home or residential home without routine nursing care	
Liaise with the community neighbourhood team and GP	
Patient/carer has contact numbers for neighbourhood teams	
Care in place	
Essential equipment at home	
Residential home with routine nursing care	
Liaise with home manager – can they support this transfer?	
Discuss plans of care, urgent needs, and options for discharge with home manager or registered nurse	
Anticipatory medications	
Medicines in place at usual place of residence? If not, has emergency department palliative prescription been done?	
Oxygen	
Complete home oxygen order form (HOOF) if oxygen required and not already in place- see also Figure 2	
Transport	
Request dedicated palliative care ambulance	
Communication and information sharing	
Give written information leaflet to patient, family, or carers	
Contact GP to ensure they are aware of transfer	
Update section 4 of ReSPECT plan	
Printed copy of ReSPECT plan including DNACPR decision must transfer with patient	

Figure 16.3 Rapid discharge checklist.

Adapted with permission from Leeds Teaching Hospitals NHS Trust Rapid Discharge from ED guideline.

Learning Point Community Palliative Care Support for Nursing and Residential Homes

Nursing and residential homes are usually privately run businesses in the UK and have their own policies and procedures for care. Residential homes do not usually have routine nursing care and experience in caring for people at the end of life will vary. It is important that staff understand ACP, including cardiopulmonary (CPR) decisions and preferred place of care and death and where to get help and palliative care support when someone wants to remain in the care home for end of life care. Community palliative care teams need to coordinate care with community (district) nursing, GPs, and nursing and residential homes and provide education and support to these groups. Local systems vary, so it is important to discuss the prescription, supply, and administration of medications and what to do when someone dies (understanding that this is an expected death) including plans for confirmation of death and certification.

Clinical Tip Principles of Prescribing At the End of Life and Individualization To Each Patient

Prescribers should consider the following principles when providing medicines for symptom control, including anticipatory medications (see Case 18, 'Coordination and Transfer of Care'):

- Check local guidelines for first- and second-line medications
- Consider appropriate route: the oral route may be lost as patients deteriorate
- Consider renal and liver function when choosing medication
- Ensure dose range is appropriate: lower doses may be required in low body weight, frail, or opioid-naïve patients

Other medications can also be given as adjuncts to reduce symptoms. Oral corticosteroids can be trialled for breathlessness or as in the clinical case, used to treat COPD exacerbations. Antibiotics should be considered according to local guidelines as part of an individualized treatment plan, where expected outcomes and duration of treatment are communicated with patients and carers. The benefits of treatment must always be balanced with burdens, for example, adverse effects of corticosteroids.[9]

Expert Comment Who Should Be a Decision-Maker? How Might Further Admissions Be Avoided?

Palliative care is provided by many professionals including teams and services for whom it is just part of their remit in addition to specialist palliative care services. It is important to remember that this means not all professionals will have the same training or remit to be decision-makers about ACP and treatment escalation plans (TEP) including decisions about transfer of care and resuscitation. In fact, it is often more junior staff, who are immediately face-to-face with patients while more senior staff are working elsewhere. It is important, therefore, to be familiar with national and local guidance and policies on who can be a decision-maker and to ensure that everyone is aware of how to get support from a decision-maker in a timely fashion if needed to avoid further admissions following the setting up of an ACP as described in this case.

Future Advances The Role of Paramedics When Responding To Urgent Palliative Care Needs

Paramedics worldwide are increasingly seeing patients with urgent palliative care needs and deciding on the appropriateness of hospital admission when patients are nearing the end of life.[10] Paramedics play a vital role in delivering palliative and end of life care in patients' homes despite their training traditionally focusing on managing life-threatening emergencies, especially in rural locations or where 24/7 palliative care services do not operate.[11, 12]

Whilst variability exists between services, UK paramedics can usually administer anticipatory medications if the medicines and a medication authorization and administration record (MAAR) chart are available in the home. They cannot replenish or adjust a syringe pump or accept verbal orders for medications, but can provide additional medications within their scope of practice; e.g. opioids or antiemetics. Initiatives such as the Macmillan End of life Care (EOLC) team, who are part of London Ambulance Service (LAS), provide palliative care education, support, and access to electronic palliative care records to empower paramedics to deliver personalized care in patients' homes.

A Final Word from the Expert

This chapter illustrates the importance of considering who might be involved in the care of a patient across the different services that make up health and social care so that effective care planning and communication occur across the system. As the case demonstrates it is also vital that professionals in both community and acute hospital settings have access to specialist palliative care advice and support for decision-making, symptom control and care planning with patients in a timely manner if patients are to receive the best possible care for their needs. It is also important that to consider the overall clinical picture, draw on available clinical evidence and individualize care plans for each patient; this includes review of any 'automatically' started interventions such as the use of oxygen as these may not be of overall benefit. Pressures on EDs can make it challenging for patients to be discharged from ED rather than admitted to acute medical units but specialist palliative care teams can still usefully help reduce length of stay and readmission even if this is the case and close working relationships with both ED and AMU can save time and other resources in addition to benefitting patients.

References

1. Grudzen CR, Stone SC, Morrison RS. The palliative care model for emergency department patients with advanced illness. *J Palliat Med* 2011; 14(8): 945–950.
2. Pennell S, Jenks A. Palliative care on the acute medical unit. *Medicine* 2017; 45(2): 65–67.
3. Dinnen T, Williams H, Yardley S, et al. Patient safety incidents in advance care planning for serious illness: a mixed methods analysis study. *BMJ Support Palliat Care* 2019; 12: e403–e410.
4. Yardley I, Yardley S, Williams H, Carson-Stevens A, Donaldson LJ. Patient safety in palliative care: a mixed-methods study of reports to a national database of serious incidents. *Palliative Med* 2018; 32 (8):1353–1362.
5. Pask S, Pinto C, Bristowe K, et al. A framework for complexity in palliative care: a qualitative study with patients, family carers and professionals. *Palliat Med* 2018; 32(6): 1078–1090.
6. Gott M, Gardiner C, Ingleton C, et al. What is the extent of potentially avoidable admissions amongst hospital inpatients with palliative care needs? *BMC Palliat Care* 2013; 12: 9.
7. Chapman S. *The Mental Capacity Act in Practice: Guidance for End of Life Care*, 1st ed. Lavenham: National Council for Palliative Care, 2008.
8. Booth S, Wade R, Johnson M, et al; Expert Working Group of the Scientific Committee of the Association of Palliative Medicine. The use of oxygen in the palliation of breathlessness. A report of the expert working group of the Scientific Committee of the Association of Palliative Medicine. *Respir Med* 2004; 98(1): 66–77.
9. Palliative Care Adult Network Guidelines plus. Anticipatory Prescribing. 2016. Available at: https://book.pallcare.info/index.php?tid = 176
10. Long D. Paramedic delivery of community-based palliative care: an overlooked resource? *Prog Palliat Care* 2019; 27(6): 289–290.
11. Carter AJE, Arab M, Harrison M, et al. Paramedics providing palliative care at home: a mixed-methods exploration of patient and family satisfaction and paramedic comfort and confidence. *CJEM* 2019; 21(4): 513–522.
12. Surakka LK, Peake MM, Kiljunen MM, Mäntyselkä P, Lehto JT. Preplanned participation of paramedics in end-of-life care at home: a retrospective cohort study. *Palliat Med* 2021; 35(3): 584–591.

CASE

17 Prescribing Review

Luke Nathaniel Hatton

Expert: Melinda Presland

Case history

David, a 75-year-old retired haematologist, presented to the emergency department (ED) with a history of increasing difficulty swallowing solid food, one-stone weight loss, and intermittent chest pain, particularly after eating. David also complained of feeling light-headed particularly when getting up from standing. On further detailed history he had been experiencing some difficulties with swallowing food for the last 3 months; this was progressive from being intermittent to continuous and with an increasing variety of food types. David also reports feeling more tired and generally 'off' their food.

David has a past medical history of type two diabetes mellitus (T2DM), hypertension, ischaemic heart disease, and a previous lobectomy for non-small cell lung cancer 4 years ago. He is an ex-smoker with a 30-pack-a-year history and drinks alcohol occasionally. He lives with his wife, in a house with stairs and drives to the supermarket. They are both independent and have no carers. Current medications, which have not changed in the past 4 years, are shown in Table 17.1. David has no known drug allergies.

David was admitted for urgent investigations and management of his symptoms. Endoscopy showed a large ulceration at the mid-level of his oesophagus, and biopsies showed an adenocarcinoma, PD-L1 negative and HER2 negative. At the endoscopy, a stent was inserted to help with swallowing issues. CT showed advanced cancer, which had spread to lymph nodes and lung metastasis present. The staging was T3, N3, M1a.

Table 17.1 List of David's current medications

Medication	Dosage
Simvastatin	40 mg OD Nocte
Ramipril	10 mg OD
Aspirin	75 mg OD
Metformin	1 g BD
Lantus® (Insulin glargine)	10 units OD Nocte
Dapagliflozin	10 mg OD
Gliclazide	80 mg BD
Amlodipine	5 mg OD
Bendroflumethiazide	2.5 mg OD
Ferrous sulphate	200 mg TDS
Multivitamins	2 tablets OD

Expert Comment Medication History and Reconciliation

Ensuring an accurate, detailed medication history is essential. It is important to check if patients are taking medications as prescribed. Changes to medications in different settings, rapid changes, a lack of information being given to patients or patients' understanding of medicines regimes, and poor adherence can all influence how patients use their medicines.

'Medicines reconciliation identifies potential in what the prescribing records say a patient should be taking, compared to the medicines the patient is, in fact, receiving and taking'.[1] Medicines reconciliation can use many sources (see Box 17.1).

GP records and discharge letters may show what has been prescribed, but it does not show what has been collected from a community pharmacy or how the patient has used the medication.

Whenever possible, the patient or their family/carers should be asked for details around medicine usage, as GP records, clinic/discharge letters, or details from community pharmacy may not always reflect what the patient takes.

Box 17.1 Source of medication information

Patient
Family or carer or place of care
Recent Prescription
Recent discharge or clinic letter
Electronic prescribing record
GP records/shared care records
Community pharmacy

David was discharged and was followed up by Oncology one week after discharge. His clinical frailty score was 3[2], performance status was one, and swallowing symptoms had improved with the stent. David still had symptoms of postural hypotension and had a postural drop of 20 mmHg when measured in clinic, with systolic blood pressure being 140 mmHg.

After going through the risk and benefits of systemic treatment, David consented to palliative oxaliplatin and fluorouracil. Before commencing chemotherapy, David's medications were reviewed, and in discussion with him it was decided to stop the statin. Given his blood pressure and symptoms of postural hypotension, it was felt that looser control of his blood pressure would be appropriate. It was decided to continue the current antihypertensive medications and review blood pressure in clinic or primary care and adjust medications based on multiple readings. With the Hb1ac being well controlled, the metformin was stopped. The changes of medications were highlighted in the clinic letter.

Learning Point Involving the Patient

The patient should always be involved in discussion around medications; the health professional should help the patient understand the risk and benefits of medications. This is especially important when patients have been on the medication for many years and a careful explanation of the change of benefit is important.

Medicines optimization is a person-centred approach that ensures our patients receive the right choice of medicines when they are needed. This approach can improve safety, adherence, and reduces waste.

Expert Comment Communication on Transfer of Care

The sharing of information about medication as a patient moves between care settings is vital and should be done as quickly as possible (ideally within 24 hours). From secondary to primary care, discharge letters are the most common form of communication around medication that GPs will receive, so ensuring that any changes, new medicines, or monitoring requirements are clearly outlined is important to avoid medicine related harm, and to facilitate timely action.

From primary to secondary care, the GP record is often used as a source for medication history and reconciliation. Ensuring this record is accurate and up to date is vital.

Clinical Tip Medication Deprescribing

Every medication has potential risks and benefits, and these change with patient need and circumstance. Some are much easier to define than others.[3] Guidelines have been developed to help aid deprescribing for example STOPP/START[4] and STOPPFrail.[5]

For example, statins have to be taken over many years to have benefit.[6] Therefore, if the patient's life expectancy is less than the expected time for benefit, patients are not likely to gain benefit but will be exposed to the potential harms.

It is important to remember clinical-acumen needs to be used when making decisions in a patient specific context.

Expert Comment Deprescribing on 'One-off' Encounters

Assessing patients and deprescribing medicines, especially those started by another clinician can be challenging, as you may not feel at liberty to make changes or feel that it is your responsibility to do so.

However, taking a patient centred approach, we should be considering what is in our patients' best interests and discussing with them as part of the consultation.

If there is an immediate need to stop a medication, due to risk or intolerable adverse effects, this should be done, e.g. parkinsonism with haloperidol for nausea (all at once approach).

If you believe changes may require additional monitoring prior to deciding on stopping, e.g. hypotension with multiple antihypertensives, there is more than one option:

- Reduce the doses of the medications and request monitoring (stepwise approach)
- Stop one or more of the medications completely and request monitoring and further deprescribing as needed (mixed approach)
- Suggest to the GP/original prescriber that changes may be required and request they consider

Any changes, monitoring requirements, or suggested changes need to be clearly documented and communicated.

David had three cycles of chemotherapy, with the last cycle showing stable disease. However, one week after having his last chemotherapy cycle, David notices that his left leg is swollen and painful. He presents to the Oncology assessment unit and undergoes an urgent ultrasound of his leg. This shows a deep vein thrombosis. David is started on anticoagulation.

In clinic, he is reviewed by his team, given the increasing burden of tiredness and nausea, which are common side effects of the chemotherapy treatment, and the deep vein thrombosis (DVT), it was discussed and agreed that further treatment was not in David's best interest.

It was felt by the oncology team that anticoagulation treatment could be stopped after 6 months, because it was a provoked DVT. Given David's background as a haematologist and his professional experience, he was keen to continue this for longer, which was taken into consideration by his oncology team. He was not particularly keen on injections and after discussion with the anticoagulation specialists' the patient was started on a direct oral anticoagulants (DOAC).

Learning Point Expert Advice

The risk of problematic polypharmacy is increasing, given the potential for overprescribing of medication, in particular 'when a condition changes and the medicine is no longer appropriate or required but is still prescribed'.[8] Thus, it is often useful to discuss with other specialities and experts in the clinical area to consider potential benefit or risk, and the rationale to continue or stop.

Expert Comment Off-label Prescribing

For medications to hold a marketing authorization (product licence) in countries, they must meet certain standards relating to safety, quality, and efficacy. As part of this process, the Summary of Product Characteristics (SmPC) details the licensed indications, routes, and doses for the medication.

The use of a medicine outside of these parameters is referred to as 'off-label' and is common practice in palliative care. This is often due to the lack of clinical trial data in the palliative care population for the given indication or route (which is required to obtain the product licence), but expert clinical practice over time has shown it to be safe and efficacious.

Before prescribing medicines off-label, the clinician must be satisfied that there are no products used within their licence which would meet the needs of the patient, that there is sufficient evidence for using the medicine outside of its licence and take responsibility for prescribing and follow-up.

The palliative care formulary[7] is an excellent guide for symptom management in palliative care, and addresses the use of medicines outside of their product licence.

David was discharged with a community palliative care team referral and appropriate social support with a preference to be admitted into the hospice in the final days of life. Over the coming months David had a steady decline in function, becoming frailer with weight loss and reduced mobility.

David is seen regularly by the palliative care nurses. David reports further dizziness upon standing and it is noted David has a significant postural drop of 30 mmHg when the blood pressure is checked. On review of the medications, it is noted David is still on antihypertensive medications. In discussion with the palliative care team at the hospice it was felt that all blood pressure control tablets could be stopped as given David's weight loss and increasingly frailty, controlling the blood pressure offered little benefit to the patient but did pose a risk of increased falls.

It was also felt that David was at increased risk of hypoglycaemia due to medication for diabetes, reduced appetite, with intermittent difficulty swallowing medications. Given this it was felt appropriate to stop the oral diabetes medications and continue the insulin with once daily blood glucose monitoring. Monitoring once a day was to ensure it did not go massively outside of range.[9]

It was felt that it could be appropriate to stop the anticoagulation for DVT, given the length of treatment time. The benefit of the DOAC was not felt to be clear cut given David was entering into the final weeks of life. However, David was keen to continue the anticoagulation given his working life as haematologist. Even though the medication tablet burden had been reduced, David was unsure if he could manage the anticoagulation tablet everyday. As not taking the DOAC everyday would reduce the effectiveness of the medication, the use of low molecular weight heparin injections was revisited, and although not a preference originally, it was now considered acceptable by David and the team.

It was felt that there was little harm in continuing the anticoagulation at present, especially given David firm views on this. It was discussed with David and explained that at some point that benefit may change, specifically towards the final days where David might be sleepy and not able to express wishes. David was happy for this.

Expert Comment Stopping Medications

It can be difficult to know what to do with certain medications, when to stop or continue. It is specific for each person, time, and place. If able, the patient should be involved in the discussion to understand their views on the medications, and a plan formulated in agreement with them.

It is useful to set time frames to review medications, for example prescribing a short course (5 days) of steroids to assess benefit and discontinuing at the review if no benefits are seen.

Learning Point Stopping Medications

It is often challenging to know whether to push for a patient to stop a medication despite their insistence to continue. Effective communication with the patient and setting review targets is often useful for the team and patient to understand each other. As always, seeking help from colleagues is good practice.

Over the next two weeks David increasingly struggled at home, with abdominal pain developing and pain with swallowing. David was initially given liquid morphine as needed, which was titrated up and switched to 40 mg MR tablets BD. For anxiety, David was given lorazepam 0.5 mg TDS as needed.

David further deteriorated and was not able to swallow liquids. David increasingly reported pain and agitation; therefore it was felt appropriate to transfer David to the hospice as per his wishes.

On admission to the hospice, the medicines were rationalized, and the remaining oral medications were stopped given the lack of oral route or appropriateness of the medicines at this time. Replacement of the oral medicines via the subcutaneous route was considered.

Given the presenting symptoms and the recent dose of oral analgesics, David was started on a syringe driver with morphine and midazolam. David did not have capacity to discuss the low molecular weight heparin injection. When his family attended, the current treatment plan was discussed with them, and it was explained David was dying and continuing the injection would be inappropriate, given the focus on symptom management and comfort.

The insulin was stopped, with once daily blood sugar monitoring agreed, and a plan to reintroduce a reduced dose after 2 days if blood glucose remains above 15 mmol/l.

Over the coming days the syringe driver was increased in accordance with David's symptoms and 'as needed' medication doses, and David died with his family at his bedside 6 days after being admitted to the hospice.

Learning Point Communication with Families

Communication is important with families, especially at the end of life. This includes communication around medications and reasons why medications are given. Explanation is often needed to help the family come to terms with why medications might be stopped and why certain medications have been started.[10]

Clinical Tip Communicating with Families

Explaining why medications have been stopped or started at the end of life is hugely important for families. An explanation such as saying we are focused on ensuring that the patient's symptoms are controlled, thus we have stopped medications as they are not helping his symptoms and are not offering any benefit currently[11] may be given.

It is also equally important to explain the reasons behind the starting of medication. For example, explaining the rationale behind the use of a syringe driver and titration of medications while minimizing the side effects.

Discussion

In summary, medication review should be considered as a constant process, to be employed at every given opportunity to ensure provision of benefit to patients without excessive side effects or burden. The benefit and harm of medications can change during the patient journey, as can the patient's view of the use of these medicines.

Open and honest discussion around the possible benefits and harms of medicine use, alongside the patient's thoughts and preferences can lead to excellent shared decision making and improved adherence to medicines and symptom management. This decision should never be set in stone and should be reviewed continuously, with the patient and/or their family and carers, throughout their journey.

There are many resources available to support the deprescribing of medicines. Seeking advice is always useful, especially with medications that are less frequently encountered or medications prescribed off-label or unlicensed.

A Final Word from the Expert

Medicines are the most common healthcare intervention, and account for up to 8% of hospital admissions, many of which may be preventable. Consideration when prescribing, reviewing, or stopping medicines is a must. Not prescribing is always an option if there is no clear indication or benefit. Impeccable communication with the patient, their family/carers and the other healthcare professionals involved in the patient's care can help support appropriate medication use, at the right time for the patient, balancing benefits and potential harms with patient goals and healthcare professional's opinions on the need for medication.

References

1. Goverment B. *Good for You, Good For Us, Good For Everyone*. D.o.H.S. Care (ed.). 2021.
2. Rockwood K, Song X, MacKnight C, et al. A global clinical measure of fitness and frailty in elderly people. *CMAJ* 2005; 173(5): 489–495.
3. Halli-Tierney AD, Scarbrough C, Carroll D. Polypharmacy: evaluating risks and deprescribing. *Am Fam Physician* 2019; 100(1): 32–38.
4. O'Mahony D, O'Sullivan D, Byrne S, O'Connor MN, Ryan C, Gallagher P. STOPP/START criteria for potentially inappropriate prescribing in older people: version 2. *Age Ageing* 2014; 44(2): 213–218.
5. Lavan AH, Gallagher P, Parsons C, O'Mahony D. STOPPFrail (Screening Tool of Older Persons Prescriptions in Frail adults with limited life expectancy): consensus validation. *Age Ageing* 2017; 46(4): 600–607.
6. Kutner JS, Blatchford PJ, Taylor DH Jr, et al., Safety and benefit of discontinuing statin therapy in the setting of advanced, life-limiting illness: a randomized clinical trial. *JAMA Intern Med* 2015; 175(5): 691–700.
7. Wilcock A, Howard P, Charlesworth S. *Palliative Care Formulary*, 7th ed. London: Pharmaceutical Press, 2020.
8. Barnett N. *Understanding Polypharmacy Overprescribing and Deprescribing* 2022. Available at: https://www.sps.nhs.uk/articles/understanding-polypharmacy-overprescribing-and-deprescribing/
9. Diabetes UK. *End of Life Guidance For Diabetes Care*. London: DK, 2021.
10. Wilson E, Caswell G, Latif A, Anderson C, Faull C, Pollock K. An exploration of the experiences of professionals supporting patients approaching the end of life in medicines management at home. A qualitative study. *BMC Palliat Care* 2020; 19(1): 66.
11. Twycross R, Wilcock A. *Introducing Palliative Care*, 5th ed. London: Pharmaceutical Press, 2021.

CASE

18 Coordination and Transfer of Care

Rosanna Hill

Expert: Adam Hurlow

Case History

Susan was a 52-year-old woman admitted to hospital with a four-week history of weight loss, fatigue, and reducing mobility, alongside increasing breathlessness and a 'dark-grainy vomit' concerning for upper gastrointestinal (GI) bleeding.

Susan was diagnosed 12 months earlier with metastatic oesophageal cancer, and after a staging computer tomography (CT) showed disease progression with new lung, liver, and bone metastases despite chemotherapy, a decision was made for best supportive care.

Susan was treated with antibiotics for community-acquired pneumonia, based on chest X-ray findings alongside raised white blood cell (WBC) count and C-reactive protein (CRP). She had normocytic normochromic anaemia (haemoglobin (Hb) 78 g/L) and was given a two-unit blood transfusion. There was no evidence of ongoing GI bleeding and her Hb improved to 85 g/L post transfusion. Other blood results showed an albumin of 19 g/L with normal renal function and mildly elevated liver enzymes. Susan was transferred to a medical ward, where she stabilized over the following week.

Despite physiotherapy and occupational therapy (OT) input, Susan's functional status remained impaired, due to overwhelming fatigue. Her Australia-modified Karnofsky Performance Status (AKPS) scale was 40%, as she was in bed more than 50% of the time.

Susan declined further investigations for her anaemia and understood that she was most likely entering the final weeks of life.

Clinical Tip Recognizing a Patient Nearing the End of Life (EoL)

The 2014 'One Chance to Get it Right' report on Care of Dying People, outlines five priorities of care: the first being recognition and communication.[1]

People approaching the EoL often exhibit non-specific signs such as anorexia, cachexia, declining mobility, and fatigue.[2] Establishing whether this reflects irreversible progression of life-limiting illness rather than potentially treatable conditions can be challenging. As an individual's health may fluctuate, the rate and degree of change in their overall condition are informative.

It is important to consider potentially treatable causes, assess the individual's likelihood of responding to treatment, and establish the person's preference regarding treatment. Persistent deterioration despite targeted interventions suggests ill-health is primarily driven by end-stage disease.

Considering this, One Chance to Get it Right focuses on recognizing unstable patients who may not recover, rather than looking to 'diagnose dying'.[1] A change in the patient's condition should trigger for a new assessment which enables patients and those important to them to participate in earlier decision-making.

Learning Point Australia-modified Karnofsky Performance Scale

The AKPS is a measure of physical function used in palliative care.[6] It is a single score between 0 and 100 based on the patient's functional ability. A score of one hundred signifies normal functional ability with no evidence of disease, with decreasing numbers showing a reducing performance status.

It can assist with clinical decision-making as a predictor of survival but also to monitor trends over time.[6]

Future Advances Biological Markers as a Predictor of Prognosis

Estimating survival is important to many patients, but clinicians' prognostication is often inaccurate, with an optimism bias.[3] There is evidence for using biomarkers as prognostic indicators, particularly in advanced cancer. The following may be abnormal in the last weeks of life and have Grade A evidence as predicters of prognosis: CRP, WBC count, serum albumin, sodium, urea, and alkaline phosphatase (ALP).[4]

Whilst there are multiple prognostic tools incorporating biomarkers, it has not been demonstrated whether they are consistently superior, or even equal to clinicians' predications of survival and the best way to use such tools remains unclear.[5] They may help provide objective underpinnings to clinical gestalt, promote consistency across teams, and support education. The application of machine learning using routine health data in electronic records may enhance prognostication beyond multiprofessional predication.[3]

In this case, we notice that the patient has a low albumin and an elevated CRP, which could be explained by her acute pneumonia. However, a trend in falling albumin and persistently elevated CRP in the absence of acute illness is suggestive of a shorter prognosis.

Evidence Base Anaemia and Blood Transfusions at the EoL

Red blood cell transfusions are commonly given for anaemia in advanced disease, despite insufficient supporting evidence. A national audit of practice in hospices, and subsequent evidence review suggests that transfusion practice remains too liberal,[7] whilst highlighting the greater risk of transfusion-associated circulatory overload in patients with advanced disease. The evidence suggests very little improvement in symptoms following transfusion, with only 18% of patients having an improvement maintained for 30 days. The literature supports personalized investigation of anaemia, with targeted interventions, with more selected use of transfusion.[8]

Susan lived with her husband Steven in a two-storey house. Although satisfied with care in hospital, she expressed a wish to be cared for and die at home. Her symptoms were well managed, and she was eating and drinking small amounts. Susan's family were supportive of her wishes but were concerned about how they would manage.

Susan understood that she would deteriorate from her cancer but might experience acute events such as another pneumonia or GI bleed. Whilst hospital-based interventions may be life-prolonging, they increase the likelihood of her deteriorating and dying in hospital. They explored the need to balance this risk against her wish to be cared for and die at home.

Steven was concerned about the management of GI bleeding at home, ensuring she was not distressed. A management approach for this was agreed.

The clinical team documented her care preferences and agreed on treatment escalation recommendations on an advanced care plan, including the recommendation for DNACPR (do not attempt cardiopulmonary resuscitation), the rationale for which the patient and her family understood and agreed with. In this case, Susan's agreed recommendations were documented on a ReSPECT (Recommended Summary Plan for Emergency Care and Treatment) form and on EPaCCS (Electronic Palliative care Coordination System).

Expert Comment

A CPR (cardiopulmonary resuscitation) recommendation (for CPR or DNACPR) is an essential element of treatment escalation planning, but it receives considerable focus at the expense of other components that logically precede it. If the antecedents of cardiopulmonary arrest are not treatable or treatment is unwanted, clinicians will not be able to prevent arrest; CPR is then unlikely to be effective or achieve anything other than short-lived return of spontaneous breathing and circulation. For patients dying at home this would entail advanced life support delivered by paramedics and transfer to hospital.

It makes sense to discuss clinical escalation for potentially treatable conditions before considering CPR, which in the context of advanced life-limiting illness is rarely effective. This re-focusses discussion to what could be achieved for potentially reversible deterioration.

Clinical Tip Advance Care and Treatment Escalation Planning

To guide care across settings, healthcare teams should encourage, empower, and enable patients to document preferences and treatment recommendations as an advanced care plan. This helps guide care in the future should they lose the capacity to participate in decisions.

An example in the UK is the nationally developed ReSPECT process.[9] Recommendations are created through discussions between the ill person, those important to them, and relevant healthcare professionals. They are based upon the person's priorities informed by realistic clinical judgement.[9]

For people going home towards the EoL, it is important to discuss, record and share recommendations concerning:

- Treatment out of hospital for anticipated problems, e.g. pneumonia or GI bleeding
- Hospital re-admission: circumstances under which it might be beneficial, or whether it is to be avoided
- Escalation in hospital
- Cardiopulmonary arrest
- Priorities of care, e.g. preferred place of death

It is essential that such plans can be accessed by all those involved in care. To enable this ReSPECT was designed as a patient-held form.

Sharing and access can be enhanced by digitally shared recommendations. Some localities have implemented digital ReSPECT, or similar initiatives, including EPaCCS.[10] Recommendations should be reviewed when there is a significant change in the person's health; their goals may change as their condition deteriorates.

EPaCCS aims to overcome some of the hurdles to digital sharing as it provides a core record, supported by data sharing agreements and standardized clinical coding to facilitate information sharing between systems.[10]

Learning Point Anticipatory Prescribing

Pre-emptively prescribed subcutaneous medication is thought to minimize treatment delay at the EoL, should symptoms arise that are unresponsive to non-pharmacological measures.[11] However, this is based on best practice guidance without robust research-evidence to support practice.[12]

Anticipatory prescriptions must consider clinical factors, including current symptom pharmacological management, renal and liver function, side effect profile, and sensitivities. They usually include:

- An opioid for pain and/or breathlessness (e.g. morphine in the absence of moderate to severe renal impairment)
- An anxiolytic sedative for anxiety or agitation (e.g. midazolam)
- An antisecretory for noisy non-tenacious airways secretions (e.g. hyoscine butylbromide)
- An antiemetic for nausea and/or vomiting (e.g. levomepromazine in the absence of seizures, Parkinson's disease, and related conditions)

Local processes must be followed, enabling community teams to administer anticipatory medications, minimizing disruption to care. It may require a community medication administration chart to be completed.

The rationale for anticipatory medications must be offered, including potential side effects, indications, and essential contact numbers. Administration for a new or deteriorating symptom should trigger a prompt clinical re-assessment.

Future research is focusing on the views and experiences of patients and their carers, clinical and cost-effectiveness, and safety.[12]

Clinical Tip Managing Bleeding at the EoL

Haemorrhage occurs in 10–20% of people with advanced cancer and may be extremely distressing.[13]

Assessment is required to establish whether urgent hospital-based management is likely to be effective. If the patient declines or is unsuitable for treatment, it is still important to reduce risk where possible, including medications that may increase the risk of bleeding. If bleeding is anticipated, this should be discussed as part of advanced care planning. In some situations, prescription of oral-antifibrinolytics such as tranexamic acid, for maintenance-control or prophylaxis may be beneficial.

There are specific considerations for managing life-threatening bleeding at the EoL:

- Non-pharmacological management: staying calm, applying direct pressure where possible, using dark towels to minimize distressing visible blood, and having emergency contacts.
- Pharmacological management: administration of a rapid-acting benzodiazepine. In an inpatient setting, this would be subcutaneous (SC) or intramuscular (IM) midazolam, or buccal midazolam if in the community.

Non-pharmacological management is most important. It is recommended not to leave a patient alone to get medications in the event of a life-threatening haemorrhage. This is more likely to exacerbate their fear and anxiety, and patients will often lose consciousness rapidly before medication is effective.[13] In addition to offering counselling about the possibility of a life-threatening bleed, a debrief should be offered to the family and any professionals involved after an event.

Following 24-hour care needs assessment and OT review, equipment was ordered including a profiling bed, and a care package was arranged.

Due to her rapid deterioration, she was felt to meet criteria for fast-track funding. Hospital discharge documentation was updated to:

- update on current clinical situation, care needs, and medication
- inform community services that a ReSPECT form and EPaCCS had been completed
- advise the Gold Standards Framework (GSF) to review her ongoing care needs

Susan was referred to the community nursing (CN) team for ongoing care and assessment, and was given a copy of her ReSPECT form. The patient and family were aware that primary care or CN teams could refer to community palliative care if she developed any needs requiring specialist involvement.

Learning Point Funding Care and Equipment

Individuals who are rapidly deteriorating and are entering a terminal phase of their illness often require timely access to care and equipment to support care outside hospital. This requires robust multiprofessional assessment of care needs, ideally without bureaucratic application and approval processes that are burdensome and may introduce delays.

In the UK this is supported with the fast-track pathway tool.[14] It is completed by a clinician who is familiar to the patient, and supports individuals to access NHS Continuing Healthcare (CHC) funding.[14] Eligibility is not limited by a specified expected prognosis, or the presence of any symptoms. The mechanism by which fast-track referrals are made and managed varies nationally, requiring an understanding of local processes.

Expert Comment

It is critical that dying people and those providing care and support in the community know who to contact if a problem arises. This varies depending upon the services involved, their local configuration, and when issues arise. Ensure contact details are provided ahead of discharge with explanation of whom to contact for what issue. Encourage early reporting of concerns before problems deteriorate into crisis, particularly 'out of hours'.

Future Advances

Some localities have implemented 'single points of contact' to coordinate end of life care (EoLC). They provide unwell people, informal carers, and professionals a single means of accessing generalist and specialist services. It is anticipated that they reduce the burden associated with navigating complex healthcare systems; ensuring the right care is delivered at the right time.

Innovative digital solutions, including person/carer-reported symptom monitoring, may enhance such models providing opportunities for proactive timely intervention. The evidence base is yet to establish what works for whom, how, in what circumstances and why, but such innovations may be an effective way of delivering proactive and coordinated EoLC in the community.

Expert Comment

Review of existing treatment recommendations is part of discharge planning. The person and those close to them should be offered the opportunity to participate in this conversation. This ensures compliance with mental capacity legislation and enables all parties to agree on what information is documented and how it will be shared.

Initial recommendations are often made at a time of stress during acute ill-health, when a person may not have fully absorbed the information or have appreciated it would be formally recorded. Friends, family, and others involved may not have participated in earlier discussions. Discussion should happen in a planned way pre-discharge rather than arising after unexpectedly receiving a copy of a treatment escalation plan just before discharge. It is also an essential part of empowering informal carers; equipping them to know what to do in event of clinical deterioration.

Learning Point Coordination and Continuity of Care

Services delivering EoLC in the community need to be able to assess for changes in someone's needs and respond effectively. Regular multiprofessional case-load reviews supported by a structured framework may help this. The GSF is one such evidence-based approach.[15] There are three steps: Identify, Assess, and Plan.[15]

It includes 'the use of the "Surprise Question"' ('Would you be surprised if this patient were to die in the next few months, weeks, days?') to help identify patients who may be approaching EoL.[16] Like 'One chance to get it right', it focuses on assessing people's needs, rather than focusing on timescales.[1,15]

Discussion

In summary, this is a case of a patient with metastatic cancer who is likely to be entering the final weeks of life and wishes to focus on care at home; prioritizing comfort over interventions to prolong life. It highlights the challenges when arranging transfer of care between services, and how to best support coordination of care for someone with palliative care needs transferring into the community.

A Final Word from the Expert

Friends, family, other unpaid carers, and the wider community are a key component of delivering EoLC. The important part they can play is often under-appreciated and may be under-utilized. Approaches that enhance self-management, better equip informal carers to comanage the challenges of community EoLC, and build on existing community assets, coupled with resourced and tailored services, may be best equipped to address the challenges facing high-quality equitable community-based EoLC.

References

1. The Leadership Alliance for the Care of Dying People. *One Chance to Get it Right.* June 2014. Available at: https://assets.publishing.service.gov.uk/government/uploads/system/uploads/attachment_data/file/323188/One_chance_to_get_it_right.pdf
2. Marie Curie. What to expect in the last weeks and days. 2022. Available at: https://www.mariecurie.org.uk/help/support/terminal-illness/preparing/what-to-expect
3. Avati A, Jung K, Harman S, et al. Improving palliative care with deep learning. *BMC Medical Inform Decis Mak* 2018; 18(4): 55–64.
4. Reid VL, McDonald R, Nwosu AC, et al. A systematically structured review of biomarkers of dying in cancer patients in the last months of life: an exploration of the biology of dying. *PLoS One* 2017; 12(4): e0175123.
5. Stone P, Vickerstaff V, Kalpakidou A, et al. Prognostic tools or clinical predictions: Which are better in palliative care? *PLoS One* 2021; 16(4): e0249763.
6. Abernethy AP, Shelby-James T, Fazekas BS, Woods D, Currow DC. The Australia-modified Karnofsky Performance Status (AKPS) Scale: a revised scale for contemporary palliative care clinical practice. *BMC Palliat Care* 2005; 4: 7.
7. Neoh K, Gray R, Grant-Casey J, et al. National comparative audit of red blood cell transfusion practice in hospices: recommendations for palliative care practice. *Palliat Med* 2019; 33(1): 102–108.
8. Neoh K, Page A, Chin-Yee N, Doree C, Bennett MI. Practice review: evidence-based and effective management of anaemia in palliative care patients. *Palliat Med* 2022; 36(5): 783–794.
9. Resuscitation Council UK. ReSPECT for healthcare professionals. Available at: https://www.resus.org.uk/respect/respect-healthcare-professionals
10. NHS England and NHS Improvement North West. *Electronic Palliative Care Coordinating Systems (EPaCCS).* Available at: https://www.england.nhs.uk/north-west/north-west-coast-strategic-clinical-networks/our-networks/palliative-and-end-of-life-care/for-professionals/electronic-palliative-care-coordinating-systems-epaccs/#: ~ :text = Electronic%20Palliative%20Care%20Coordination%20Systems,people's%20discussions%20about%20their%20care
11. NHS Scotland. *Scottish Palliative Care Guidelines, Anticipatory Prescribing.* June 2014. Available at: https://www.palliativecareguidelines.scot.nhs.uk/guidelines/pain/anticipatory-prescribing.aspx
12. Bowers B, Ryan R, Kuhn I, Barclay S. Anticipatory prescribing of injectable medications for adults at the end of life in the community: A systematic literature review and narrative synthesis. *Palliat Med* 2019; 33(2):160–177.
13. NHS Scotland. *Scottish Palliative Care Guidelines, Anticipatory Prescribing.* April 2014. Available at: https://www.palliativecareguidelines.scot.nhs.uk/guidelines/palliative-emergencies/Bleeding.aspx
14. Department of Health and Social Care. *Fast Track Pathway Tool for Continuing Healthcare.* December 2018. Available at: https://www.gov.uk/government/publications/nhs-continuing-healthcare-fast-track-pathway-tool
15. National Gold Standards Framework Centre, The Gold Standards Framework. 2022. Available at: https://goldstandardsframework.org.uk/
16. The Gold Standards Framework Centre. *The GSF Prognostic Indicator Guidance.* October 2011. Available at: https://www.goldstandardsframework.org.uk/cd-content/uploads/files/General%20Files/Prognostic%20Indicator%20Guidance%20October%202011.pdf

CASE

19 Giving Remote Advice to Families and Other Professional Providers

Shaun Peter Qureshi, Philippa Guppy, and Georgina Osborne

Expert: Rasha Al-Qurainy

Case history

Pam is a 79-year-old woman with a diagnosis of metastatic breast cancer. She has a one-week history of worsening pain associated with her right breast for which her general practitioner (GP) prescribed 10 mg modified release oral morphine twice daily (with *pro re nata (PRN)* immediate release oral morphine). After two days, Pam's pain had not improved, limiting her sleep, and the GP had called the hospice duty doctor for advice.

Learning Point Remote Advice and Consultations

Palliative care healthcare professionals are often required to provide remote advice to other healthcare professionals as well as patients and their significant others (Figure 19.1). For the purposes of this case, we have defined advice and consultations separately.

Advice is remote whenever the consulted healthcare professional is not in the immediate presence of the patient; the patient may not be previously known to them, and advice may be sought from healthcare professionals from multiple sites/services covering a wide geographical area. Several healthcare professionals may seek remote advice including GPs, district nurses, paramedics, and healthcare professionals from other clinical disciplines or palliative care services.

Remote consultations involve direct contact between healthcare professionals and patients / their significant others via telephone or video; they have become increasingly common since the COVID-19 pandemic.

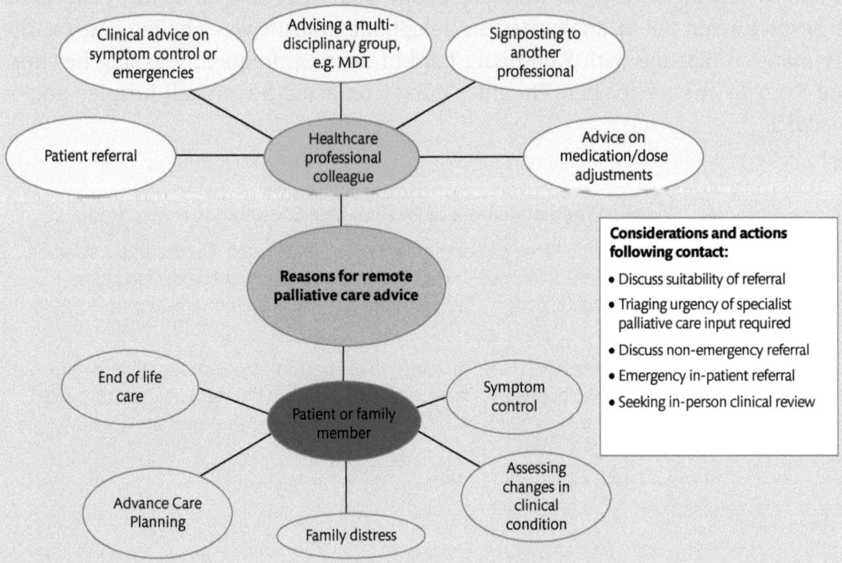

Figure 19.1 Examples for reasons for remote palliative care advice.

Expert Comment

The COVID-19 pandemic caused all healthcare professionals to re-evaluate how we approach patient interactions. Remote consultations evolved to protect patients and staff from viral transmission[1] and are now an accepted part of clinical practice in mainstream medical care.[2] Feedback suggests that patients have welcomed this modality.[3] It is therefore vital for all palliative care healthcare professionals to be competent in providing remote consultations and emerging variations of telemedicine.

Clinical Tips Giving Remote Advice to Healthcare Professionals

Palliative care healthcare professionals may be consulted for remote advice for various reasons. The following are key in guiding the advice given:

- Role of the person seeking advice
- Purpose of the desired consultation
- Urgency of situation

Clinical Tips Utilizing Different Sources to Support Your Assessment

Several information sources can be utilized to gain a greater understanding of a patient's case including:

- Patient
- Significant others (including relatives, carers, residential or nursing home staff)
- Healthcare professionals who have reviewed the patient–verbal handover or written documentation
- Electronic patient records including primary and secondary care
  - Clinic letters
  - Discharge summaries
  - Blood results and imaging
- Electronic palliative care coordination systems (EPaCCS)
  - Advance care plans
  - Resuscitation status and Treatment Escalation Plans (TEP)

Information gathered from these sources can support decision-making and the advice given.

Expert Comment Managing Risk When Giving Remote Advice to Healthcare Professionals

One must consider the quality of information being relayed by the healthcare professional, especially if the patient is unknown to the palliative care team. The palliative care healthcare professional should focus their questions, ensuring they have the breadth of clinical information they need to support the caller with decision-making. If the caller is unable to provide salient information, a specific decision may not be possible. In this instance one could advise the caller to seek out the additional information or provide generic advice with caveats. Keeping contemporaneous notes is advised either via a shared electronic record or by emailing a locally agreed proforma via an encrypted email platform.

The GP submitted a non-urgent referral to the hospice's community care team on a Friday afternoon and the patient was subsequently allocated for Monday morning triage by a community palliative care nurse.

Over the weekend, Pam's breast pain worsened, and she became distressed that 'nothing was being done' and 'worrying about what this could all mean'. Pam called the hospice team about analgesia; the telephone consult was challenging for the duty nurse to manage with Pam being hard-of-hearing, frequently asking her husband Peter to answer for her. The duty nurse contacted the on-call hospice doctor for advice.

Learning Point Triaging Whether Remote or Face-to-Face Consultation is Required

Patients have diverse clinical needs. Many clinical problems can be managed via remote consultation, whereas others will need an in-person consult; the consultation format should be decided on a case-by-case basis, incorporating the patient's needs, nature and context of presenting problem, and clinical judgement.

Professional medical organizations have issued guidance to aid decision-making regarding remote versus face-to-face consultation, though this is not exhaustive, and does not replace applying clinical reasoning to determine the assessment needs of individual patients; there is no 'one size fits all' approach (Tables 19.1 and 19.2).[1,4,5]

Table 19.1 Adapted General Medical Council Guidance for determining whether remote consultations are appropriate[1,4,5]

Remote consultations may be appropriate when:	Remote consultations may be inappropriate when:
• The patient's clinical need is straightforward	• The patient has complex needs
• You have access to the patient's medical records	• There is no access to medical records
• Patient examination is not required	• You need to examine the patient
• You can give the patient all required information	• There are doubts about patient capacity
• A safe system exists to prescribe remotely	• There are safe-guarding concerns
• The patient has the capacity to decide about treatment	• High risk treatment is being discussed or potentially needed
• You can provide a robust management plan remotely	• The patient cannot use technology or does not have access to technology

Source: data from NHS England (2020). *Clinical guide for the management of remote consultations and remote working in secondary care during the coronavirus pandemic.* https://www.rcslt.org/wp-content/uploads/2021/10/NHS-England-clinical-guide-for-the-management-of-remote-consultations-and-remote-working-in-secondary-care-during-the-coronavirus-pandemic.pdf; Royal College of General Practitioners (2020). *Remote versus face-to-face: which to use and when?.* https://elearning.rcgp.org.uk/pluginfile.php/154305/mod_page/content/13/Remote%20versus%20face-to-face_Nov%202020.pdf; and General Medical Council (2020). *Remote consultations flowchart.* https://www.gmc-uk.org/ethical-guidance/learning-materials/remote-consultations-flowchart.

Table 19.2 Emerging indications for remote consultations in palliative care

Remote consultations may be appropriate to:	Remote consultations may be inappropriate to:
• Triage urgency of clinical issue	• Conduct routine first assessment
• Review stable patients	• Discuss advance care planning
• Review non-urgent issues	• Review complex symptoms
• Review non-complex symptoms	• Review of acute symptoms that necessitate examination and investigation
• Review medication changes	
• Form part of virtual ward service	
• Multidisciplinary/family meetings	

Often a remote consultation will be held first to identify the issue and establish whether this can be addressed entirely remotely or if it requires a face-to-face consultation, and if so, who is the most appropriate healthcare professional to conduct this.

The hospice doctor sought further information about Pam before returning the call. She did not have access to the local hospital records but reviewed the referral including medication history and clinical letters. The doctor called Pam to see if a video consultation was possible; she confirmed she had a portable computer device and was able to navigate it sufficiently.

Learning Point Advantages and Disadvantages of Remote Consultations

Advantages	Disadvantages
• Convenience for patients who can avoid travel costs and time.	• Digital inequity—relies on patients access to technology and their ability and competency in using it.
• Ease of access for patients with comorbidities, limited mobility, and or lack of carer.	• Challenges for patients with visual, hearing, and cognitive impairments.
• More inclusive for family members (including those who are not close geographically) to join consultations.	• Limited physical assessment.
• Potential for more frequent and regular contact.	• Lack of visual cues—it is more difficult to assess non-verbal cues and emotion remotely.
• Increased service responsiveness	• Challenges in addressing sensitive issues including breaking bad news and complex advance care planning discussions.
• More inclusive for healthcare professionals to join consultation with patient	

Clinical Tips Technical Aspects of Remote Consultations

Conducting remote consultations requires access to technology, both for the palliative care professional and the patient. As a minimum, this requires telephone access, but video consultations may be preferable given the added benefit of additional visual cues and therapeutic presence (particularly helpful for sicker patients or those with complex communication needs).

Technical preparation*

- Environment
  - *Try to re-produce an environment that replicates a real clinical setting*
  - Ensure privacy and quiet as much as possible
  - Prearrange the consultation time with the patient where possible (provides reassurance)
- Technology and software available
  - *Use a desktop or laptop computer with high quality audio-visual capabilities*
  - *Consider a trial run of technology with a 'buddy'—video settings, volume, microphone and camera, internet coverage, power.*
  - *Ensure internet access is secure; use strong passwords and encryption technology*
  - Use NHS-approved tools and avoid using personal devices
- Ensure you have remote access to the relevant IT systems
  - Remote access to NHS IT systems and clinical records
  - Remote access to palliative care/hospice IT systems and clinical records

Initiating the consultation

- Establish who the patient is, identifying name, and date of birth
- Help the patient with the technical set-up, check 'can you hear me?' or 'can you see me?' and guide them if required
- Be mindful of the patient's environment; the same privacy/confidentiality is required as a face-to-face consult: Check where the patient is and if anyone else is present e.g. "Who else can hear our conversation?", "Are we able to speak openly?"
- Gain consent for the consultation
- Agree a contingency plan in the event of technology failure: check patient phone number in case connection fails
- Formal introduction including, name, role, and the reason for the consultation
- Provide context to help build rapport e.g. 'we met/spoke last week'

Closing the consultation

- Summarize key points; be aware of the possibility that something could have been missed due to technical interference
- Be clear on anything that has not been followed up on and plan for when these will be addressed.
- Advise the patient you are going to end the call and say goodbye before doing so. Invite the patient to disconnect first, removing concern the consult was interrupted by a technical issue.
- Ensure accurate, contemporaneous documentation

* Text in *italics* refers to video consultations only.

Adapted with permission from Burke K. et al. (2021) Advanced Telecommunications Course Mastering sensitive conversations via remote consultations v.1. [unpublished]. Clinical Education, University College London Hospitals NHS Foundation Trust, UK.

Expert Comment How to Build Rapport During Remote Consultations

Remote consultations present challenges for healthcare professionals in establishing a rapport, addressing sensitive issues, and conveying empathy with patients and significant others. Many principles of good verbal and non-verbal communication skills are transferrable from face-to-face settings, but some require careful consideration to ensure effective remote consultations.

- Use simple, unambiguous language.
- Consider your tone of voice, particularly when unable to use non-verbal communication.
- Demonstrate engagement and active listening with brief verbal affirmations.

- During video consultations, keep your attention on the screen and look directly at the patient.
- Inform the patient when you are otherwise occupied e.g. writing notes.
- In the absence of being able to gauge someone's understanding by observing their non-verbal cues, pauses hold greater significance, allowing the opportunity for patients to ask questions.
- Recognition of emotions in virtual environments often requires verbal acknowledgement, compared with non-verbal reassurance which is often used in face-to-face settings.
- When discussing sensitive issues, silence can be used in place of offering a tissue or an understanding touch.

During the video consultation, Pam was fully conversant and able to engage more in a conversation than via phone. Her pain was intermittent, located in the right breast, fluctuating in severity, with a 'gnawing' character. Pam was not distressed, acutely unwell, nor showing obvious signs of opioid toxicity. The doctor was also able to observe her home environment to a limited extent. Pam confirmed that the PRN morphine 'helped a little bit for an hour or so'; it was clear that she was uncertain about medication doses and was not taking her long-acting morphine consistently. The doctor rediscussed how to take immediate-release PRN morphine and long-acting regular morphine, checking her understanding. She ensured Pam that had the 24-hour advice line should her symptoms worsen and arranged for a telephone follow-up after the weekend.

Clinical Tip Clinical Assessment in Remote Consultations

Limited physical examination of patients using video consultation is possible, adding value to your overall assessment in informing your management plan.[7]

- General appearance
- Conscious level
- Skin colour changes, including pallor, cyanosis, and jaundice
- Facial expressions, including grimaces which may indicate pain severity
- Breathlessness, including respiratory rate, and ability to complete sentences
- Tremor or jerking movements

Discussion

Consulting remotely can create an environment where discussion with colleagues is less opportune. Be mindful of still needing to gain opinions of the wider multidisciplinary team (MDT) where necessary. Occasionally patient cues and concerns may be more difficult to pick up on, therefore consider a lower threshold in escalating to face-to-face. It is also important to consider the patient pathway in its entirety, noting the last time a face-to-face visit was conducted. This is to ensure patients are not 'missed' by consecutive remote contacts by all involved in their care. It is advisable for units to set up processes to avoid this.

Expert Comment Managing Risk When Undertaking Remote Consultations

Consideration must be given to the unique challenges provided by remote consultations, ensuring that medico-legal standards are met and minimizing the risks to patient safety. The principles of the UK General Medical Council's 'Good Medical Practice' must continue to be applied, i.e. it is necessary to obtain adequate patient consent, ensure confidentiality, keep contemporaneous notes, perform an appropriate assessment of the patient's symptoms, communicate with other doctors to ensure continuity of care, and have appropriate indemnity in place.[8]

Learning Point Education and Support

As remote consultations become increasingly common, it is important to consider training for healthcare professionals on how to conduct them and the key considerations. Specific tips include:

- Remote consulting can feel isolating. Take opportunities to share cases alongside participation in regular team catch-ups.
- Appraisal: Consider double headset mode with your supervisors for workplace-based assessments/ other learning opportunities, with patient consent.
- Clinicians adapt to new systems at varying rates, with some requiring longer periods of support.
- The Royal College of General Practitioners provides useful guidance, e-learning modules, and resources.[9]

Future Advances

The need for palliative care is projected to increase, as populations age.[10] Despite this, there is a shortage of palliative care consultants and nursing staff.[11] To meet this increasing need, creative ways of working will be necessary to ensure services can be delivered. Technology can widen access for community-based care, improving responsiveness whilst decreasing travel times for patients (with potential quality-of-life benefits) and healthcare professionals (aiding service efficiency).[12] Beyond remote consultations, virtual ward models are evolving allowing step down from hospital care and complementing the existing suite of hospice and community services.

Virtual MDMs (multidisciplinary meetings) are fast emerging to combat the staffing challenges and can enable palliative care teams to manage patients with complex needs more flexibly and in areas where specialist input has traditionally been less available. NHS and third sector partnership working with companies such as Supportive Care UK are demonstrating the value of remote consultant input.[13]

Evidence Base

Remote consultations and telemedicine are rapidly evolving fields in healthcare, prompted by the COVID-19 pandemic.[14] They are now an accepted part of clinical practice,[2] with increasing evidence of its benefits and use in wider healthcare delivery. Feedback suggests patients have welcomed this modality,[15, 16] with over 90% experiencing a positive interaction and 80% stating they would use it again.[3] Patients prefer video consultations to those without, if available to them.[16] Research initially focused on primary care settings but increasingly is addressing telemedicine's role in palliative care services,[12, 17] with case reports supporting its use in hospice services through the implementation of remote visits, virtual ward rounds, and MDTs.[13, 14]

A Final Word from the Expert

As remote consultations become increasingly embedded in clinical practice, it is important for healthcare providers to consider how they utilize them to best support their services, patients, and other healthcare professionals. When used appropriately, remote consultations provide many advantages enabling timely assessment and/or implementation of management plans to improve care. There are also complexities and challenges in conducting remote consultations, particularly in being able to develop a rapport with patients which is key in palliative care, though simple strategies can be used to mitigate these. As healthcare providers and professionals become more confident with remote consultations, we are likely to further develop what can be offered remotely which will be beneficial in enabling palliative care specialists to share their expertise across numerous sites and a wider geographical area. Building on the strong reputation of palliative care for personalized care, remote input should form part of a blended offer for patients and the wider healthcare family.

References

1. NHS England, NHS Improvement. Clinical guide for the management of remote consultations and remote working in secondary care during the coronavirus pandemic. 2020. Available at: https://www.rcslt.org/wp-content/uploads/2021/10/NHS-England-clinical-guide-for-the-management-of-remote-consultations-and-remote-working-in-secondary-care-during-the-coronavirus-pandemic.pdf
2. Horton T, Jones B. Three key quality considerations for remote consultations. The Health Foundation. 2020. Available at: https://www.health.org.uk/news-and-comment/blogs/three-key-quality-considerations-for-remote-consultations
3. Nash A, Gadd B. What patients and staff really think about remote consultations. 2021. NHS Providers. Available at: https://nhsproviders.org/news-blogs/blogs/what-patients-and-staff-really-think-about-remote-consultations

4. Royal College of General Practitioners. Remote versus face-to-face: which to use and when?. 2020. Available at: https://elearning.rcgp.org.uk/pluginfile.php/154305/mod_page/content/13/Remote%20versus%20face-to-face_Nov%202020.pdf
5. General Medical Council. Remote consultations flowchart. 2020. Available at: https://www.gmc-uk.org/ethical-guidance/learning-materials/remote-consultations-flowchart
6. Burke K, Chitale A, Delgado S, et al. Advanced Telecommunications Course Mastering sensitive conversations via remote consultations v.1. [unpublished]. Clinical Education, University College London Hospitals NHS Foundation Trust. June 2021. [available by email: uclh.clinicaleducation@nhs.net]
7. British Medical Journal. Covid-19 remote consultations. 2020. Available at: https://www.bmj.com/sites/default/files/attachments/resources/2020/04/cv19-remote-web-v1.3_1.pdf
8. General Medical Council. Good medical practice. 2019. Available at: https://www.gmc-uk.org/ethical-guidance/ethical-guidance-for-doctors/good-medical-practice
9. Royal College of General Practitioners. Remote consultations and triaging. Available at: https://elearning.rcgp.org.uk/mod/page/view.php?id = 10551#RCGP
10. Bone AE, Gomes B, Etkind SN, et al. What is the impact of population ageing on the future provision of end-of-life care? Population-based projections of place of death. *Palliat Med* 2018; 32(2): 329–336.
11. Kamal AH, Bull JH, Swetz KM, et al. Future of the palliative care workforce: preview to an impending crisis. *Am J Med* 2017; 130(2): 113–114.
12. Keenan J, Rahman R, Hudson J. Exploring the acceptance of telehealth within palliative care: a self-determination theory perspective. *Health Technol* 2021; 11: 575–584.
13. Supportive Care UK. *Case Studies: Ellenor Hospice, Gravesend*. Available at: https://www.supportive.care/case-studies/ellenor-hospice
14. eHospice. *Hospice Care Goes Virtual in Response to Covid-19*. 2020. Accessed at: https://ehospice.com/uk_posts/hospice-care-goes-virtual-in-response-to-covid-19/
15. Healthwatch, National Voices, Traverse. The doctor will zoom you now: getting the most out of the virtual health and care experience. 2020. Available at: https://www.nationalvoices.org.uk/sites/default/files/public/publications/the_dr_will_zoom_you_now_-_insights_report-min.pdf
16. NHS Providers. What patients and staff really think about remote consultations. 2021. Available at: https://nhsproviders.org/news-blogs/blogs/what-patients-and-staff-really-think-about-remote-consultations
17. Hawkins JP, Gannon C, Palfrey J. Virtual visits in palliative care: about time or against the grain? 2020. Accessed at: https://spcare.bmj.com/content/10/3/331.citation-tools

CASE

20 What to Expect with a Death at Home

Tammy Oxley

Expert: Catherine Malia

Case history

Sophie, a 63-year-old female with metastatic pancreatic cancer, was treated with six cycles of palliative chemotherapy. Repeat scans showed disease progression despite chemotherapy, therefore a decision was made for best supportive care.

A few weeks later Sophie's husband David rang their general practitioner (GP) as he was concerned she had further deteriorated.

On review, the GP found Sophie was now bedbound, eating and drinking very little, and spending most of the day sleeping. The GP identified no reversible factors and explained they felt Sophie was approaching the end of her life. Sophie had no uncontrolled symptoms, but her husband was struggling to manage her reduced mobility and incontinence.

The GP sensitively initiated advance care planning discussions. A Recommended Summary Plan for Emergency Care and Treatment (ReSPECT) form was completed, recording Sophie's wishes: she did not want any further investigation or escalation to hospital, and her preferred place of death was home. The ReSPECT form documents personalized recommendations for a person's care in the event that they become unable to make or express choices (see Case 18, 'Coordination and Transfer of Care', for further detail).

Expert Commentary Communication

Where it is recognized that a person is entering the last days of life, health professionals should provide:

- Clear communication, establishing the extent to which the patient wishes to be involved in discussion and decision-making
- Clear information about prognosis and what is likely to happen as death approaches
- Opportunities for the patient and relatives to express any goals, wishes, fears, or worries
- Information about who to contact for help in and out-of-hours

Decisions and discussions should be recorded in the patient's record and, with consent, shared with relevant health professionals.[1, 2]

Evidence Base Trends in Patients Dying at Home

The number of patients dying at home is rising; data from England and Wales demonstrate an annual increase from 2005 (*n*=94 245) to 2020 (*n*=166 576), with the exception of 2009.[3] There has been a significantly larger increase in 2020 and early 2021, thought to be an indirect consequence of COVID-19.[3] Whilst it is unknown whether this steep increase will continue, research pre-pandemic projected that the number of patients dying at home will continue to rise.[4] One projection suggested, that if overall deaths increase by 27% from 2014 to 2040, the number of home deaths will increase by 88.6%.[4]

Learning Points Home as Preferred Place of Death

Place of death is often used as a proxy measure for the quality of death and effectiveness of services.[5] Dying at home has previously been used as a marker of a 'good death', based on the assumption that this would be a patient's preference. It is therefore essential to clarify patients' preferences regarding place of death; achieving this preference is what matters. Research is ambiguous. A recent systematic review found, when missing data was excluded, home was the preferred place of death for the majority of respondents in 53/65 reports.[6] However, when missing data was included the results were less clear and preferred place of death was home for the majority of respondents in only 36/65 reports.[6] Decisions around preferred place of death are complex and patients may seek advice from those important to them and from health professionals. Preferences may change over time, and it is imperative than an up-to-date preferred place of death is clearly documented.[4] Lack of timely or accurate communication of advance care planning decisions was the most commonly reported incident in an analysis of advance care planning episodes resulting in patient safety incidents.[7]

Expert Comment What is Home?

It is recognized that home assumes increased significance as people near death. Research exploring the meaning of 'home' to dying patients highlights that it is more than a physical address. Instead, home is somewhere safe, a place of refuge and freedom. At home, people can focus on living as well as dying, be in control, and attend to their own affairs. Having 'the right people around you' enables people to feel connected to those they love. For some, returning home at end of life is not about a building but a spiritual reconnection to the place they come from.[5, 8]

It is argued that death is seen as a discrete event happening at one point in time, however dying is a dynamic process. The concept of 'placing work' describes the ongoing efforts of staff to ensure a dying person's environment feels as safe and meaningful to them as possible, highlighting that in order to make a place suitable for dying, spaces often have to be altered both physically and symbolically due to the changing relationship between a person and their environment as death approaches.[9]

Learning Points Barriers and Facilitators to Dying at Home

National Institute for Clinical Excellence (NICE) guidance in the UK states, where possible, that patients' preferences for place of death should be supported.[1] Achieving this preference is not always feasible. One study found only 23% of patients known to palliative care services, whose preference was home, died in this setting.[10] Factors that increase a person's likelihood of dying at home include: living with others, receiving home care and support from extended family.[8, 10] There is conflicting evidence about the effect of functional status on dying at home; one study suggests a high functional status is a facilitator, whilst another suggests the converse.[8, 10] Three key factors considered by professionals when assessing feasibility of dying at home are; disease-specific factors (such as risk of bleeding), carer participation/availability and relationships/priorities of both the patient and their family.[11]

Learning Points Support for Patients Dying at Home

Dying patients may require generalist palliative care (in the UK this is usually provided by GPs and community district nursing teams), specialist palliative care (provided by community palliative care teams generally consisting of clinical nurse specialists, doctors, and other members of the multidisciplinary team) or a combination of the two. NICE guidance stipulates that adults approaching the end of life should be provided with access to a health professional or advice line, available at all times.[1] However, geographical variation exists in support available to patients dying at home in the UK, both in-hours and out-of-hours.

Within the UK, individuals approaching the end of life may be eligible for funding which enables swift access to necessary care or equipment for individuals with a rapidly deteriorating condition that may be entering a terminal phase.

Expert Comment Informal Support for Patients Dying at Home

Death and dying have become increasingly medicalized in western society resulting in a loss of societal knowledge, skills, and confidence to support people dying at home. Whilst largely managed by healthcare systems, the bulk of caring falls to the dying themselves, family, and friends.[2] In response, a growing global compassionate communities movement is bringing together local networks that build capacity to identify and support those who are dying, caring or grieving in local communities.[2] The role of a 'death doula' is gaining popularity. Duties vary according to the needs of the patient but typically involve advocacy, provision of emotional and spiritual support, as well as help with practical tasks.

Learning Point Medications for Patients Dying at Home

Access to anticipatory medication is key for effective symptom management in the dying phase. An individualized approach to prescribing is recommended.[12, 13] Availability of medication may reduce avoidable and unwanted hospital admissions in crisis situations.[13] Specific medications may be necessary for patients at risk of particular emergencies, such as bleeding or seizures. NICE advises patients approaching the last days of life should have access to pharmacy services with a supply of necessary medications.[1] However, research has identified frequent problems with access in the community.[13] Difficulties can occur at any point in the process: including getting a prescription written, lack of community stock of medications and patients or relatives struggling to access/collect medication out-of-hours.[13] Many different services are involved and communication between these can be problematic.[13] These issues may be complicated by medications required frequently being controlled drugs, such as opioids and benzodiazepines. Health professionals should be aware of these potential issues and attempt to mitigate by planning ahead.

Future Advances Carer Administration of Subcutaneous Anticipatory Medications

Traditionally, subcutaneous anticipatory medications have been administered by health professionals. In some areas, carers are being trained to administer these medications. One randomized control trial assigned patients at home, in the last weeks of life, to an intervention group (where their carers were trained to administer injections) or control group (usual care).[14] Benefits included: a reduction in time to symptom relief; symptoms improved to an acceptable level within 30 minutes in 88.8% of patients in the intervention group compared with 26.7% in the control group. Time to medication administration was lower in the intervention compared with control group: a median of 5 and 105 minutes respectively. By study completion, carers' self-reported confidence level for administering medications was high. However, there were some concerns from health professionals regarding screening and selection of suitable participants.[14] This exciting advance may help improve symptom management for patients who die at home.

Expert Comment Supporting Caregivers

Supporting a loved one to die at home can be a source of comfort and satisfaction, but can also be a stressful experience fraught with uncertainty, isolation, exhaustion, and financial strain. The impending loss of a loved one is combined with taking on a role for which carers feel underprepared. Carer support has been linked with better bereavement outcomes, improved quality of care, and increased likelihood of achieving home death.[15]

Assessing carers' needs is important, consider:

- Practical training including how to safely move a loved one, provide skin or mouth care
- Equipment to help at home
- Financial support
- Emotional support

In the UK, carers are entitled to a free carer's needs assessment which is accessed via the local council. A number of third sector organizations offer advice, information, and support.

A care package was instigated and a hospital bed and commode delivered, enabling Sophie to live downstairs.

Unfortunately, Sophie began hallucinating and became agitated. David called the district nurse (DN), who administered a haloperidol injection which reduced her distress. They referred to the community palliative care team.

On review, the palliative care clinical nurse specialist (CNS) recognized that Sophie was terminally agitated and dying. This was sensitively explained to David. She had been given multiple doses of haloperidol with benefit; therefore, a continuous subcutaneous infusion was started. The CNS arranged for night sitters and provided contact details for specialist palliative care advice out-of-hours.

Sophie's agitation settled. She continued to deteriorate and died at home two days later with her husband present. The DN attended to verify Sophie's death and the GP completed the Medical Certificate of Cause of Death. Her CNS arranged for bereavement support for David.

Clinical Tip Management of Terminal Agitation

Terminal restlessness, also referred to as terminal agitation, is delirium with features of agitation, which develops in the last days of life.[16] It is common; features of delirium are seen in 88% of dying patients.[16] Management generally adopts a step-wise approach, starting with recognition. Patients should be reviewed to ensure there is no reversible cause which may benefit from specific intervention, for example urinary retention, which may require a catheter. Sensitive explanation to the family, including a recognition that the patient is dying, is key. Non-pharmacological management includes orientation of the patient and reassurance. Pharmacological management may be considered if the patient continues to be distressed. Options include antipsychotics (such as haloperidol) and benzodiazepines (such as midazolam). These may need to be administered subcutaneously if the patient is unable to take oral medications. Unfortunately, symptoms may be refractory to this initial management and require further intervention.[16]

Expert Comment Process After Death at Home

The need for individualized, compassionate care that respects a person's expressed wishes continues after death. Where a patient's next of kin was absent, they should be informed. Support should be provided to those close to the deceased, as well as the opportunity to undertake any rituals or preparation of the body. Religious and cultural wishes should be considered. Members of local faith communities may attend to the deceased and support those bereaved.[17] Verification of death, the formal process in which death is confirmed, is recommended within four hours following death at home. Relatives should be advised that the official time of death may differ from when the person stopped breathing.[18] Relatives should be directed to contact the GP to issue the required death certificate. The doctor must have seen the deceased in the 28 days prior to death.[19] Clinicians should be aware of circumstances that require referral to a coroner, and relatives should be informed where this is necessary.

It is important to provide relatives with information about next steps, including contacting a funeral director and registering the death.

Evidence Base Quality of Death at Home

The National Survey of Bereaved People (VOICES) provides evidence of bereaved relatives' views of their lived experience of end of life care provided for adults in England.[20] The most recent available data from 2015 included experiences by place of death, as detailed in Tables 20.1 and 20.2.[20]

Table 20.1 Responses to questions about experience in the last two days of life categorized by place of death

	Strongly agree/agree		Neither agree/disagree		Disagree/strongly disagree	
	Any setting	Home	Any setting	Home	Any setting	Home
Had sufficient pain relief	80.9%	80.2%	8.9%	8.0%	10.3%	11.7%
Had enough help to meet personal care needs	79.5%	78.7%	8.1%	7.8%	12.4%	13.5%
Had enough help with nursing care	79.3%	77.8%	8.3%	8.5%	12.5%	13.8%

Relatives were questioned about the support received at the time of death, as detailed in Table 20.2.

Table 20.2 Responses to the question, 'Were you or his/her family given enough help and support by the healthcare team at the actual time of his/her death?' categorized by place of death[20]

Yes definitely		Yes to some extent		No not at all	
Any setting	Home	Any setting	Home	Any setting	Home
58.7%	55.4%	27.1%	24.0%	14.2%	20.6 %

These results suggest that, generally sufficient analgesia and care is provided for patients dying at home; and is comparable with other settings. However, support from health professionals specifically at the time of death was less available for those dying at home.

It should be noted that data was collected from relatives, therefore is a proxy measure of patients' experiences. Secondly, it is collected four to eleven months after bereavement, so recollections of events may have changed.

Discussion

In summary, this case considers a patient approaching the end of her life, whose wish was to die at home. Input from a wide variety of health professionals was required to facilitate this. Key actions included recognition of dying, good communication with both the patient and relative, clear documentation of expressed wishes, provision of anticipatory medication, funding for care and equipment, and contact details for support and information. Support after death was also provided: both logistical (verification of death) and supportive (bereavement care for family).

A Final Word from the Expert

The number of people dying at home is rising and likely to rise further. In order to facilitate patients' preferences to die at home, it is vital to consider facilitators and address a number of identified barriers. The growth of innovative approaches such as compassionate communities may help to rebalance death and dying as a normal part of life occurring in and supported by local neighbourhoods who are trained and experienced in end of life care, leading to better outcomes for patients and relatives.

References

1. National Institute for Health and Care Excellence (NICE). NICE Guideline: End of life care for adults: service delivery. 2019. Available at: https://www.nice.org.uk/guidance/ng142
2. Sallnow L, Smith R, Ahmedzai S, et al. Report of the Lancet Commission on the value of death: bringing death back into life. *Lancet* 2022; 10327(399): 837–884.
3. Office for National Statistics, Deaths registered in private homes, England and Wales: 2020 final and January to June 2021, provisional, 2021. Available at: https://www.ons.gov.uk/peoplepopulationandcommunity/birthsdeathsandmarriages/deaths/articles/deathsinprivatehomesenglandandwales/2020finalandjanuarytojune2021provisional#deaths-in-private-homes-2001-to-2021
4. Bone A, Gomes B, Etkind S, et al. What is the impact of population ageing on the future provision of end-of-life care? Population-based projections of place of death. *Palliat Med* 2018; 32(2): 329–336.
5. Collier A, Phillips J, Iedema R. The meaning of home at the end of life: a video-reflexive ethnography study. *Palliat Med* 2015; 29, (8): 695–670.
6. Hoare S, Morris Z, Kelly M, et al. Do patients want to die at home? A systematic review of the UK literature, focused on missing preferences for place of death. *PLoS One* 2015; 10(11): e0142723.
7. Dinnen T, Williams H, Yardley S, et al. Patient safety incidents in advance care planning for serious illness: a mixed-methods analysis. *BMJ Support Palliat Care* 2019; 12(e3): e403–e410.
8. Gomes B, Higginson I. Factors influencing death at home in terminally ill patients with cancer: systematic review. *BMJ* 2006; 7540 (332): 515–521.
9. Driessen A, Borgstrom E, Cohn S. Placing death and dying: making place at the end of life. *Soc Sci Med* 2021; 291: 113974.
10. Higginson I, Daveson B, Morrison RS, et al. Social and clinical determinants of preferences and their achievement at the end of life: prospective cohort study of older adults receiving palliative care in three countries. *BMC Geriatr* 2017; 17(1): 271–285.
11. Sathiananthan M, Crawford G, Eliott J. Healthcare professionals' perspectives of patient and family preferences of patient place of death: a qualitative study. *BMC Palliat Care* 2021; 20: 147.
12. National Institute for Health and Care Excellence (NICE). NICE Guideline: Care of dying adults in the last days of life, 2015. Available at: https://www.nice.org.uk/guidance/ng31/resources/care-of-dying-adults-in-the-last-days-of-life-pdf-1837387324357
13. Ogi M, Campling NB, Birtwistle J et al. Community access to palliative care medicines—patient and professional experience: systematic review and narrative synthesis. *BMJ Support Palliat Care* 2021, doi:0.1136/bmjspcare-2020-002761.
14. Poolman M, Roberts J, Wright S et al. Carer administration of as-needed subcutaneous medication for breakthrough symptoms in people dying at home: the CARiAD feasibility RCT. *Health Technology Assessment* 2020; 24(25): 1–150.
15. Grande G, Austin L, Ewing G et al. Assessing the impact of a Carer Support Needs Assessment Tool (CSNAT) intervention in palliative home care: a stepped wedge cluster trial. *BMJ Support Palliat Care* 2017; 7(3): 326–334.
16. Lacey J, Cherny N. Management of the actively dying patient. In *Oxford Textbook of Palliative Medicine*, edited by Cherny N, Fallon M, Kaasa S, et al. 6th ed. Oxford: Oxford University Press, 2021, ch. 18.3.
17. Hospice UK. *Care after Death; Guidance for Staff Responsible for Care After Death*, 3rd ed. 2020. Available at: https://professionals.hospiceuk.org/what-we-offer/clinical-and-care-support/clinical-resources
18. Hospice UK and National Nurse Consultant Group (Palliative Care). *Care After Death: Registered Nurse Verification of Expected Adult Death Guidance*, 4th ed. 2021. Available at: https://professionals.hospiceuk.org/docs/default-source/What-We-Offer/Care-Support-Programmes/Care-after-death/rnvoead-special-covid-19-edition-final_2.pdf?sfvrsn = 2

19. NHS England. Coronavirus Act expiry: death certification and registration easements from 25 March 2022. 2022. Available at: https://www.england.nhs.uk/coronavirus/wp-content/uploads/sites/52/2022/03/C1566_-coronavirus-act-expiry-death-certification-and-registration-easements-from-25-march.pdf
20. Office for National Statistics. National Survey of Bereaved People (VOICES) 2015 edition of this dataset. 2016. Available at: https://www.ons.gov.uk/peoplepopulationandcommunity/healthandsocialcare/healthcaresystem/datasets/nationalsurveyofbereavedpeoplevoices

CASE

21 Individualized End of Life Care Plans

Stephanie Hicks

Expert: Ben Bowers

Case history

Patrick, a 54-year-old man with a background of recurrent, metastatic squamous cell carcinoma (SCC) of his left oropharynx, was admitted to hospital following a three-week history of progressive dysphagia and a two-day history of fevers. His oncological background included left neck dissection and subsequent salvage surgery, radiotherapy, and chemotherapy. A recent restaging CT scan showed progressive lung metastases and the head and neck multidisciplinary meeting outcome was that his condition would not improve with further surgery or systemic anticancer therapy. He had been referred to his local CPCT.

Regular medications included fentanyl 50 microgram/hour patch applied 72 hourly and omeprazole 20 mg OD. Patrick lived alone and had no formal care package or equipment at home, although had become increasingly weak in recent weeks and was spending >50% of his day in bed. His next of kin was his brother and he had two nieces, all of whom lived locally.

On examination he had a fever of 38.4°C, an elevated respiratory rate, and tachycardia. He had coarse crackles at his right base. Investigations demonstrated raised inflammatory markers, with white cell count (WCC) 15.6×10^9/L and C-reactive protein (CRP) 182. COVID-19 PCR was negative. His albumin was low at 16 g/L and his estimated glomerular filtration rate (eGFR) was 63. His chest X-ray showed patchy consolidation in the right base. He was commenced on intravenous (IV) antibiotics for aspiration pneumonia and IV fluids. A treatment escalation plan was established by his responsible team, in discussion with Patrick and his brother, to include ward-based treatment of reversibility, but that escalation to intensive care or use of ionotropic support, ventilation, or dialysis would not be appropriate. A Do Not Attempt Cardiopulmonary Resuscitation (DNACPR) form was completed. During admission, he was reviewed by the Speech and Language Therapy team and found to have significant oropharyngeal dysphagia and high risk of aspiration. Patrick declined enteral feeding options and chose to continue sips of thin fluids, accepting the risk of aspiration.

On day 2 of admission, his IV antibiotics were escalated, on the advice of microbiology, due to rising inflammatory markers and ongoing haemodynamic instability. By day 4, there had been further clinical and biochemical deterioration. Patrick was bedbound and drowsy, although able to engage in short conversation. He was breathless, maintaining target saturations on 4 L oxygen and had persistent crackles in his right lower zone. His oral cavity was dry and he had reduced skin turgor, with cool peripheries and reduced capillary refill time. He had no audible respiratory secretions and no peripheral oedema.

Learning Point Diagnosing Dying

It can be difficult to be certain that a person is dying and there is insufficient evidence for any specific prognostic tools to guide this judgement precisely for any given individual person. Recognition that someone may be entering the last days of life is the essential first step to ensuring individualized end-of-life care.[1] National Institute for Health and Care Excellence (NICE) (UK) guidance suggests changes that could occur in a person entering the last days of life include:

- Changes in communication, deteriorating mobility, or performance status, or social withdrawal
- Increased fatigue, progressive weight loss, and reduced appetite
- Reduced consciousness, mottled skin, noisy respiratory secretions, and Cheyne–Stokes breathing[2]

These signs and symptoms are often best taken in context of an assessment of clinical changes over time, as well as consideration of potential for reversibility. They should ideally be made by a senior clinician who knows the patient, with involvement from the multidisciplinary team (MDT). The individual should be regularly reassessed for changes that may suggest improvement.

Patrick's responsible consultant, with input from the MDT, identified he was likely entering the last hours to days of life. His understanding of recent events was explored and he wanted to know information about his prognosis, in the presence of his brother. His brother urgently visited to discuss plans for care, and they agreed to a referral to the HPCT. A discussion was facilitated to explore what Patrick's priorities would be at the end of life, with his brother's input, with a view to formulating an individualized end of life care plan.

Evidence Base One Chance to Get It Right

In July 2013, an independent review of use of the Liverpool Care Pathway for the Dying Patient (LCP) in the UK was published.[3] The LCP, developed during the 1990s, was a widely implemented clinical tool to facilitate caring for dying patients and aimed to emulate hospice care within all care settings. However, the review found evidence of both good and poor practice in end of life care being delivered through its application and its use was discontinued across the UK. A subsequent multicentre cluster randomized trial in Italy found no significant difference in overall quality of care between wards which implemented the LCP and those that did not.[4]

The Leadership Alliance for the Care of Dying People was established to set out the future approach to end of life care and published One Chance to Get It Right in 2014.[1] This document proposed **five priorities of care for the dying person**, based on expert consensus:

'1. This possibility is recognized and communicated clearly, decisions made and actions taken in accordance with the person's needs and wishes, and these are regularly reviewed and decisions revised accordingly.
2. Sensitive communication takes place between staff and the dying person, and those identified as important to them.
3. The dying person, and those identified as important to them, are involved in decisions about treatment and care to the extent that the dying person wants.
4. The needs of families and others identified as important to the dying person are actively explored, respected, and met as far as possible.
5. An individual plan of care, which includes food and drink, symptom control, and psychological, social, and spiritual support, is agreed, coordinated, and delivered with compassion'.[1]

Expert Comment

Individualized end of life care plans should meet and reflect the needs and wishes of the patient and those important to them. Care plans should include:

- Ongoing communication and involving patients and families in clinical decision-making
- Personal goals and wishes (e.g. emotional, psychological, social, spiritual, cultural, and religious needs)

- Preferred place of care and death
- Preferences for physical and symptom management, including hydration and nutrition
- Anticipating and meeting likely symptom control needs
- Requirements for care after death
- Resources needed

Care planning conversations should not routinely be a one-off event. Plans need to be kept under regular review and revisited with patients and those important to them as their situations, priorities, and wishes change.[2]

Expert Comment

The withdrawal of the Liverpool Care Pathway (LCP) in the UK had profound repercussions for person-centred end of life care, many of which are still being experienced. The international palliative care community has largely responded to the crisis experienced in the UK by rationalizing that the tool failed only where it was poorly implemented and interpreted. The episode also highlighted the dangers of an application of a standardized pathway that was largely based on palliative care values and aspirations in a cancer population, without a robust evidence base.[1,3,5]

Figure 21.1 demonstrates the key areas identified as being important to Patrick and his family and enabled the team to develop an individualized end of life care plan. Patrick's preference for privacy and ongoing care in hospital, where he was familiar with staff and felt safe, led to him being prioritized for a side room. His family were allowed to visit at any time and a fold-out bed was organized. This enabled his brother to stay with him overnight. Classical music could be played in his room through a portable radio. A referral was made to the hospital chaplaincy team; who visited him on the ward.

Patrick was struggling with oral medications due to dysphagia and drowsiness and these were rationalized. He had been experiencing intermittent pain over his left jaw, which had

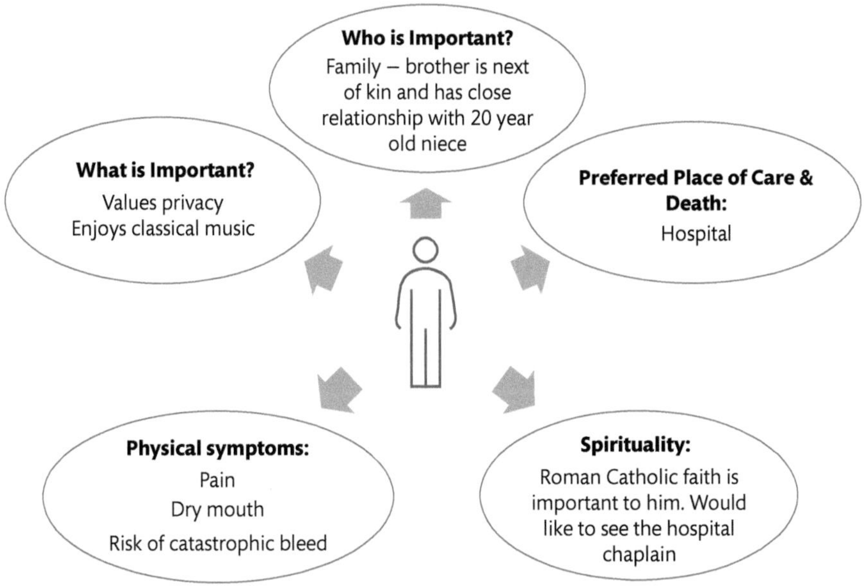

Figure 21.1 A visual representation of Patrick's needs and wishes in the last days of life.

> **Expert Comment**
>
> Anticipatory prescribing started as part of the LCP and remains recommended best practice internationally.[2, 5] Care is based primarily on clinicians' perceptions and experiences that anticipatory medications offer reassurance to all and facilitate effective symptom control.[5] However, anticipatory medications are simultaneously reassuring and a source of unease to patients and families;[6] prescriptions need careful, open discussion and tailoring to their preferences and experience. The clinical effectiveness, cost-effectiveness, and safety of prescribing anticipatory medication have been inadequately investigated.[5]

previously responded well to immediate release oral morphine liquid PRN, in addition to his background Fentanyl patch. The palliative care team recommended continuation of his Fentanyl 50 microgram/hour patch and use of PRN subcutaneous morphine 10 mg (maximum hourly) for breakthrough pain: approximately $1/6^{th}$ of his background total opioid. They recommended prescribing PRN subcutaneous anticipatory medications for symptoms that might occur in the last days of life, including agitation, nausea/vomiting and respiratory secretions as per their local guidelines. The CT scan results indicated that Patrick's cancer was in the proximity of large blood vessels, including the carotid artery. Therefore, he was at risk of a catastrophic haemorrhage. This risk was sensitively explained to Patrick, his family, and ward staff, and an anticipatory, PRN once only dose of intramuscular (IM) Midazolam 10 mg was prescribed should haemorrhage occur.

> **Expert Comment**
>
> Injectable anticipatory medications should be considered for common symptoms at the end of life. Possible symptoms include pain, breathlessness, nausea and vomiting, agitation, and noisy respiratory secretions.[2, 5] It is important to take an individualized approach to anticipatory prescribing and consider patient preferences, the likelihood of specific symptoms occurring, the benefits and harms of prescribing or not prescribing medications, the care setting, and the time it would take to obtain medications.[2] Choice of medications and dosing need to consider local guidelines, opioid naivety, comorbidities, and presence of organ dysfunction (particularly renal and/or liver failure).

> **Clinical Tip Management of Catastrophic Haemorrhage**
>
> Catastrophic haemorrhage is an uncommon emergency, but one which can have a significant impact on patients, families, and healthcare professionals.[7] It is important to identify those at risk, such as those with large head and neck cancers, large centrally located lung cancers, severe thrombocytopenia, haematological malignancies, and those with coagulopathy, in order to appropriately prepare for its occurrence.[8] Management includes supportive measures, such as ensuring someone stays with the patient, call for assistance, apply pressure, place the patient in the lateral position and use dark towels to camouflage blood loss.[7] The use of 'crisis medication' is aimed at reducing awareness/distress of the individual in the context of death being anticipated within minutes. Most commonly, this includes the use of a sedative +/- anxiolytic such as SC/IM/IV/buccal midazolam 10 mg.[9] However, given the speed at which death may occur and the time it takes to prepare and administer injectable medication, crisis medication may be ineffective and should not be prioritized over remaining with the patient.[7]

> **Expert Comment**
>
> For patients at risk of catastrophic haemorrhage whose preference is for end of life care at home, it is important to have sensitive, realistic conversations about managing acute haemorrhage with all involved in care. Preparation should include access to dark towels, crisis medication and advice on who the family should call: a paramedic via 999 may be most appropriate given the requirement for immediate support.[10]
>
> Psychological support for family and professional caregivers, including bereavement counselling and the opportunity to debrief, should be offered following a catastrophic haemorrhage.

> **Evidence Base Clinically Assisted Hydration at the End of Life**
>
> CAH at the end of life, involving the administration of intravenous or subcutaneous fluids, is often an emotive subject. An individual's inability to tolerate oral hydration has been shown to be associated with high levels of emotional distress in bereaved relatives.[11, 12] However, a recent systematic review found insufficient evidence regarding the impact of CAH on either symptoms or survival for patients

in the last days of life.[13] Therefore, when CAH is being considered, an individualized approach must be used which considers the dying person's preferences, level of consciousness, thirst, comfort, risk of pulmonary oedema, and potential for temporary recovery.[2] Conversations should be anticipated and pre-emptively conducted, rather than waiting for questions to arise, and should discuss the uncertainty around the benefit of CAH and whether it prolongs life or extends the dying process. It is essential to review the effectiveness of CAH at least every 12 hours and monitor for adverse effects, including increased respiratory secretions and oedema.[2]

On clinical examination, Patrick had dry mucus membranes and reduced skin turgor. Although drowsy, he nodded when asked if he felt thirsty. As part of his individualized end of life care plan, he received regular mouth care. This included supporting him with sips of fluids when awake enough, using a soft toothbrush to gently clean his teeth, gums, tongue, and palate, and applying a water-based lip balm to keep his lips moist.[11] Clinically assisted hydration (CAH) was discussed with Patrick and his family, including potential benefits and risks. Their preference was to trial CAH and it was agreed to be clinically appropriate to start one litre 0.9% sodium chloride subcutaneously over 24 hours. After 24 hours, his hydration status was re-reviewed. Patrick was unconscious and had a moist mouth. He had no peripheral oedema but did have audible respiratory secretions. It was explained to his family that, in view of the new development of respiratory secretions, the risks of continuing CAH now outweighed its potential benefits. The decision was made to stop subcutaneous fluids. Patrick died peacefully 36 hours later with his brother present.

Future Advances Clinically Assisted Hydration at the End of Life

Definitive studies are urgently needed to determine whether CAH has any impact on patients' survival or symptoms in the final days of life.[13] Decisions about CAH may impact on other preferences at the end of life, such as staying in hospital to receive hydration.[13] Whilst some areas have local guidance on the use of SC fluids in the community, trained staff, equipment, and infrastructure may not always be readily available. Future research and guidance on the provision of CAH in community settings would be invaluable.

Discussion

In summary, this is a case of a patient with recurrent, metastatic SCC of his left oropharynx admitted to hospital with aspiration pneumonia. Despite ward-level treatment of reversibility with IV antibiotics and fluids, his condition continued to deteriorate and he was identified as being in the final days of life. This was communicated to him and his family and enabled the cocreation of an individualized end of life care plan.

His preferences included a desire for end of life care in hospital. Arrangements were made to support family visiting and a relaxing, familiar environment. His spiritual care needs were supported with the input of the hospital chaplaincy team. Anticipation of symptoms included a need to consider how to best manage his risk of having a catastrophic haemorrhage. It was also essential that this risk was carefully explained to him, his family and ward staff in order to prepare for what might happen. Given he had symptoms of dehydration and wished to trial CAH, subcutaneous fluids were administered. He subsequently developed respiratory secretions and it was appropriately identified as a potential side effect of the fluids, which were stopped prior to his death. The case highlighted the importance of an individualized, holistic approach to care at the end of life and clear, pre-emptive communication with patients and families.

A Final Word from the Expert

There are numerous uncertainties in planning for and managing dying. Hospital-based cultures and clinicians' priorities for facilitating home deaths and withdrawing active treatments, including CAH, do not always match with patients and families' expectations and wishes. Sometimes hospital can feel the safest place to be at the end of life. This case highlights the importance of actively exploring patients' and families wishes and concerns, then cocreating individualized care plans and regularly revisiting these as situations and needs change.

References

1. Leadership Alliance for the Care of Dying People. *One Chance To Get It Right*. London: UK Government, 2014. Available at: https://assets.publishing.service.gov.uk/government/uploads/system/uploads/attachment_data/file/323188/One_chance_to_get_it_right.pdf
2. National Institute for Health and Care Excellence (NICE). Care of dying adults in the last days of life: NICE guideline [NG31]. 2015. Available at: https://www.nice.org.uk/guidance/ng31/resources/care-of-dying-adults-in-the-last-days-of-life-pdf-1837387324357
3. Neuberger J. More care, less pathway: a review of the Liverpool Care Pathway. 2013. Available at: https://assets.publishing.service.gov.uk/government/uploads/system/uploads/attachment_data/file/212450/Liverpool_Care_Pathway.pdf
4. Costantini M, Romoli V, Di Leo S, et al. Liverpool Care Pathway for patients with cancer in hospital: a cluster randomised trial. *Lancet* 2014; 383: 226–237.
5. Bowers B, Ryan R, Kuhn I, Barclay S. Anticipatory prescribing of injectable medications for adults at the end of life in the community: a systematic literature review and narrative synthesis. *Palliat Med* 2018; 33(2): 160–177.
6. Bowers B, Pollock K, Barclay S. Simultaneously reassuring and unsettling. Patient, informal caregiver and clinician perspectives of community anticipatory medication prescriptions: a longitudinal qualitative study. *Age Ageing* 2022; 51(12): 1–11.
7. Harris DG, Noble SIR. Management of terminal hemorrhage in patients with advanced cancer: a systematic literature review. *J Pain Sympt Manage* 2009; 38: 913–927.
8. Prommer E. Management of bleeding in the terminally ill patient. *Haematology* 2005; 10(3): 167–175.
9. Watson M, Armstrong P, Back I, Gannon C, Sykes N. *Palliative Adult Network Guidelines*, 4th ed. Lisburn, NI: Tricord, 2016, p. 199.
10. Ubogagu E, Harris DG. Guideline for the management of terminal haemorrhage in palliative care patients with advanced cancer discharged home for end-of-life care. *BMJ Support Palliat Care* 2012; 2: 294–300.
11. Royal College of Nursing. *Mouth Care Matters in End-of-Life-Care*. 2021. Available at: https://www.rcn.org.uk/professional-development/publications/mouth-care-matters-in-end-of-life-care-uk-pub-009-921
12. Yamagishi A, Morita T, Miyashita M, et al. The care strategy for families of terminally ill cancer patients who become unable to take nourishment orally: recommendations from a nationwide survey of bereaved family members' experiences. *J Pain Symp Manage* 2010; 40: 671–683.
13. Kingdon A, Spathis A, Brodrick R, et al. What is the impact of clinically assisted hydration in the last days of life? A systematic literature review and narrative synthesis. *BMJ Support Palliat Care* 2021; 11: 68–74.

CASE

22 Depression in Life-limiting Illness

Felicity Wood

Expert: Annabel Price

Case history

Angela was a 58-year-old lady of Black African origin with ovarian cancer and metastatic peritoneal disease. She had increasingly been struggling with low mood over the last few months. This was picked up during a clinical interview by a clinical nurse specialist working with community palliative care services who were trying to manage her pain.

At the time of diagnosis, she already had metastatic disease which was not amenable to treatment with curative intent. Prior to diagnosis she had been experiencing abdominal bloating and reduced appetite for several months but hadn't sought medical advice. She had dismissed her symptoms as insignificant until abdominal pain made it difficult for her to work as a cleaner.

Learning Point

Depression is common at the end of life with prevalence ranging from 24% to 70%.[1] It is frequently underdetected and undertreated.[2]

It is associated with emotional suffering, fatigue, increased pain, decreased treatment adherence, disability, poorer prognosis, and higher mortality.[3]

Learning Point

The patient had been seeing the palliative care team for the management of her pain and had not reported or sought help for her low mood. Patients don't always volunteer their psychiatric symptoms, and we might not always look for them, so it is important to proactively screen for them.

One of the following screening tools may be useful in addition to clinical judgement:

- HADS (Hospital Anxiety and Depression scale)
- BEDS (Brief Edinburgh Depression Scale)
- A generic symptom assessment scale that includes one or more questions about depression, e.g. the Palliative care Outcome Scale (POS)

Expert Comment

There are disparities in the access to palliative care services for people from ethnic minorities. Various reasons for this unmet need include cultural and communication issues.[4] As the population ages, the proportion of older people from ethnic minority backgrounds and their end of life care needs will increasingly grow. Research, in association with practice and policy is important to adapt services for those from ethnic minorities.[4]

Once the diagnosis was made, Angela struggled to come to terms with this. Her mood deteriorated over the course of 6 months. At the time it was picked up, she was experiencing fatigue, reduced appetite, and poor sleep. She struggled with concentration when trying to read or watch television. She had lost pleasure in her daily activities.

Expert Comment

Good palliative care is an important factor in helping to prevent the development of depression.[3] Good communication and providing appropriate information and psychosocial support can help people cope with stress. Identifying those at higher risk of developing depression is important so additional support can be offered as needed.

Clinical Tip

ICD-10[5] criteria are used to diagnose and rate the severity of depression. Biological symptoms of depression are difficult to distinguish from cancer-related symptoms.[6] Endicott[7] proposed substituting psychological symptoms for the biological symptoms of depression in those who are physically unwell to improve diagnostic accuracy (see Table 22.1).

Another challenge when recognizing depression is the difficulty distinguishing it from fear and sadness. Terminally Ill Grief or Depression Scale (TIGDS) may be useful differentiating depression from grief in palliative care when this is unclear.

Learning Point Risk Factors for Depression in Palliative Care

- Personal or family history of depression[3]
- Life stressors
- Lack of social support
- Younger age
- Advanced disease at diagnosis
- Poorly controlled symptoms
- Poor performance status or disabilities

Expert Comment

Although faith can often be protective, sometimes it can lead to the opposite feelings when the cultural expectation is different from the lived experience.

Expert Comment

Wish for hastened death has been defined as either a passive wish for death without active plans, a request for help to hasten death, or a plan for suicide.[8] Wish for hastened death is strongly associated with depression in palliative populations.[9] This highlights the importance of identifying and effectively managing depression in those with advanced disease.

Clinical Tip Alternative Diagnoses to Consider

Delirium: acute onset with prominent cognitive impairment especially inattention

Dementia: slower onset with prominent memory and functional impairment

Drug reactions: onset linked to a new drug starting

Table 22.1 Endicott criteria

Biological symptom	Psychological symptom
Change in appetite/weight	Tearfulness, depressed appearance
Sleep disturbance	Social withdrawal, reduced talkativeness
Fatigue/ loss of energy	Brooding self-pity, pessimism
Reduced concentration	Lack of reactivity

Reproduced with permission from Endicott J. (1984). Measurement of depression in patients with cancer. *Cancer*. 15(53): 2243–2248. DOI: 10.1002/cncr.1984.53.s10.2243.

Angela lived with her husband and 24-year-old son. Prior to becoming unwell she worked as a cleaner and was very active, describing herself as 'always on my feet'. Her husband worked long hours doing shift work, so she had always been in control of family life and took pride in looking after her family. She described her husband as a good man but not very good at 'the emotional stuff'. She said that he found it very hard to talk about the prospect of losing her and she felt guilt about the prospect of being a burden on him as her health deteriorated. Her son was doing temporary office work and she was concerned about how he was going to cope with her disease progression. She described him as a 'late bloomer' who had always been quite reliant on his family. She worried a lot about how her husband and son would cope without her after her death.

She has always had a busy life; she was an active member of her local church, sang in church choir, and often spent time with friends. A few weeks after her diagnosis she began withdrawing from her social activities and avoided seeing her friends.

She felt guilty about feeling so low as everyone around her was encouraging positivity. As a result, she did not reveal any of her feelings to her friends and tried to mask it. She was aware that she had not genuinely smiled for several months. This led to further social withdrawal which exacerbated her low mood further.

On mental state examination she was tearful, had slowed movements, and reduced eye contact. She was emotionally flat. There were no psychotic symptoms, and she was cognitively intact. She had some insight into the impact her physical illness was having on her mood.

In terms of risk, she did not feel suicidal but often wished she wouldn't wake each morning. This was at odds with her cultural beliefs as she felt a pressure to live as long as possible. Her friends would tell her to 'keep fighting'. This made her feel worse as she felt she ought to want to fight her illness, but she felt no motivation for this.

Angela did not have a previous history of any mental health problems. She did not drink alcohol often or ever use illicit substances. She thought her mother may have experienced depression but had never sought help for this. She thought a great uncle ended his own life, but this was not talked about openly in the family.

Investigations were carried out to rule out a metabolic or biochemical reversible cause of her depressive symptoms. She was not on steroids. Her calcium and thyroid function were normal. The possibility of frontal brain metastases leading to frontal apathy was considered but her CT head scan was normal.

Figure 22.1 shows her bio-psycho-social formulation. She was struggling with the experience of many different losses in her life. Her change in physical functioning had led to her not being able to work as a cleaner any longer. She was used to

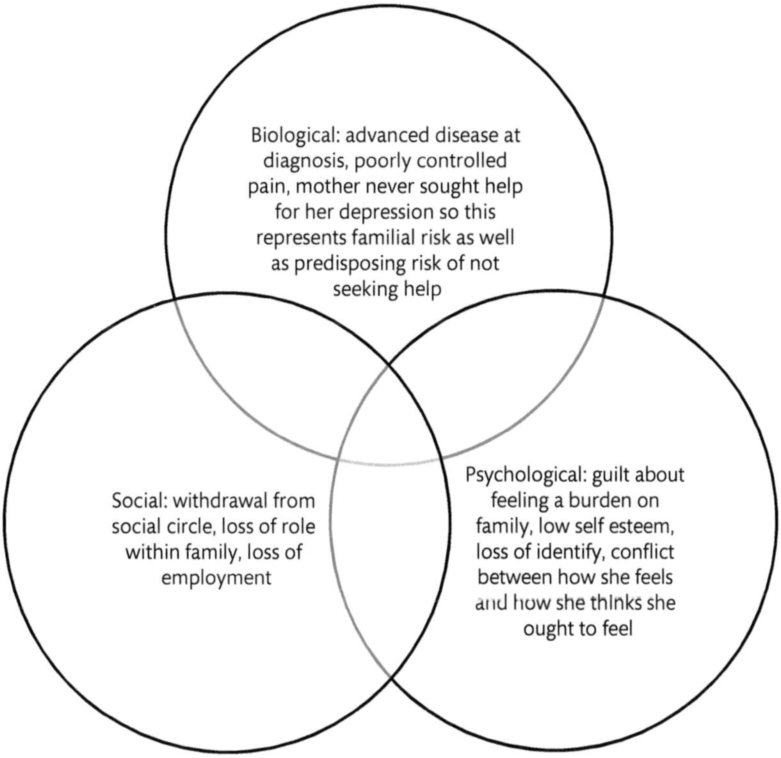

Figure 22.1 Angela's bio-psycho-social formulation.

being busy and active and this was no longer possible. She felt that her identity was stripped from her because she felt she had lost some of her key roles, both at work and within the family. This led to intense feelings of guilt that she was putting too much extra responsibility onto her husband and son. Her focus in life had always been to care for others so she was struggling to accept help herself. She also felt that she had lost her circle of friends as she felt alienated from them. She felt no motivation to socialize and felt exhausted from constantly masking her true feelings. Due to reduced energy levels and motivation, she was struggling to get washed and dressed. This, however, further exacerbated her low mood as she experienced this as another loss of self.

The palliative care team made a referral to the local liaison psychiatry service. She was assessed and diagnosed with a moderate depressive episode. Management options were explored with her using a bio-psycho-social approach. She was keen to access complementary therapy and her husband was referred to the family support team.

Medication options were discussed with her. She was initially unsure about taking medication for her mood. She was given written information and options were fully explained to her. She agreed to start antidepressants and mirtazapine was started in the hope that it may also contribute towards improved appetite, and sleep. She was reviewed for side effects within the first week of treatment, but she was tolerating the medication well. Her symptoms were then reviewed every 2 weeks and she continued to take mirtazapine at 30 mg daily.

Expert Comment

Liaison psychiatry services can provide invaluable support for palliative care teams; caring for patients, providing education, and engaging in research.[10]

Evidence Base

A systematic review[1] has shown antidepressants to be effective in reducing depressive symptoms and improving quality of life. There is less evidence available about specific antidepressant choices, but mirtazapine and citalopram have been shown to be effective in palliative care.[11] Antidepressants may be beneficial even when prognosis is short,[12] so it is important to consider appropriate treatment. The Maudsley Guidelines[13] provide useful guidance for prescribing in psychiatric illness at the end of life.

Psychological therapy options were discussed with her. She was offered a course of cognitive behavioural therapy (CBT) to focus on her depressive symptoms. This focused on her core beliefs; the role of her 'inner critic' and feelings of guilt. She practised ways of connecting with the present moment.

The combination of medication and psychological therapy helped to improve her mood and she felt able to cope better with her situation. She identified her key values as positive relationships with her family and friends and her Christian faith. She was able to identify what thoughts and behaviours moved her closer to her values. She felt more motivated to engage with a close friend and found this relationship supportive. She recognized that the guilt she was feeling about her family was further drawing her away from them. The palliative care team were able to offer family support sessions to her husband and son who found it a useful space to acknowledge their feelings. They also provided support to her and her husband to think about her future wishes and plans including funeral arrangements. With her increased motivation, she felt able to make a memory box for her son and found it helpful writing letters to her family and close friends. She collected photographs and wrote down favourite recipes so she could feel more connected with family life going forwards. She linked up with a support group and found it validating to talk more authentically with people who understood what she was going through. She started attending a hospice day therapy craft group, giving her a chance to be productive whilst maintaining positive relationships with others. She met with the spiritual care team at the hospice who provided her a space to express her distress, she found this a supportive way to connect with her faith and she found peace and comfort through this.

Learning Point

When starting antidepressants, it is important to review frequently for side effects and effectiveness and get up to a therapeutic dose as quickly as is safely possible, especially when time is likely to be short.

Clinical Tip

When swallowing issues are present, consider alternative preparations:

- Most standard-release antidepressants can be crushed and administered via nasogastric tube if required
- Many are available as oral solutions for those who have difficulty taking tablets: mirtazapine, fluoxetine, sertraline, and paroxetine
- Mirtazapine and fluoxetine are available as dispersible tablets
- Citalopram and escitalopram are available as drops

Future Advances

Whereas conventional psychological treatments work towards problem-solving, this can often be a challenging approach in life-limiting illness where there are often complex psychological issues with no simple solution. Acceptance and Commitment Therapy (ACT) is flexible and trans-diagnostic allowing patients to tolerate distress and aim to live in the present.[16, 17] This is a novel third-wave CBT and evidence on its effectiveness in this population is being gathered.[18]

Evidence Base

Although access to psychological professionals in UK hospices has improved, many hospices feel that their overall psychological services were not adequate.[14] Links with mental health services are felt to be crucial in improving access to specialist care.

The National Institute for Health and Care Excellence (NICE) recommends that people with advanced illnesses with significant levels of psychological distress should be offered prompt access to specialist psychological care.[15]

A systematic review on the evidenced-based management of depression in palliative care[1] showed there to be significant benefit from the following non-pharmacological treatments: counselling, clinical hypnosis, dignity therapy, cognitive therapy, CBT, music intervention therapy, guided imagery, progressive muscle relaxation, acupuncture, mindful breathing, and short-term review psychotherapy.

Angela's health deteriorated over a few weeks and after discussion with her and her family it was agreed that she would try to remain at home. Her husband and son managed well with support from the community palliative care team, and until the end of her life she enjoyed the company of her family and friends. She continued to take the antidepressant until she became too drowsy to continue oral medications about a week before her death.

Learning Point

Sometimes stopping antidepressants can cause symptoms which may include dizziness, nausea, paraesthesia, anxiety, and headaches.[3] All antidepressants can cause discontinuation symptoms, particularly if stopped suddenly, however this is more likely in drugs with a shorter half-life, such as paroxetine or venlafaxine. If it is not possible to taper the dose gradually, if someone is in the last days of life, consideration can be given to benzodiazepines to manage any associated agitation or restlessness.

Discussion

In summary, this is the case of a 58-year-old lady with metastatic cancer and depression. She experienced low mood, anhedonia, loss of interest with reduced concentration and motivation. She also presented with reduced appetite and poor sleep but her physical illness impacted on these features too, making them less specific for depression. She struggled with feelings of guilt and withdrew from her usual social contact. The advanced state of her illness at diagnosis, combined with uncontrolled physical symptoms added to her risk of developing mood disorder.

A combination of antidepressant medication and psychological therapy helped to improve her mood. Her family benefited from targeted support. As a result, she felt able to connect better with her family and friends and was able to draw more value from her activities and interactions with others.

A Final Word from the Expert

Identifying and managing depression in people with advanced disease can make a huge difference to patient experience, quality of life and relationships but it is easy to miss, especially when patients don't volunteer their symptoms, or we have less cultural expectation of this as a problem. Building active detection of depression into routine patient assessment ensures early diagnosis and opportunities to provide evidence-based, effective interventions.

References

1. Perusinghe M, Chen KY, McDermott B, Evidence-based management of depression in palliative care: a systematic review. *J Palliat Med* 2021; 24(5): 767–781.
2. Stiefel R, Trill MD, Berney A, et al. Depression in palliative care: a pragmatic report from the Expert Working Group of the European Association for Palliative Care. *Support Care Cancer* 2001; 9(7): 477–488.
3. Rayner L, Higginson IJ, Price A, Hotopf M. *The Management of Depression in Palliative Care: European Clinical Guidelines*. London: Department of Palliative Care, Policy & Rehabilitation.
4. Calanzani N, Koffman J, Higginson IJ. *Palliative and End of Life Care for Black, Asian and Minority Ethnic groups in the UK*. Marie Curie. 2013. Available at: https://www.mariecurie.org.uk/globalassets/media/documents/who-we-are/diversity-and-inclusion-research/palliative-care-bame_full-report.pdf
5. World Health Organization (WHO). *The ICD-10 Classification of Mental and Behavioral Disorders: Clinical Descriptions and Diagnostic Guidelines*. Geneva: World Health Organization, 1992.
6. Lawrie I, Lloyd-Williams M, Taylor F. How do palliative medicine physicians assess and manage depression. *Palliat Med* 2004; 18(3): 234–238.
7. Endicott J. Measurement of depression in patients with cancer. *Cancer* 1984; 15(53): 2243–2248.
8. Hudson PL, Kristjanson LJ, Ashby M, et al. Desire for hastened death in patients with advanced disease and the evidence base of clinical guidelines: a systematic review. *Palliat Med* 2006; 20(7): 693–701.
9. Price A, Lee W, Goodwin L, et al. Prevalence, course and associations of desire for hastened death in a UK palliative population: a cross-sectional study. *BMJ Support Palliat Care* 2011; 1(2): 140–148.
10. Irwin SA, Ferris FD. The opportunity for psychiatry in palliative care. *Can J Psychiatry* 2008; 53(11): 713–724.
11. Rayner L, Price A, Hotopf M, Higginson IJ. Expert opinion on detecting and treating depression in palliative care: a Delphi study. *BMC Palliat Care* 2011; 10: 10.

12. Rayner L, Lee W, Price A, et al. The clinical epidemiology of depression in palliative care: systematic review and meta-analysis. *Palliat Med* 2011; 25(3): 36–51.
13. Taylor D, Barnes T, Young A. *The Maudsley Prescribing Guidelines in Psychiatry*, 14th ed. Oxford: Wiley Blackwell, 2021, pp. 829–830.
14. McInnerney D, Candy B, Stone P, et al. Access to and adequacy of psychological services for adult patients in UK hospices: a national, cross-sectional survey. *BMC Palliat Care* 2021; 20(1): 31.
15. National Institute for Clinical Excellence (NICE). Improving supportive and palliative care for adults with cancer. 2004. Available at: https://www.nice.org.uk/guidance/csg4/resources/improving-supportive-and-palliative-care-for-adults-with-cancer-pdf-773375005
16. Hayes SC, Luoma JB, Bond FW, et al. Acceptance and commitment therapy: model, process and outcomes. *Behav Res Ther* 2006; 44(1): 1–25.
17. Burian H, Böge K, Burian R, et al. Acceptance and commitment-based therapy for patients with psychiatric and physical health conditions in routine general hospital care—development, implementation and outcomes. *J Psycho Res* 2021; 143: 110374.
18. Low J, Serfaty M, Davis S, et al. Acceptance and commitment therapy for adults with advanced cancer (CanACT): study protocol for a feasibility randomised controlled trial. *Trials* 2016; 17: 77.

SECTION 4

Interface between palliative care and mental health

CASE 23 Hoarding and Associated Disorders

Manraj Bhamra

Expert: Khalida Ismail

Case history

An 82-year-old woman, Helga, called her GP stating that she was unable to move due to severe pain, and was unable to attend the surgery. She was screaming and crying down the phone, exclaiming that she was very frightened.

On reviewing Helga's medical records, she had not attended the practice in five years, including for routine health checks. She was last seen with non-specific symptoms and 'total body pain' shortly after her husband died five years ago. Her previous records noted diagnoses of hypertension and obesity, but otherwise suggested limited patient contact.

The GP carried out an urgent home visit. On knocking, the GP heard shouts, but was unable to gain entry to the house. The police and fire brigade were called for assistance and the door was broken down. An overpowering stench of rotten food and excrement was noted in what appeared to be an extreme state of neglect. There was evidence of extensive hoarding. The home was completely filled with boxes and piles of books and clothes in a disorganized manner, obstructing all views, and presenting a significant fire risk.

She was found to be lying on a sofa and was unable to move herself. There appeared to be marked weight loss compared with the past history of obesity. She was surrounded by empty packets of food, empty bottles, bags, and the room was full of flies. Faeces were noted beside her and staining her clothes.

Helga refused to move from the sofa despite gentle prompting and refused to attend hospital, stating that she only needed painkillers for her abdominal pain. There was concern that her significant state of physical decline and neglect was impacting on her ability to make decisions. Following a multidisciplinary assessment and discussion by professionals at the scene, she was deemed to lack capacity to consent to further investigations and management of her pain under the Mental Capacity Act 2005. A best-interest decision was made to transfer her to hospital on an orthopaedic stretcher, with the fire brigade and paramedics supporting this.

Clinical Tip Differential Diagnosis of Hoarding

Hoarding behaviour may represent a discrete disorder or can be a symptom that is a manifestation of another psychiatric disorder, most commonly obsessive-compulsive disorder (see Figure 23.1). These may be distinguished by the individual's intentions behind hoarding and their ability to discard objects. Where hoarding is a symptom of a psychiatric disorder, it may occur without purpose or intention and individuals can discard items without distress. Where hoarding is a result of a primary discrete disorder, the behaviour is intentional and impairing. Discarding items is associated with significant distress.[1]

Additionally, those with a primary discrete hoarding disorder are more like to suffer from comorbid psychiatric disorders, most commonly depression, generalized anxiety disorder, and social anxiety.[2]

It is therefore even more pertinent to facilitate the comprehensive assessment and management of individuals to identify the functional and motivational components of their disorder (see [1] for further reading on a comprehensive approach to doing this and further discussion about the complex interacting components of the symptoms of hoarding) (see Table 23.1).

Table 23.1 Differential diagnosis of psychiatric disorders that feature hoarding behaviour

Diagnosis (ICD-11 code)	Hoarding manifestation	Differentiation from hoarding disorder
Hoarding disorder (6B24)	Object accumulation occurs due to repetitive urges or behaviours which may be passive or active in nature. Distress associated with discarding items	N/A
Psychotic disorders (6A2)	Object accumulation is driven by delusions	Individuals often display other psychotic symptoms such as thought disorder and hallucinations
Mood disorders (6A7, 6A8)	Object accumulation occurs secondary to depressive (low energy, poor motivation, apathy) or manic symptoms (excessive spending)	Individuals display no distress associated with discarding items Hoarding occurs without purpose or interest in depressive disorders Manic episodes are often of insufficient duration to allow significant clutter to develop
Obsessive-compulsive disorder (6B20)	Individuals accumulate excessive amounts of objects (compulsive hoarding)	Accumulation often occurs in order to neutralize obsessional thoughts and is unwanted and distressing Accumulation in hoarding disorder may be pleasurable
Dementia (6D8)	Object accumulation occurs due to progressive cognitive deficits and behavioural symptoms (repetitive behaviour, disinhibition) or an inability to discard items	Hoarding occurs without purpose or interest and individuals often display no distress associated with discarding items. Individuals may display severe behavioural and personality changes

Learning Point Hoarding in the Elderly

Studies suggest that the prevalence of hoarding in older adults is nearly three times higher compared to younger adults and increases linearly by 20% with every five years of age.[3, 4]

Given its chronic and progressive course, the consequences of hoarding are more distressing and impairing with age due to the accumulation of objects over time and an increased inability to discard items. Hoarding in the elderly is associated with social isolation, self-neglect, environmental risks, and comorbid psychiatric and physical disorders.[5, 6] Additionally, older adults remain more resistant to treatment, making early diagnosis crucial.[7]

Depressive and anxiety disorders are the most common comorbid mental disorders in older adults with hoarding disorder. Late-life onset hoarding behaviour may be associated with dementia.[5]

Expert Comment Assessing Capacity in an Individual Who Resists Help

On a home visit, assessments should consider the extent of hoarding, the level of risk, physical and mental health, and mental capacity. All attempts should be made to engage an individual and gain their trust. Urgent intervention should be taken if needed, for example, transfer to hospital. Where immediate action is not required, a multiagency case conference should be held with relevant professionals attending.

When intervention or treatment is refused, consider if the patient has a psychiatric illness and utilize the relevant local mental health/capacity frameworks (here, this would be the Mental Health Act as she resides in England). On initial review in this case, it is as of yet unclear if she is suffering from a psychiatric illness and there is no known past psychiatric history, and so the Mental Health Act would not be an appropriate framework. An assessment of her capacity using the Mental Capacity Act 2005 should be made. Here, she is deemed to lack capacity to consent to further investigations and treatment as she does not appear to be able to weigh up the benefits and risks of intervention (including prevention of further serious deterioration of physical health), and is unable to communicate this. Decisions can be made about intervention in her best interest.

On admission, a full medical assessment was undertaken, and a large pelvic mass found clinically. Helga was amenable to imaging which confirmed a stage IV ovarian carcinoma with metastases to the liver. There was no evidence of brain metastases or cerebral atrophy on MRI brain imaging.

Liaison psychiatric assessment was requested due to poor engagement with staff, agitation, and resistance to interventions. On mental state examination, Helga presented as withdrawn with low mood, tedium vitae (loathing of life), and low self-worth. She reported further symptoms of depression, including anergia, anhedonia, and anorexia. The Montreal Cognitive Assessment (MoCA) was utilized as a screening tool for cognitive impairment. This found a reduced score of 22/30, which was indicative of mild cognitive impairment. A diagnosis was made of a depressive episode with associated features of hoarding and cognitive impairment.

A reassessment of her capacity to consent to investigations and treatment was performed. Helga was not able to retain, weigh up, or communicate information due to her depressive illness and cognitive impairment, and thus was deemed to lack capacity to make these decisions.

Through several assessments, Helga was able to give an account of her personal history, including a background of childhood domestic violence relating to her father, who suffered from low mood and alcohol problems. This pattern was eventually repeated by her husband who at times became violent towards her and her son when he drank alcohol. He had a stroke at the age of 65 and she became his primary carer until he died five years ago. Her son lived in California, and they had had no regular contact in the past 4 years.

Sociocultural assessment noted that she lived alone in her own home without any support. She was previously fully independent with activities of daily living prior to her husband's death but now struggled with tasks due to poor energy and fatigue. She was unable to prepare food or use the toilet due to compromised kitchen and bathroom access. She had been surviving on dried foods with little appetite. She had had a limited social network since the death of her husband, and recently had not left the house for some weeks.

Her case was discussed at the gynae-oncology MDM and anticancer treatment was not felt to be indicated as she had widespread metastases and a poor performance status. Palliative care was recommended. Helga expressed a fear of dying, hopelessness, and increased anxiety with disease progression. She was initially reluctant to commence an antidepressant but was eventually agreeable. Sertraline was commenced as an inpatient and titrated up slowly, to which she responded with a significant improvement in mood. Her cognitive impairment resolved with a repeat MoCA score of 28/30. She was also referred to the inpatient psychology team for anxiety and low mood, and cognitive behavioural therapy techniques were incorporated into these sessions.

Her preferred place of care and death was her own home. Initially she was resistant to any interventions at home, including deep cleaning. Her hospital admission was therefore prolonged whilst her condition progressed, as it was not deemed safe for her to be discharged home. As her mood and cognition improved, she subsequently began to engage with social services who were able to facilitate a deep clean of her home in due course without any significant distress. Although preparations were being made for discharge home with a robust package of care and close monitoring by the community palliative care team, her condition unfortunately deteriorated, with resulting increase in her care needs, and she instead agreed to be discharged to a nursing home for end of life care.

Expert Comment Pseudodementia

This term was first coined in 1961 to describe cases which closely mirrored dementia.[8] It is now widely used to describe the cognitive deficits occurring in various psychiatric disorders, particularly depression in older adults. This often presents with a diagnostic dilemma as cognitive impairment may be seen in depression and dementia can manifest with depressive symptoms. It is important to note the absence of a neurodegenerative process in these disorders, which would usually be associated with progressive cognitive deterioration. These cognitive deficits are therefore technically reversible if the underlying psychiatric disorder is treated. In cases of depression in older adults presenting with cognitive impairment in the absence of an underlying neurodegenerative process (a pseudodementia picture), treatment of the mood disorder with pharmacotherapy and psychological therapy would expect to see a resolution of these cognitive deficits. In this case, effective treatment of the patient's depression with sertraline has resolved the cognitive impairment noted on initial assessment.[9-11]

Discussion

In summary, this is a case of a patient whose presenting symptom of pain revealed extensive hoarding, squalid living conditions, and self-neglect on an urgent home visit. Assessment in hospital noted examination and imaging findings consistent with metastatic ovarian carcinoma. A comprehensive psychiatric assessment was undertaken, which concluded that she did not have a primary diagnosis of a hoarding disorder but instead her hoarding was a symptom secondary to depression with associated cognitive impairment.

Functional assessment indicated a gradual decline in functional ability and increasing self-neglect since the death of her husband. This was likely multifactorial and secondary to symptoms associated with malignancy, depression, and cognitive impairment.

Treatment was supportive due to the advanced nature of her disease. She demonstrated significant improvements in mood and cognition with sertraline, to the extent that she was able to engage with psychosocial interventions. Inpatient psychology addressed her anxiety and fear of dying related to her newly diagnosed life-limiting illness. Patient wishes and preferred place of death were considered in the discharge planning process. The unsafe living conditions associated with her hoarding behaviours were resolved through removals and deep cleaning. Multidisciplinary working was critical to the therapeutic alliance here.

Unfortunately, despite an improvement in her mental state, her physical condition deteriorated, and she could no longer be discharged back to her own home. This highlights that there is a subgroup of patients that do not come into contact with services until it is often too late for significant intervention. It is therefore crucial to differentiate between hoarding related to a psychiatric disorder and a primary hoarding disorder.

Clinical Tip Diagnosis of Hoarding Disorder

The diagnosis of hoarding disorder is often made when other diagnoses that result in hoarding have been excluded (see Figure 23.1 for details).[12]

International classification of diseases (ICD-11) diagnostic criteria for hoarding disorder (6B24):

1. Accumulation of possessions that results in cluttered living spaces, compromising their use or safety. Accumulation occurs due to repetitive urges or behaviours which may be passive or active in nature, and difficulty discarding possessions due to a perceived need for them and distress associated with discarding them.
2. Symptoms result in significant distress or impairment in personal, family, social, educational, occupational, and other areas of functioning.

Additional clinical features:

- Assessment may also include collateral information and visual inspection of the home.
- Items are often hoarded due to their emotional significance, perceived characteristics, or values.
- Individuals may be unable to find important items, move around or exit their home, prepare food, or use appliances or furniture.
- Individuals may have chronic physical comorbidities such as obesity, limited mobility, and are exposed to numerous environmental risks because of their hoarding.

Expert Comment Hoarding in Palliative Care

Treatment of hoarding in palliative care patients presents additional challenges, given limited timeframes and numerous barriers to care. The first step is to establish whether this is a discrete disorder in its own right or a symptom secondary to another psychiatric disorder (Figure 23.1). In this case, hoarding behaviour is a manifestation of the patient's depressive illness. Object accumulation has occurred without purpose or interest secondary to symptoms of low energy, poor motivation, apathy, and cognitive impairment. There appears to have been minimal distress associated with the deep clean. Symptoms related to her ovarian carcinoma are likely to be further contributing to object accumulation and an inability to discard items.

Approaches used in these settings include harm reduction, developing a therapeutic rapport with the patient and trauma-informed care and treatment of associated psychiatric disorders if present. Harm reduction acknowledges chronic difficulties with hoarding and aims to reduce its impact by minimizing environmental risks and hazards and returning control to the patient. Motivational interviewing is a focused counselling style and may be helpful to assess and support readiness to change, acknowledging ambivalence to change, weighing up the options (parting with possessions or allowing a deep clean versus continuing to suffer with pain and other symptoms) and level of insight. Trauma-informed care recognizes traumatic experiences that may have precipitated hoarding disorders and aims to provide an environment in which the individual feels safe and can develop trust in order to 'let go' of their possessions.

Special considerations for hoarding in palliative care include assessing for hoarding routinely in reviews, recognizing timeframes and illness severity, mental capacity assessment, the level of risk, trauma-informed care to improve practice, carer education, and multiagency collaboration.

For further information on the treatment of hoarding disorder specifically, see [13-16].

Evidence Base Future Directions in Hoarding Research

Research on hoarding disorder has increased significantly since its recognition as a distinct disorder. Much of this has recently focused on cognitive dysfunction as a potential aetiological factor in the development and maintenance of hoarding, as well as emotional features such as a lack of insight in many patients.[17] Future studies aim to understand impairments associated with hoarding and comorbid psychiatric conditions.

Whilst cognitive and behavioural techniques (CBT) have been shown to be effective in hoarding, current treatments are not as robust as for other psychiatric disorders.[17] Technology-supported hoarding interventions, cognitive rehabilitation treatment, compassion-focused therapy, motivational interviewing, and harm reduction have all shown promise.[18] Treatment effects with antidepressants may not be sufficient. The use of novel agents, such as stimulants and cognitive enhancers, or augmentation of psychological therapies with medications, may be future options. Further studies and more effective treatments are required for this disabling condition.

A Final Word from the Expert

This case recognizes the complex journey that individuals with hoarding often experience. It is unfortunate that this lady disengaged from health services and social networks following the death of her husband, likely due to the onset of a depressive illness. Associated symptoms of low energy, poor motivation, apathy, and cognitive impairment are likely to have facilitated hoarding through the passive accumulation of objects and an inability to discard them. Additionally, her depressive illness and underlying malignancy will have contributed to progressive functional deterioration and further social isolation. As a result, she is discovered in a state of squalor, requiring urgent medical and psychiatric assessment and treatment in her best interest. Diagnoses of ovarian carcinoma, depression, and cognitive impairment are made. Rapid and effective treatment of her depression resulted in significant improvement in her mental and cognitive state, and recovery of mental capacity. This allowed her to engage with a care plan.

This case demonstrates a good outcome for hoarding and depressive illness through pharmacological, psychological, and social interventions, despite a deterioration in her physical health. Trauma-informed care and multiagency collaboration are key components of this.

References

1. Maier T. On phenomenology and classification of hoarding: a review. *Acta Psychiatr Scand* 2004; 110: 323–337.
2. Frost RO, Steketee G, Tolin DF. Comorbidity in hoarding disorder. Depress Anxiety 2011; 28: 876–884.
3. Samuels JF, Bienvenu OJ, Grados MA, et al. Prevalence and correlates of hoarding behavior in a community-based sample. *Behav Res Ther* 2008; 46: 836–844.
4. Cath DC, Nizar K, Boomsma D, et al. Age-specific prevalence of hoarding and obsessive compulsive disorder: a population-based study. *Am J Geriatr Psychiatry* 2017; 25: 245–255.
5. Ayers CR, Saxena S, Golshan S, et al. Age at onset and clinical features of late life compulsive hoarding. *Int J Geriatr Psychiatry* 2010; 25: 142–149.
6. Koenig TL, Chapin R, Spano R. Using multidisciplinary teams to address ethical dilemmas with older adults who hoard. *J Gerontol Soc Work* 2010; 53: 137–147.
7. Pertusa A, Gaston RL, Choudry A. Hoarding revisited: there is light at the end of the living room. *BJPsych Advances* 2019; 25: 26–36.
8. Kiloh LG. Pseudo-dementia. *Acta Psychiatr Scand* 1961; 37: 336–351.
9. Frost RO, Hartl TL. A cognitive–behavioral model of compulsive hoarding. *Behav Res Ther* 1996; 34: 341–350.
10. Iervolino AC, Perroud N, Fullana MA, et al. Prevalence and heritability of compulsive hoarding: a twin study. *Am J Psychiatry* 2009; 166: 1156–1161.

11. Timpano KR, Exner C, Glaesmer H, et al. The epidemiology of the proposed DSM-5 Hoarding Disorder: exploration of the acquisition specifier, associated features and distress. *J Clin Psychiatry* 2010; 72: 780–786.
12. World Health Organization (WHO). *ICD-11: International Classification of Diseases* (11th revision). Geneva: World Health Organization; 2019.
13. Tolin D, Frost RO, Steketee G, et al. Cognitive behavioural therapy for hoarding disorder: a meta-analysis. *Depress Anxiety* 2015; 32: 158–166.
14. Tolin DF. Understanding and treating hoarding: a biopsychosocial perspective. *J Clin Psychology* 2011; 67: 517–526.
15. Saxena S, Brody AL, Maidment KM, et al. Paroxetine treatment of compulsive hoarding. *J Psychiatr Res* 2007; 41: 481–487.
16. Saxena S, Sumner J. Venlafaxine extended-release treatment of hoarding disorder. *Int Clin Psychopharmacol* 2014; 29: 266–273.
17. Davidson EJ, Dozier ME, Pittman JOE, et al. Recent advances in research on hoarding. *Curr Psychiatry Rep* 2019; 21: 91.
18. Bratiotis C, Muroff J, Lin NXY. Hoarding disorder: development in conceptualization, intervention and evaluation. *Focus* 2021; 19: 392–404.

CASE

24 Delirium

Kitty Jackson

Expert: Felicity Wood

Case history

Michael was a 77-year-old gentleman with metastatic non-small cell lung cancer, who was admitted to a hospice inpatient unit for pain management. Past medical history included chronic kidney disease and benign prostatic hypertrophy. He wore glasses and hearing aids. He smoked and did not drink alcohol.

Michael described pain in his chest wall, in keeping with a site of metastatic bone disease. He was taking amitriptyline and oxycodone modified release (MR) and using as-required oxycodone immediate release (IR) liquid. He had urinary frequency and was taking senna and opening his bowels daily. He described falling asleep during the day and difficulty concentrating. No specific assessment of his risk of developing delirium was carried out and no preventative measures were enacted. Delirium screening was not undertaken.

Learning Point

NICE delirium guidelines promote individual patient risk assessment with application of a personalized multicomponent non-pharmacological intervention for those deemed at risk.[1]

Predisposing risk factors for delirium[2]:

- Age over 65 years
- Cognitive impairment
- Multiple comorbidities
- Significant injuries (e.g. hip fracture)
- Functional impairment
- Iatrogenic events (e.g. bladder catheterization, polypharmacy, or surgery)
- History of, or current, alcohol excess
- Sensory impairment (e.g. visual impairment or hearing loss)
- Poor nutrition
- Terminal phase of illness

The risk of delirium is increased by the number of factors present.

Non-pharmacological multicomponent interventions to prevent delirium focus on reducing or eliminating several risk factors for delirium. Details of common intervention components are in Table 24.1. A systematic review assessing this approach in hospitalized (non-ICU) patients shows they reduce the occurrence of delirium by 43% compared to usual hospital care.[3] There is no clear evidence any medication is effective in preventing delirium.[4]

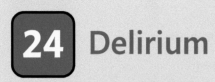

Table 24.1 Non-pharmacological interventions to prevent delirium[1, 5, 6] (The same interventions can be used to manage delirium)

Orientation	Appropriate lighting Clear signage Clock and calendar Reorientate to time, place, and person Cognitively stimulating activities Facilitate visits from family and friends
Address sensory impairment	Hearing aids and glasses Resolve cause of impairment where possible
Optimize sleep-wake patterns	Avoid unnecessary procedures during sleeping hours including medication rounds Reduce noise and light during sleep periods
Optimize mobility	Mobilize as patient's performance status allows Appropriate walking aids Active range-of-motion exercises
Optimize the patient's physiology	Optimal hydration and nutrition Bladder and bowel function Supplementary oxygen, if appropriate
Address infection	Look for and treat infection Avoid unnecessary catheterization Implement infection control procedures
Address pain	Assess for pain, including looking for non-verbal signs of pain Start or review pain management
Medication review	Complete a medication review for people on multiple medications and de-prescribe where possible

One week after admission Michael became confused. He was difficult to rouse from sleep. He struggled to hold a conversation and kept losing his train of thought and falling asleep. He was disoriented and couldn't recall conversations from the day before and appeared to be responding to unseen stimuli. Hypoactive delirium was diagnosed.

Evidence Base

Delirium is common in the palliative care setting: 58.8–88% of patients have delirium in the weeks or hours preceding death.[7] Within an inpatient palliative care unit, 60% will have delirium at some point during their inpatient stay.[8]

It is associated with worse patient outcomes including prolonged hospitalization, increased mortality, and higher likelihood of discharge to long-term care.[5] It can lead to complications such as falls and pressure sores.[9] Delirium is distressing to patients, family, carers, and nursing staff.[10] Delirium, and its treatment with sedating medications, interferes with patient communication.[11]

Learning Point

Delirium is a condition characterized by acute onset of fluctuating levels of cognition and a disturbance in attention and awareness. It occurs when a disturbance in a person's physical health affects their cognitive function, and develops over a short period of time.[12] In practice this means

Expert Comment

Diagnosing delirium can be challenging, especially the hypoactive subtype. It is commonly missed or misdiagnosed, for example as dementia or depression. Therefore, guidelines advocate delirium screening using a validated tool to identify patients with probable delirium.[6] Multiple validated tools exist, the particular tool you use should be guided by local guidelines and your own familiarity with individual tools. Examples include the 4AT tool, Confusion Assessment Method (CAM), and the Single Question in Delirium (SQUID).

patients may present with confusion, disorientation, hallucinations, doing or saying things that are out of character, restlessness and agitation, drowsiness, becoming withdrawn and less active, difficulty concentrating, and day-night reversal. These symptoms can be subtle and easy to miss.

Expert Comment

Delirium can be divided into three psychomotor subtypes:

- Hyperactive patients are agitated, hyperalert and restless
- Hypoactive patients are drowsy and slow to respond
- Patients with the mixed subtype have features of both. In palliative care, hypoactive and mixed subtypes are the most common.

Assessment for reversible causes was undertaken: medication review showed that amitriptyline and oxycodone doses had been increased. A review of Michael's charts showed a catheter had been inserted. He hadn't opened his bowels for six days.

A complete physical examination revealed no new findings and no evidence of opioid toxicity. A collateral history from the family revealed that his hearing aid was lost and that he usually used nicotine patches in hospital. Blood tests showed no evidence of infection, electrolyte disturbance, or organ dysfunction.

Where possible, the reversible causes of delirium were managed. Oxycodone doses were reduced without the patient's pain worsening. Constipation was treated, nicotine patches prescribed, and a hearing aid acquired.

Learning Point

Initial management of delirium relies on clinical assessment and treatment for reversible causes of delirium. In patients with advanced cancer, 50% of delirium is reversible and multiple precipitants are common.[13,14] This means a systematic assessment evaluating all common reversible factors is important. Key reversible causes of delirium include:

- **Drugs and polypharmacy**: opioids, benzodiazepines, corticosteroids, tricyclic antidepressants, anticonvulsants, antimuscarinics and others
- **Drug withdrawal**: alcohol, nicotine, illicit substances, benzodiazepines, opioids
- **Uncontrolled symptoms**: urinary retention, constipation, pain
- **Metabolic disturbance**: electrolyte abnormalities, dehydration, hyper/hypoglycaemia
- **Organ failure**: renal failure, liver failure, respiratory failure
- **Other physiological disturbance**: hypoxia, anaemia
- **Infection**
- **Brain pathology**: primary brain tumour, brain metastases, leptomeningeal disease
- **Changes in environment**: unfamiliar faces, room, or routines, loss of visual/hearing aids

Expert Comment

The patient's stage of illness, likely reversible causes of delirium, and the patient and caregivers' preferences should all be considered when deciding what to investigate and treat. Some reversible factors are always appropriate to assess and treat, e.g. urinary retention or pain. Some factors may technically be reversible, but not be appropriate to do so - for instance, undertaking an invasive procedure in a dying patient. There may also be irreversible underlying causes of delirium. Delirium in advanced illness can be an indicator of poor prognosis and is often a part of the dying process.

Non-pharmacological management measures for delirium were undertaken. A clock and calendar were placed in view of Michael. Staff introduced themselves and oriented him. Pain was regularly assessed as he was thought unlikely to self-report pain. Michael was also provided with extra time and assistance at mealtimes to optimize hydration and nutrition.

Over the next five days improvement was seen: Michael was more often awake and alert, although he continued to be disoriented. However, the next day, he was more confused, agitated, and distressed. He was incoherent and believed he was imprisoned. He was lashing out if staff approached and was responding to unseen stimuli. He was pulling at his catheter and trying to climb out of bed. It was not possible to safely approach him. Nursing staff were unsure if this was worsening delirium or if he was now terminally agitated. On medical review, hyperactive delirium was diagnosed.

Learning Point

The mainstay of delirium management is non-pharmacological. The aims of non-pharmacological management are to promote brain recovery, assess and treat agitation and distress, prevent complications of delirium (e.g. immobility, falls, pressure sores, dehydration, malnourishment, isolation) and to support patients and carers.[6]

Non-pharmacological management of delirium is broadly similar to non-pharmacological prevention of delirium (Table 24.1). Additional elements include communication with patients and relatives about the diagnosis of delirium, and detecting, assessing, and treating distress.

Expert Comment

A common source of confusion regarding delirium in palliative patients is the relationship between 'terminal agitation' and 'delirium'. The terms are distinct and not interchangeable (Figure 24.1). Terminal agitation is any agitation occurring in the last few days of life.

Dying patients who have a hyperactive delirium with agitation have both 'delirium' and 'terminal agitation'. Dying patients can be agitated for a reason other than delirium, such as uncontrolled symptoms, or emotional distress.

It is useful to identify the presence or absence of delirium in a patient with terminal agitation as this may alter management.

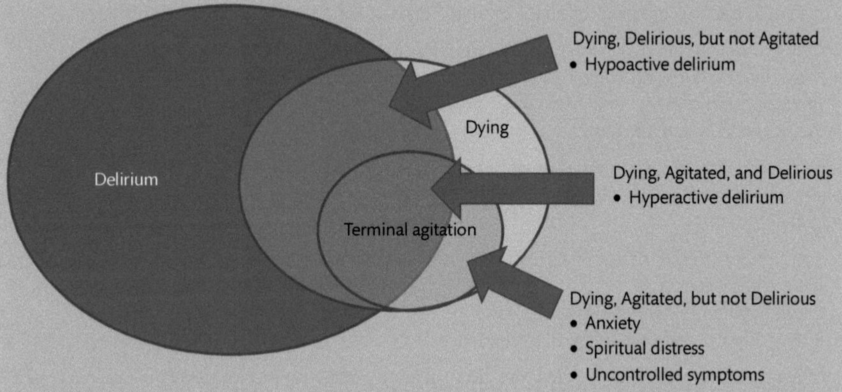

Figure 24.1 The relationship between delirium and terminal agitation. This figure explains the relationship between delirium and terminal agitation. It shows how these terms are not interchangeable but do overlap in some patients.

Given Michael's severe agitation and distress, and the risk to staff and patient safety, it was agreed that medication would be administered with the aim of safely carrying out a physical assessment. Michael refused to take oral haloperidol 0.5 mg and subcutaneous haloperidol 0.5 mg was administered with family assistance to distract Michael. Thirty minutes after this, it was possible to perform an examination.

Learning Point

Pharmacological management of delirium can be considered in specific circumstances[1]:

- Patient is a danger to themselves or others
- Distress: severe agitation or distressing hallucinations

The decision to treat with medication should be made in consultation with the patient (if possible) and their family as, even in these circumstances, sedation may not be a desirable outcome for some patients.

If a medication is to be used, an 'as required' approach, with low starting doses, should be taken. Regular medication should not be prescribed in the first instance. Any prescribed medications should be reviewed regularly, used short-term, and not continued once the delirium has resolved.[1, 6]

Learning Point

A patient lacking capacity to consent to pharmacological management of delirium should be treated under the appropriate national legal framework (in this case the Mental Capacity Act 2005,[15] which would require a best interest decision to be made).

A best interest decision about pharmacological treatment in delirium should ideally involve a family member or patient advocate, nursing staff that know the patient, the healthcare professional prescribing the medication and a pharmacist. Options for treatment can then be discussed, including continuing non-pharmacological management, oral, or subcutaneous medication. If the patient refuses medication, options including patient restraint or covert medication may be considered, but these are only appropriate in exceptional circumstances. It is important to follow the least restrictive option that would maintain patient safety. The agreed treatment plan should be recorded and regularly reviewed.

Clinical Tip

Local policy should guide your medication choice. However, haloperidol (an antipsychotic) is generally accepted as the first-line medication for delirium.[1] Risks of antipsychotic medications include[16]:

- Cause or exacerbate parkinsonism—haloperidol is contraindicated in Parkinson's disease
- Increased stroke risk and death, especially in the elderly with dementia
- Predisposition to arrhythmia through QT prolongation
- Reduction in seizure threshold

If haloperidol has proved ineffective, or is inappropriate, a benzodiazepine could be used as an alternative.[17] Sublingual lorazepam would be the first-line choice. Risks of using benzodiazepines include[16]:

- Sedation, which can increase falls risk
- Increased confusion
- Cardiorespiratory depression
- Risk of physical and psychological dependence

In a dying patient with refractory delirium, taking a more sedative approach to delirium management may be appropriate to relieve patient and family distress. In this case, using a sedating antipsychotic such as levomepromazine alone, or in conjunction with a benzodiazepine such as midazolam, may be appropriate.[17]

Evidence Base

The evidence of benefit from any medication in the treatment of delirium is lacking.

Several Cochrane reviews look at drug therapy in delirium. They conclude that in hospitalized, non-ICU patients antipsychotics do not reduce the severity of delirium, resolve symptoms, or lower the risk of dying[18] and that available evidence doesn't support the routine use of benzodiazepines.[19]

Michael was febrile with a palpable bladder. He was diagnosed with a catheter associated urinary tract infection, a blocked catheter, and urinary retention. The catheter was removed and oral cefalexin prescribed. A discussion was held with his family to explain the diagnosis of delirium and the precipitating factors, and to give advice on how to interact with him.

Clinical Tip

Hallucinations are common in delirium and do not always require pharmacological management. Listening to patients, without contradicting what they are experiencing, and validating their distress is supportive. Explanation about the cause of the hallucinations and the wider context of delirium to both patients and carers can be reassuring. Patients may benefit from distraction activities. If significant distress persists despite these measures, then management with haloperidol can be considered.

Clinical Tip

Given the impact of delirium on patients and families it is vital they are informed, supported, and involved in decision-making regarding delirium management. Communicate with patients and families[6]:

- If a patient is at risk of delirium
- If a patient develops delirium
- At discharge following an episode of delirium

These conversations should explain[6]:

- What delirium is and what the symptoms are; ensure you use the word 'delirium'
- What causes delirium
- How families can be involved in supporting their relative both to prevent and manage delirium

Over the next week Michael became less agitated, more alert, and less confused. However, some symptoms of delirium persisted, including intermittent disorientation, poor short-term memory, and daytime somnolence. His condition stabilized at this new baseline, and he was discharged home with a package of care and ongoing community palliative care support.

Expert Comment

In a palliative care population, many patients will never regain their pre-delirium cognitive function before they die.

Recovery from delirium can be a prolonged process, especially in older adults. In up to 65% of older adults, some symptoms of delirium persist for at least 12 months.[20] Most palliative care patients have a shorter prognosis than this and are therefore likely to die without full resolution of their delirium symptoms.

This has implications for care needs, decision-making, and ongoing patient or carer distress, which need to be considered when planning future care.

Discussion

In summary, a patient with metastatic lung cancer was admitted to a hospice for symptom management. Screening for delirium on admission would have revealed multiple risk factors and some subtle signs of delirium. Addressing these and implementing a personalized non-pharmacological intervention may have helped prevent development of a more severe and enduring delirium.

Multiple factors, including medication, constipation, sensory deprivation, nicotine withdrawal, blocked catheter, and urinary tract infection contributed to the development of initially hypoactive, and subsequently hyperactive delirium. Precipitating factors were reversed, where possible, and non-pharmacological delirium management was undertaken, although this could have been more comprehensive. The use of haloperidol was appropriate to maintain patient safety and to allow clinical assessment. Despite treatment of the causes of delirium, some symptoms persisted to discharge.

A Final Word from the Expert

This case demonstrates the complex factors that can contribute to delirium; in palliative care there are often many potential contributing factors. In this case, Michael experienced both hypoactive and hyperactive phases of illness. Hypoactive delirium is often mistaken for depression, so it is always important to consider delirium as a differential diagnosis. As there is limited evidence for pharmacological treatment, prevention and non-pharmacological management should be the focus. Psychoeducation for patients and families is important as delirium is likely to reoccur. Doing this effectively will help patients to seek help appropriately in future and can ease the burden on families through better understanding of the condition.

References

1. National Institute for Health and Care Excellence (NICE). Delirium: prevention, diagnosis and management. (Nice Guideline CG103). Available at: https://www.nice.org.uk/guidance/cg103
2. Clinical Knowledge Summary (CKS). Delirium: What are the risk factors?: National Institute for Health and Care Excellence (NICE). 2021. Available at: https://cks.nice.org.uk/topics/delirium/background-information/predisposing-factors/
3. Burton JK, Craig LE, Yong SQ, et al. Non-pharmacological interventions for preventing delirium in hospitalised non-ICU patients. *Cochrane Database Syst Rev* 2021; 7: CD013307.
4. Siddiqi N, Harrison JK, Clegg A, et al. Interventions for preventing delirium in hospitalised non-ICU patients. *Cochrane Database Syst Rev* 2016; 3: Cd005563.
5. LeGrand SB. Delirium in palliative medicine: a review. *J Pain Symptom Manage* 2012; 44(4): 583–594.
6. Scottish Intercollegiate Guidelines Network (SIGN). Risk reduction and management of delirium. 2019. Available at: https://www.sign.ac.uk/our-guidelines/risk-reduction-and-management-of-delirium/
7. Hosie A, Davidson PM, Agar M, Sanderson CR, Phillips J. Delirium prevalence, incidence, and implications for screening in specialist palliative care inpatient settings: a systematic review. *Palliat Med* 2013; 27(6): 486–498.
8. Watt CL, Momoli F, Ansari MT, et al. The incidence and prevalence of delirium across palliative care settings: a systematic review. *Palliat Med* 2019; 33(8): 865–877.
9. O'Keeffe ST, Lavan JN. Clinical significance of delirium subtypes in older people. *Age Ageing* 1999; 28(2): 115–119.
10. Breitbart W, Gibson C, Tremblay A. The delirium experience: delirium recall and delirium-related distress in hospitalized patients with cancer, their spouses/caregivers, and their nurses. *Psychosomatics* 2002; 43(3): 183–194.
11. Bruera E, Fainsinger RL, Miller MJ, Kuehn N. The assessment of pain intensity in patients with cognitive failure: a preliminary report. *J Pain Symptom Manage* 1992; 7(5): 267–270.
12. American Psychiatric Association. *Diagnostic and Statistical Manual of Mental Disorders*, 5th ed. Washington DC: American Psychiatric Publishing, 2013.
13. Bush SH, Tierney S, Lawlor PG. Clinical assessment and management of delirium in the palliative care setting. *Drugs* 2017; 77(15): 1623–1643.
14. Lawlor PG, Gagnon B, Mancini IL, et al. Occurrence, causes, and outcome of delirium in patients with advanced cancer: a prospective study. *Arch Intern Med* 2000; 160(6): 786–794.
15. Mental Capacity Act 2005, c.9, HMSO.
16. Twycross R, Wilcock A, Howard P. *Palliative Care Formulary*, 7th ed. London: Pharmaceutical Press, 2020.
17. Hosker CMG, Bennett MI. Delirium and agitation at the end of life. *BMJ* 2016; 353: i3085.
18. Burry L, Mehta S, Perreault MM, et al. Antipsychotics for treatment of delirium in hospitalised non-ICU patients. *Cochrane Database Syst Rev* 2018; 6(6): Cd005594.
19. Li Y, Ma J, Jin Y, et al. Benzodiazepines for treatment of patients with delirium excluding those who are cared for in an intensive care unit. *Cochrane Database Syst Rev* 2020; 2(2): CD012670.
20. Cole MG, McCusker J. Delirium in older adults: a chronic cognitive disorder? *Int Psychogeriatr* 2016; 28(8): 1229–1233.

CASE

25 Dementia

Kirsty Tolmie

Expert: Karen Harrison Dening

Case history

An 84-year-old man, David, was referred by his GP to the community specialist palliative care service. He presented with a history of weight loss, hoarseness, and dysphagia. CT revealed a large supraglottic tumour extending to the right tongue base and several enlarged level II and III cervical lymph nodes. Lymph node biopsy confirmed a poorly differentiated squamous cell carcinoma and the disease was staged as T4aN2bM0.

David had a past medical history of Alzheimer's disease diagnosed at memory clinic five years earlier. His cognitive function had declined rapidly over three years and he was experiencing significant memory impairment, poor executive functioning, and word-finding difficulties. Despite being informed of his dementia and cancer diagnoses he had been unable to retain much of the information shared with him and had little insight into his medical problems.

The regional specialist ear, nose, and throat (ENT) multidisciplinary team discussed the case and due to the extent of the malignant disease and the diagnosis of moderate to severe dementia recommended a best supportive care approach.

David was reviewed by a community palliative care nurse specialist. With prompting he was able to report or was observed to have a number of physical symptoms, including pain, fatigue, loss of appetite, and dysphagia.

He became resistive to care, pushing away attempts to support personal care, especially involving his head and neck. Co-codamol 30 mg/500 mg caused worsening confusion and constipation, and was replaced by paracetamol 1 g four times daily. David rarely self-reported pain and never requested PRN analgesia, but if offered, accepted oral morphine (immediate release) solution 2.5 mg from a spoon.

David's daughter reported a change in his mood and behaviour. His sleep pattern was altered to the extent that he woke nightly and often paced from room to room. When his daughter attempted to provide comfort he would become increasingly agitated and distressed. He often removed the dressing from his neck wound, causing it to bleed, and he had become incontinent of urine and faeces. If he could be persuaded to take additional analgesia, his agitation and distress reduced significantly. Given the likelihood that pain was driving the behavioural changes, particularly overnight when he was receiving no background analgesia, he was commenced on a long-acting opioid, morphine sulphate (modified release) 5 mg BD. Morphine was titrated in increments to 20 mg BD, and to reduce tablet burden and risk of

Expert Comment

Comprehensive assessment of changes in functional ability is vital when trying to understand the needs of patients with dementia. Numerous studies have attempted to identify prognostic indicators or indices that may guide clinicians in adopting a more palliative approach to care.[1] Assessment tools must however be used with some caution as they may be more reliable at identifying people with dementia at low risk of dying rather than those at higher risk of death.[2]

non-adherence was subsequently converted to a transdermal (12 microgram/hour) fentanyl patch.

Learning Point

Impaired cognition and the inability to communicate the experience of pain presents a challenge for healthcare professionals when managing complex symptoms. Literature suggests people with advanced dementia have a symptom burden comparable to those with cancer, experiencing pain, breathlessness, and anorexia.[3] Pain is however often under-detected and undertreated, with some studies reporting prescribed doses of opioids being as much as three times lower in people with cognitive impairment compared to those who are cognitively intact.[4]

Clinical Tip

Where communication has become a problem avoid PRN prescriptions but use routine administration for pain relief. A trial of regular analgesia resulting in an improvement in behaviour and a reduction in distress can be considered a diagnostic tool in itself.

Expert Comment

Acknowledging pain in oneself requires a high degree of comprehension; where the pain is, the nature of the pain and memories of having experienced pain in the past. The 'gold standard' for pain assessment is self-reporting and many patients with moderate to severe dementia can still report pain reliably. However, for many, as the illness advances they begin to lose high-level executive functioning, comprehension, and judgement. They may fail to recognize their experiences as being pain related and responses are in the form of behaviours, using this way to communicate distress. This often places the emphasis on those around them to 'witness' the pain and how it is manifested.

Learning Point

Pain Assessment Tools

Assessment scale	Intended use	Domains	Scoring
The Abbey Pain Scale	6 behavioural observational domains Measures changes in behaviour so requires repeated measurements	Vocalization Facial expression Change in body language Behavioural changes Physiological changes Physical changes	0–2 no pain 3–7 mild pain 8–13 moderate pain 14+ severe pain
The Pain Assessment in Advanced Dementia Scale (PAINAD)	Five-point observational scale Sensitive to both active and non- active states	Breathing Negative vocalization Facial expression Body language Consolability	1–3 mild pain 4–6 moderate pain 7–10 severe pain
Disability Distress Assessment Tool (DisDAT)	Not specific for pain rather observes distress behaviours Nine appearance and behaviour categories	Appearance Jaw movement Appearance of eyes Skin appearance Vocal sounds Speech Habits and mannerisms Body posture Body observations	Compares identified signs and behaviours and their severity with previous observations
Doloplus 2	Observation of ten pain related behaviours	Somatic reactions (5 subcategories) Psychomotor reactions (2 subcategories) Psychosocial reactions (3 subcategories)	Score > 5 indicates pain

Source: data from Lichtner V. et al. (2014). Pain assessment for people with dementia: a systematic review of systematic reviews of pain assessment tools. *BMC Geriatr.* 17:14:138. DOI: 10.1186/1471-2318-14-138.

Clinical Tip

Behavioural observation tools can be used to gain a baseline from which pain and distress behaviours can be better understood. For example, if a person with dementia is admitted into a hospital ward or care home, collateral history on how the person reacted to and managed their pain historically, combined with observational tool indicators, can establish their personal norm and support management plans.

Despite titration of opioids and the addition of neuropathic adjuvant analgesics, David's pain control remained suboptimal. A request for hospice admission was made and the case was discussed at the admissions MDT. A multi-professional holistic needs assessment was completed to establish personal care requirements, home routine, environmental stressors and distress triggers, and carer needs. Preadmission planning also sought to build confidence, knowledge, and skills amongst hospice staff and aided person-centred care planning.

Learning Point

The decision to admit a person with dementia into a hospice is influenced by a number of factors:

- Dementia is associated with prognostic uncertainty and is characterized by a prolonged and dwindling disease trajectory. Attempting to understand when the person stops 'living' with dementia and starts 'dying' with dementia can pose a challenge and impacts on decisions about where patients should be cared for.[6]
- It is well known that a change in environment can cause disorientation and worsen the behavioural and psychological symptoms of dementia. The benefits of moving the person into an unfamiliar environment, and the risk of future moves must clearly outweigh any potential detrimental effects.[7]
- Patient preferences should always be taken into account. Lack of early anticipatory care planning and communication difficulties in the later stages of the illness means the wishes of the person may be unknown or misunderstood.[8]
- Although there is a significant crossover between palliative care and dementia care, hospices may not possess all the specialist resources required to meet the needs of a person with advanced dementia.[9]

On admission to the hospice, the Abbey pain scale was used to determine David's baseline, and over time to identify any subtle changes in his behaviour which may be due to the effects and experiences of pain. Opioid analgesia was titrated and neuropathic adjuvants were added with good effect.

Non-pharmacological care focused on goal setting and sensory stimulation. Completion of meaningful and pleasurable activities such as painting and taking a bath were offered and he received aromatherapy and hand massage. Carer engagement was encouraged and the care plan was reviewed regularly at family meetings. Intervention with medication was reserved for episodes of severe agitation and distress.

Learning Point

75% of patients with dementia will experience behavioural and psychological symptoms of dementia (BPSD) at some stage of the illness.[11]

BPSD include:

- Agitation
- Aggression
- Abnormal vocalizations
- Delusions
- Hallucinations
- Wandering
- Disinhibition

Caution should be observed as many of the signs and symptoms of BPSD are similar to those of pain and distress in a person with communication difficulties. Diagnostic overshadowing of a diagnosis of dementia may lead to a misinterpretation of attempts to communicate pain as BPSD.

Expert Comment

There is growing interest in spirituality and spiritual care, which are seen increasingly as essential components in person-centred care and in maintaining the quality of life of people with dementia, especially towards the end of life when capacity may be lost. Namaste Care is an example of a systematic, multisensory care programme that is aimed specifically at meeting the spiritual needs of people with advanced dementia who are no longer able to participate in social or group activities. Namaste Care does not require verbal communication and can help foster people's sense of connection with themselves and families/friends/caregivers.[10]

Learning Point The Non-pharmacological Management of Behavioural and Psychological Symptoms of Dementia

Non-pharmacological interventions should be favoured in the first instance over pharmacological interventions when managing BPSD, taking both a patient-centred and carer-centred focus. Despite a limited and somewhat weak evidence base for the use of non-pharmacological therapies, longstanding patient and clinical experience strengthens the value of this evidence. Validation therapy, cognitive stimulation therapy, and reminiscence therapy are all patient-centred techniques aimed at improving mood and reducing BPSD. Sensory stimulation including music therapy and aromatherapy can positively affect mood, irritability, and disruptive behaviour, however these effects are not sustained beyond the time when the intervention is being delivered. Specialist nursing to meet unmet care needs, physical activity, and the effective management of concomitant pain and depression have also all been shown to improve BPSD.[12]

Learning Point The Pharmacological Management of Behavioural and Psychological Symptoms of Dementia

There is some evidence that cholinesterase inhibitors may have a positive effect on BPSD in mild and moderate stages of dementia.

Antipsychotics are associated with increased mortality and risk for cerebrovascular events and should be reserved for cases of extreme distress and where there is a risk of harm. Risperidone is the only antipsychotic licenced for the short-term management of resistant aggression in people with dementia, and there may be a role for the use of haloperidol in the management of delirium. However, NICE guidance recommends antipsychotics should only be initiated under specialist supervision, such as, by an old age psychiatrist.

Benzodiazepines are associated with worsening cognitive symptoms in people with dementia and their use should therefore be reserved for the management of distress and agitation in the dying phase of the illness.[13]

David's mental capacity was assessed using the appropriate local legal framework (in this case, The Adults with Incapacity Act—see learning point), and the multidisciplinary team concluded that his deteriorating cognitive function meant he was no longer able to make informed decisions about his medical treatment. He and his family continued to participate in the decision-making process, allowing his past and present preferences to be incorporated into his care plan. A Do Not Resuscitate (DNACPR) decision was agreed and a care plan focused on providing comfort, reducing symptom burden, and avoiding excessive medical interventions or hospital admissions. A best-interests meeting concluded that artificial feeding was unlikely to improve David's quality of life, and risked causing unnecessary distress and suffering. He was supported to continue to eat and drink when he was alert enough to do so.

Learning Point

Across the UK, capacity legislation exists to protect people who lack mental capacity and support legally valid decisions to be made about finances, welfare, or medical treatment. All legislation is predicated upon the presumption an individual has capacity until an assessment proves otherwise. In Scotland the Adults with Incapacity Act 2005 (AWIA) states interventions must be the best interpretation of the will and preferences of the person. In England and Wales the Mental Capacity Act 2005 (MCA) is based on a best interests decision using the least restrictive option. In Northern Ireland, the Mental Capacity Act (NI) 2016 bears many similarities to the MCA.[14]

Evidence Base

Researchers have sought to understand thresholds at which a person with impaired cognitive function can still reliably make decisions relating to an advanced care plan.[15] Using the Mini mental state examination (MMSE), a score of 18–20 was considered to be a reliable threshold, however, the tool was not designed to assess the capacity to make decisions, so scoring below this threshold should not exclude people with dementia from taking part in future planning conversations.

Expert Comment

Dementia can affect a person's ability to make decisions because it can affect the parts of the brain involved in remembering, understanding, and processing information. However, this does not necessarily mean that a person with a diagnosis of dementia lacks the capacity to make all decisions.

Personal autonomy should always be promoted and a person's capacity maximized. Capacity legislation states mental capacity is both 'decision-specific' and 'time-specific', meaning that the principles of mental capacity law must be applied each time that a decision needs to be made.

As the patient approached end of life the holistic approach to care continued with non-pharmacological interventions delivered alongside small doses of subcutaneous medication to control distressing symptoms. After 5 weeks, David died peacefully with family and hospice staff present.

Discussion

There are estimated to be 944,000 people living with dementia in the UK and indications that this will increase to 1 million people by 2025 and 2 million by 2051.[16] Dementia is currently the leading cause of death in the UK and one of the major causes of disability and dependency among older people.[17]

People with dementia experience a similar spectrum of symptoms to those with cancer, but often experience them for longer and to a greater severity. Despite this, patients with dementia, especially those who live alone, are less likely to see their GP or have contact with district nurses, and are less likely to be referred to specialist palliative care services.[18]

This case explores some of the challenges, barriers, and facilitators, which exist for people with dementia, their carers, and the healthcare professionals supporting them. It is a good example of how comorbidity impacts on treatment and care decisions and demonstrates the role of specialist palliative care in advanced dementia.

Evidence Base

The European Association of Palliative Care's (EAPC) white paper defines palliative care in dementia using evidence and expert consensus to present 11 domains and 57 recommendations for optimal care. It suggests that dementia is regarded as a terminal illness and that palliative care is fundamental to all dementia treatment and care. It also recommends the delivery of person-centred care, goal setting, continuity, prognostication, symptom control, carer support, education, and training.[19]

Future Advances

An EAPC taskforce is currently developing recommendations specifically to conceptualize advance care planning (ACP) in dementia. It aims to provide a definition and identify how ACP may differ in people where decision-making capacity is likely to be lost at an early point in the disease process compared with illnesses such as cancer.[20]

A Final Word from the Expert

Multi morbidity is common in people with dementia. The most common comorbidity experienced in people with dementia is cancer. Whilst dementia is itself a life limiting condition, many people with dementia will die from the effects of another comorbid condition before they reach the advanced stages of dementia. The symptom burden at end of life in dementia is not dissimilar to those in the advanced stages of cancer, with pain being the most experienced. However, pain in dementia is often under recognized, poorly assessed, and so under managed. This is often due to the impaired communication as a result of the cognitive and capacity changes brought about by dementia. This places the emphasis on clinicians to better understand how pain and other distressing symptoms may be manifested in a person with dementia, and to make best interest decisions on their management.

References

1. Sampson EL, Harrison Dening K. Chapter 27: Palliative and End-of-life Care. In: Dening T, Thomas A, Stewart R, Taylor JP, editors. *Oxford Textbook of Old Age Psychiatry*, 3rd ed. Oxford: Oxford University Press, 2021, pp. 395–396.
2. Van der Steen JT, Ooms ME, van der Wal G, Ribbe MW. Withholding or starting antibiotic treatment in patients with dementia and pneumonia: prediction of mortality with physicians' judgment of illness severity and with specific prognostic models. *Med Decis Making* 2005; 25(2): 210–221.

3. McCarthy M, Addington-Hall J, Altmann D. The experience of dying with dementia: a retrospective study. *Int J Geriatr Psychiatry* 1997; 12(3): 404–409.
4. Morrison RS, Siu AL. A comparison of pain and its treatment in advanced dementia and cognitively intact patients with hip fracture. *J Pain Symptom Manage* 2000; 19(4): 240–248.
5. Lichtner V, Dowding D, Esterhuizen P, et al. Pain assessment for people with dementia: a systematic review of systematic reviews of pain assessment tools. *BMC Geriatr* 2014; 17(14): 138.
6. Wong WM (2018). P2-320: How to do better prognostication in advanced dementia. *Alzheimer's & Dementia* 14: P805–P805.
7. Bakker R. Sensory loss, dementia, and environments. *Generations* 2003; 27: 46–51.
8. Detering K, Fraser, SA, Whiteside K, Silvester W. O-71 Not competent but not silent – a pilot study of ACP with dementia patients. *BMJ Support Palliat Care* 2015; 5: A22–A23.
9. Midtbust MH, Alnes RE, Gjengedal E, Lykkeslet E. Perceived barriers and facilitators in providing palliative care for people with severe dementia: the healthcare professionals' experiences. *BMC Health Serv Res* 2018; 18(1): 709.
10. Simard J. *The End-of-Life Namaste Care™ Program for People with Dementia*. Baltimore, MD: Health Professions Press, 2013.
11. National Collaborating Centre for Mental Health. Dementia: the NICE-SCIE guideline on supporting people with dementia and their carers in health and social care. 2007. Available at: http://www.scie.org.uk/publications/misc/dementia/dementia-fullguideline.pdf
12. Abraha I, Rimland JM, Trotta FM, et al. Systematic review of systematic reviews of non-pharmacological interventions to treat behavioural disturbances in older patients with dementia. *BMJ Open* 2017; 7: e012759.
13. Management of non-cognitive symptoms associated with dementia. *Drug Ther Bull* 2014; 52: 114–118.
14. Ruck Keene A, Ward A. With and without 'best interests': the Mental Capacity Act 2005, the Adults With Incapacity (Scotland) Act 2000 and constructing decisions. *Int J Ment Health Capacity Law* 2016; 17.
15. Dening KH, Jones L, Sampson EL. Advance care planning for people with dementia: a review. *Int Psychogeriatr* 2011; 23(10): 1535–1551.
16. Wittenberg R, Knapp M, Hu B, et al. The costs of dementia in England. *Int J Geriatr Psychiatry* 2019; 34(7): 1095–1103.
17. Office for National Statistics (ONS 2020). Deaths registered in England and Wales: 2020. Available at: https://www.ons.gov.uk/peoplepopulationandcommunity/birthsdeathsandmarriages/deaths/bulletins/deathsregistrationsummarytables/2020
18. Lloyd-Williams M, Payne S, Dennis M. Specialist palliative care in dementia: patients with dementia are unable to access appropriate palliative care. *BMJ* 2005; 330(7492): 671–672.
19. Van der Steen JT, Radbruch L, Hertogh CM, et al. White paper defining optimal palliative care in older people with dementia: a Delphi study and recommendations from the European Association for Palliative Care. *Palliat Med* 2014; 28(3): 197–209.
20. Van der Steen JT et al. Advance care planning in dementia: conceptualisation and recommendations for practice, policy and research. Available at: https://www.eapcnet.eu/eapc-groups/task-forces/advance-care-planning-in-dementia/

CASE

26 Learning Disabilities

Jamie Richardson

Expert: Valerie Potter

Case history

Andrew was a 67-year-old male with a moderate learning disability (LD). He had lived in a residential home for four years following the death of his mother. He was prescribed risperidone 500 micrograms BD and atorvastatin 20 mg ON. Andrew was non-verbal but used basic signs to communicate his needs. He required assistance with all personal care and support in the community. He attended a day centre four days a week and enjoyed drives to the airport to watch planes land.

Clinical Tip Communication

Patient-specific communication difficulties can prevent people with learning disabilities (PwLD) engaging effectively with health services.[1] Poor communication between healthcare professionals, patients, and carers contribute to excess death rates seen in PwLD.[2] While everyone is an individual, approaches to adapting communication for PwLD may include:

- With the individual
  - Adapted language (e.g. short sentences, frequent pauses)
  - Use of Makaton and other sign-based languages
  - Easy-read documentation
  - Visual and symbolic communication aids (e.g. Picture Exchange Communications System (PECS®))
- Between professionals and carers
  - Hospital passports, including personal information, communication style, etc.
  - Care planning meetings
  - Best interest meetings when a patient lacks capacity

Future Advances Hospital Passports

Hospital Passports have been available for over a decade. Despite extensive use, little evidence exists to show the impact on health outcomes, while the content of passports can vary between hospitals. Future research will need to focus on the effectiveness and standardization of these documents.

While initially settled, over a six-month period Andrew became more distressed, self-injurious, and began throwing objects. Over this period, Andrew lost 8 kg in weight.

Expert Comment

Healthcare professionals (HCPs) need to listen to the person's family and/or usual carers who are often the first to notice a change in a behaviour compared to baseline, which may indicate an underlying problem requiring investigation. Distressed or 'challenging' behaviours can be the means of patients communicating physical illness. Carers must be supported in having the confidence to raise such concerns.

It is important to have baseline knowledge of the person and the use of tools to identify distress can be helpful. For example, the Disability Distress Assessment Tool (DisDAT) helps to identify distress cues in people with limited communication by recording signs and behaviours of contentment, enabling distress to then be identified more clearly.[3]

Expert Comment

When assessing PwLD, it is often extremely useful to have a family member/carer present, to reduce the person's anxiety about what is happening and to provide information on the person's usual presentation helping in the interpretation of the new behaviours.

At an appointment with his GP, the doctor attempted an abdominal examination, but as they palpated Andrew's abdomen, he became distressed and slapped the GP. Following this incident, the GP prescribed Lorazepam 1 mg as required and made an urgent referral to the community LD team for assessment of Andrew's behaviours.

Evidence Base Diagnostic Overshadowing

Diagnostic overshadowing is a tendency to attribute a change in behaviour to a condition such as LD without considering other biopsychosocial causes, risking potentially worrying diagnoses being missed.[4] This can lead to inappropriate referrals, delays in treatment, and excess mortality. Data shows PwLD are at increased risk of a variety of physical health conditions[5] and are three times more likely to die from avoidable medical causes.[2] When health checks are completed, half of adults with LD have an unmet medical need.[6] For children with LD, missed early symptoms are a factor in excess deaths rates, while most excess deaths in young adults with Mild LD are potentially avoidable.[7] The more severe the LD, the higher the risk of premature death.[8]

Ways to reduce the risk of diagnostic overshadowing include communicating directly with the patient, paying attention to behaviour change and non-verbal communication, adjusting the physical environment to make it as comfortable as possible, and taking advice from the people who know the patient best to understand their baseline.[9]

Before being seen by the community LD Team, Andrew had a generalized tonic-clonic seizure. With no history of epilepsy, an ambulance was called. Post-ictal on assessment, he was transferred to hospital.

In the emergency department, Andrew became distressed and aggressive, requiring security to restrain him. With advice from Liaison Psychiatry, he was administered IM Lorazepam 1 mg. He settled enough to allow observations to be completed before being admitted to a side room under the Acute Medicine Team.

Clinical Tip Reasonable Adjustments

Reasonable adjustments are legal requirements placed upon public organizations such as the NHS to make services accessible to people with disabilities including LD.[10] The General Medical Council (GMC) has produced five simple adjustments clinicians could make for PwLD[11]:

1. Offer extra time for appointments, or split appointments to allow the patient time to digest important information.
2. Tailor communication to the patient, taking care to avoid jargon.
3. Check understanding frequently, considering capacity when understanding is in doubt.
4. Offer early appointments or at quieter times to avoid busy waiting rooms.
5. Demonstrate examinations or procedures on yourself or a carer before attempting it on the patient.

This list is not exhaustive and rather a good starting point. Everyone is an individual, and individual adjustments may be needed.

Following admission Andrew had a second seizure, and the medical team requested a CT head scan. In the radiology department, Andrew became distressed when asked to lie on the bed and the procedure was abandoned.

Expert Comment

The style of communication used must be tailored to the individual and be non-technical and non-threatening. Written information should be offered in an Easy Read format; there are booklets available from several sources covering different medical investigations and treatments. It is helpful to have the patient's usual carer present during any procedures and for the person to visit the unfamiliar environment in advance if possible. Consider adjustments such as relaxation therapies, graded exposure, or if thought to require sedation, seeking help from other hospital specialities such as the learning disability nurse or the anaesthetic team.

A further scan under general anaesthetic was arranged following a best interest meeting. This found a 5 cm mass in his left frontal lobe. A scan of his chest, abdomen, and pelvis found a mass in his thoracic spine and enlarged lymph nodes in his left axilla. The primary site could not be determined. Andrew was referred to the Cancer of Unknown Primary (CUP) Multidisciplinary Team (MDT) for discussion.

Expert Comment

All new patients with a CUP will be presented at CUP MDT to discuss and decide upon the best treatment plan. There should be a palliative care presence at all cancer MDTs to contribute to the decision-making process and to explore issues such as the person's symptom control, advance care planning considerations, and relevant psychosocial factors.

Expert Comment

It is important that PwLD are helped to understand their diagnosis, likely symptomatic course, and prognosis so they have the opportunity to plan ahead and have their wishes and preferences known. Understanding what is causing their symptoms helps reduce anxiety of the unknown and can help them cope with any treatments.

Before the MDT, a carer noticed a Recommended Summary Plan for Emergency Care and Treatment (ReSPECT) form by Andrew's bed. The form stated Andrew was not for resuscitation in the event of cardiac arrest. It contained no details of a discussion with Andrew or carers and cited 'Learning Difficulties' as the rationale for the decision. The carer raised this with the ward sister and consultant, who agreed it was inappropriate and withdrew the form pending the CUP MDT.

Learning Point Do Not Attempt Cardiopulmonary Resuscitation and Learning Disability

Decisions regarding cardiopulmonary resuscitation (CPR) can be complex and are covered in more detail in Case 46. For PwLD, decisions regarding escalation of care should be taken in the same way as the general population, consulting the patient and/or family and carers as appropriate. Reviews have found that 73% of adults with LD had a DNACPR decision at the time of death, with decisions more likely for patients with moderate, severe, or profound LD and for those over 65.[2]

However, of the decisions in place, 29% were incorrectly completed with the three main reasons being;

- No evidence of a decision-making process
- Documentation problems such as missing signatures or incorrect patient details
- Inappropriate rationale for the decision such as LD without qualification

This last point is particularly concerning. PwLD are more likely to experience poor health[5, 12] which may be an appropriate reason for not escalating care. LD alone should never be considered an appropriate rationale and clinicians should be prepared to challenge such decisions if they occur.

At the CUP MDT, it was agreed Andrew had advanced cancer which would require further investigation to actively treat. Given Andrew's distress with investigations thus far, alongside the advanced nature of disease and his deteriorating performance status, it was agreed Andrew would not tolerate burdensome treatment and was for best supportive care. This was discussed with Andrew and his care staff. It was unclear how much Andrew understood.

Learning Point End of Life Planning

Children begin to understand death is a permanent, irreversible state from the age of five.[13] For PwLD, this understanding may be delayed, if it develops at all. With a limited understanding of death, it may be difficult to discuss end of life care. However, evidence suggests these discussions can be completed effectively, with 79% of discussions about death with PwLD described as 'comfortable/somewhat comfortable' in one study,[14] and while the fear of death did not increase, anxiety symptoms improved significantly.

Barriers to involving PwLD in end of life decisions includes patients not being aware of the terminal diagnosis, assumptions around capacity, communication difficulties, and resorting to a third-party decision maker.[15] Potential solutions to these problems include link nursing between LD and palliative services, training in non-verbal communication, longer appointment times, use of screening tools for physical symptoms, and adjustments such as relaxing of visiting hours.[16]

Expert Comment

It is important to involve PwLDs in developing their awareness of death. This should start before a diagnosis of a life limiting condition with conversations encouraged which normalize dying. Events such as deaths in the media or of family members or friends can be used to start these discussions as can campaigns such as Dying Matters Awareness week. This helps PwLD to be more prepared for the death of those they are close to and ultimately for their own.[17]

The palliative care team spoke to Andrew about his preferences for care. Using the example of his mother's death, they discussed dying and where this could occur. Andrew's preference was to return to his residential home.

Expert Comment

Advance care planning (ACP) is the term used to describe the conversation between people, their families, and their carers about their future wishes and priorities for care. Some groups are less likely to have the opportunity to plan for a 'good death' and this includes PwLD. It is vital PwLD are offered the opportunity to engage with the ACP process allowing them to make choices for their end of life care and to make clear their preferences. If the person does not have capacity to fully participate in such discussions, it remains important to open up honest conversations about the future and to support them to identify and share their wishes. This may require the use of different formats to adapt the process to that which works best for them and there are toolkits available developed specifically to support PwLD with ACP. It is important to involve those close to the person and to document (in an accessible format), regularly review, and share the plan with relevant HCPs.

With the support of his community palliative care team and an increased care package and equipment from social care, Andrew was discharged a month later. Andrew deteriorated further once home with increased fatigue, weakness, and reduced oral intake. End of life symptoms included moderate terminal agitation and upper respiratory tract secretions which were managed by the community palliative care team in conjunction with Andrew's GP and home staff. He died after four weeks at home.

Expert Comment

It can be particularly difficult for PwLD to adjust from their usual, familiar environment to another. PwLD must be supported to remain at home if this is their preferred place of care and death, which it often is. To achieve this, supported living environments and residential units need to ensure they can provide continuity of care up to and including the dying phase. This requires care providers to develop their staff's knowledge and confidence in caring for people at end of life as well as providing effective support and supervision.

Vital to remaining at home is access to community specialist palliative care services. The Confidential Inquiry into premature deaths of people with a learning disability (CIPOLD)[18] found that for many PwLD who were dying, end of life care was not coordinated and the support for the person and their families could have been improved. It also identified that PwLD were less likely to have access to specialist palliative care services and opioid analgesia than a comparison group of people without a learning disability.[17] It is imperative PwLD who have palliative and/or end of life needs are referred in a timely manner to their local palliative care team and that palliative care specialists are competent and confident in delivering care to PwLDs.

Expert Comment

A lack of collaborative working between learning disability and specialist palliative care services is recognized with PwLD having reduced access to specialist palliative care. An established relationship between the two services does not traditionally exist which leads to a poor understanding of each other's role and the services each provides, and for PwLD, a poor referral rate to palliative care.[16] Joined-up working, with cross-sector training, is required to ensure staff working in learning disability services have an understanding of the role and how to access palliative and end of life care, and that those working within palliative and end of life care services receive learning disability training.[17]

Discussion

Medical care for PwLD is the same as the general population. As we have seen with Andrew's case, it is the patient journey which may deviate from the norm for a variety of patient, clinician, and institutional factors. Aiming to address these factors, be it through training, reasonable adjustments, or structural reforms, we can hope to improve care for PwLD at what can be a confusing and distressing time in their lives.

A Final Word from the Expert

This case demonstrates the challenges and barriers that PwLD and a terminal diagnosis often experience. There was a delay in diagnosis when a change in Andrew's behaviour from baseline should have prompted further investigation. In hospital, reasonable adjustments were not initially made to facilitate the necessary investigations and then to explain the findings together with the MDT outcome. The DNACPR form was completed to an unacceptable standard citing learning disabilities as the reason CPR would be inappropriate. It is essential that the communication format is tailored to suit the individual so that they can understand the information provided and are offered the opportunity to engage with ACP discussions. Once home, a collaborative approach between the person, family, carers, LD, and palliative care team is paramount to ensure that high quality and equitable end of life care is delivered to PwLD.

References

1. Backer C, Chapman M, Mitchell D. Access to secondary healthcare for people with intellectual disabilities: a review of the literature. *J Appl Res Intellect Disabil* 2009; 22(6): 514–525.

2. University of Bristol; The Learning Disabilities Mortality Review (LeDeR) Programme Annual Report 2020; University of Bristol; 2021. Available at: https://leder.nhs.uk/images/annual_reports/LeDeR-bristol-annual-report-2020.pdf
3. St Oswald's Hospice; Distress and Discomfort Assessment Tool (DisDAT); St Oswald's Hospice. Available at: https://www.stoswaldsuk.org/how-we-help/we-educate/education/resources/disability-distress-assessment-tool-disdat/
4. Neurotrauma Law Nexus; Neuroglossary; Neurotrauma Law Nexus; 2022. Available at: https://www.neuroglossary.com/neuroglossary
5. Liao P, Vajdic C, Trollor J, Reppermund S. Prevalence and incidence of physical health conditions in people with intellectual disability – a systematic review. *PLoS One* 2021; 16(8): e0256294.
6. Baxter H, Lowe K, Houston H, et al. Previously unidentified morbidity in patients with intellectual disability. *Br J Gen Pract* 2006; 56(523): 93–98.
7. Hirvikoski T, Boman M, Tideman M, Lichtenstein P, Butwicka A. Association of intellectual disability with all-cause and cause-specific mortality in Sweden. *JAMA Netw Open* 2021; 4(6): e2113014.
8. Abuga JA, Kariuki SM, Kinyanjui SM, et al. Premature mortality, risk factors, and causes of death following childhood-onset neurological impairments: a systematic review. *Front Neurol* 2021; 12: 627824.
9. Blair J. *Diagnostic Overshadowing: See Beyond the Diagnosis; University of Hartfordshire.* Available at: http://www.intellectualdisability.info/changing-values/diagnostic-overshadowing-see-beyond-the-diagnosis
10. NHS England. Reasonable adjustments; NHS England. Available at: https://www.england.nhs.uk/learning-disabilities/improving-health/reasonable-adjustments/
11. General Medical Council; Learning disabilities; General Medical Council. Available at: https://www.gmc-uk.org/ethical-guidance/ethical-hub/learning-disabilities
12. Cooper SA, McLean G, Guthrie B, et al. Multiple physical and mental health comorbidity in adults with intellectual disabilities: population-based cross-sectional analysis. *BMC Fam Pract* 2015; 16: 110.
13. Marie Curie. How grief may affect children. Marie Curie. 2020. Available at: https://www.mariecurie.org.uk/help/support/bereaved-family-friends/supporting-grieving-child/grief-affect-child
14. Stancliffe RJ, Wiese MY, Read S, et al. Does talking about end of life with adults with intellectual disability cause emotional discomfort or psychological harm? *J Appl Res Intellect Disabil* 2020; 34(2): 659–669.
15. Kirkendall A, Linton K, Farris S. Intellectual disabilities and decision making at end of life: a literature review. *J Appl Res Intellect Disabil* 2016; 30(6): 982–994.
16. Adam E, Sleeman KE, Brearley S, et al. The palliative care needs of adults with intellectual disabilities and their access to palliative care services: a systematic review. *Palliat Med* 2020; 34(8): 1006–1018.
17. Palliative Care for People with Learning Disabilities (PCPLD) Network; Delivering high quality end-of-life care for people who have a learning disability; NHS England. 2017. Available at: https://www.england.nhs.uk/publication/delivering-high-quality-end-of-life-care-for-people-who-have-a-learning-disability/
18. Confidential Inquiry into Premature Deaths of People with Learning Disability (CIPOLD); Final Report; University of Bristol. 2013. Available at: http://www.bristol.ac.uk/cipold/reports/

CASE

27 Delivering Palliative Care to the Patient with Severe Mental Illness

Daniel Hughes

Expert: Maggie Bisset

Case history

Yusuf (50 years old) moved to the UK with his parents aged six. After a difficult childhood, with a physically violent alcohol-dependent father, Yusuf started working in construction. His first episode of psychosis was in his mid-twenties, when he started to hear voices and believed his co-workers were plotting his assassination. He was diagnosed with paranoid schizophrenia. Subsequently, Yusuf's engagement with mental health teams was intermittent, and he required psychiatric admissions regularly, predominantly under the Mental Health Act (MHA). Yusuf has been under the community mental health team, treated with various oral and long acting intramuscular (depot) antipsychotics.

Clinical Tip

All references to MHA refer to the Mental Health Act of England and Wales (1983), separate (although not dissimilar) legislature exists for Scotland and Northern Island. The same is true of the Mental Capacity Act (2005). Internationally, there are many variations of similar legal approaches to the treatment of mental disorders and those who lack capacity.

Learning Point Schizophrenia

Schizophrenia is a psychotic illness characterized by disturbances in thinking, self-experience, cognition, affect, and behaviour. Core features include delusional beliefs, hallucinations (a perception in the absence of external stimulus) and disordered thinking (demonstrated by disordered speech). Symptoms must have been present for at least a month and not be due to another health condition or psychoactive substances. Some experience a relapsing and remitting illness course, whilst others have enduring symptoms.[1]

Learning Point Severe Mental Illness (SMI)

SMI refers to a group of debilitating mental illnesses that severely impair one's ability to engage in functional and occupational activities. It includes schizophrenia, schizoaffective disorder, and bipolar affective disorder.

After Yusuf's mother died suddenly, he stopped attending clinic, and taking his medications, denying he was mentally unwell. Yusuf accused neighbours of breaking into his flat and was seen shouting to himself. He was self-neglecting, losing considerable weight. Yusuf was admitted to a psychiatric ward on a section two of the MHA. He initially declined physical examination and bloods. Yusuf smoked 40 cigarettes a day and appeared breathless on mild exertion.

Expert Comment Social Isolation

People with SMI often have few or no social contacts[2] which may enhance their vulnerability as they approach end of life.

Evidence Base Parity of Esteem

People with SMI die between 15 and 20 years earlier than those without.[3] This is multifactorial; including late presentation, delayed diagnosis, insufficient treatment of physical illnesses, pharmacological interactions of antipsychotic medication and associated unhealthy lifestyle (including poor diet, high smoking rates, excessive alcohol consumption, and lack of exercise).[4] Increased rates of suicide also contribute towards this mortality gap.[5] Comorbid SMI and physical health diagnoses can lead to unnoticed somatic symptoms, and complex pharmacological interactions may lead to undetected side effects or complications.

Physical illnesses that may typically be treated by palliative care teams are commonly seen in those with SMI, and often have worse outcomes. Cancer screening rates are lower.[6] Evidence regarding incidence of various cancers in SMI is highly variable; prostate and colorectal cancer appear to be less

Expert Comment Diagnostic Overshadowing

First described in intellectual disabilities, diagnostic overshadowing occurs when symptoms of physical illness are attributed to a patient's mental illness, resulting in misdiagnosis, and delayed treatment.

prevalent, whilst breast, and lung cancers have a higher incidence. The evidence for higher mortality rates in those diagnosed with cancer alongside SMI is unequivocal.[5]

Other non-oncological conditions which may benefit from a palliative care approach are also thought to be more prevalent in an SMI population, with increased rates of chronic obstructive pulmonary disease,[6] heart failure,[7] and dementia[8].

Learning Point Mental Health Act (MHA)

Detaining under a section two (for assessment, lasting up to 28 days) or section three (for treatment, lasting up to six months initially) requires two doctors (one of whom must be 'section 12 approved') and an approved mental health practitioner (AMP). Such sections cannot be used in public places or in A&E. In emergencies, shorter sections can be applied by one doctor (S5(2), for up to 72 hours) or one nurse (S5(4), up to six hours). Most sections can be transferred between hospitals (e.g. psychiatric to physical health wards).

For more information, see: https://www.nhs.uk/mental-health/social-care-and-your-rights/mental-health-and-the-law/mental-health-act/

Yusuf had recently presented at his general practice reporting his neighbours had tampered with his medication, resulting in diarrhoea, and stomach-ache. This was ascribed to mental illness. Once on the ward, Yusuf was restarted on antipsychotics, with some reduction in symptom intensity. He continued to voice persecutory delusions regarding his neighbours and so was placed on a section three once his section two expired.

Learning Point Persecutory Delusion

A delusional belief is not based in reality, is fixed, and not in keeping with someone's educational or cultural background.[9] Persecutory delusions are the most frequent delusion, typically involving the belief that someone is being interfered with from the outside.[10] It is important to be aware of the patient's emotional response to a persecutory delusion with a focus on your concern for their wellbeing. It is rarely helpful to overtly challenge a patient's delusion, but rather try to understand why the person believes what they do whilst being open about your own understanding of these beliefs.

On the ward, Yusuf was found collapsed, tachycardic, but normotensive. After transfer to the local acute hospital, he accepted blood tests demonstrating low haemoglobin (55 g/dL) and deranged liver function tests. On examination, there was a palpable left lower quadrant mass. CT scan showed suspected Stage IVB colorectal tumour with liver metastases. Surgical and oncological Multidisciplinary Teams (MDTs) agreed operating would not be in his best interests, but that palliative chemotherapy could be offered. Yusuf was referred to the hospital palliative care team for symptomatic management.

Clinical Tip Palliation in a Psychiatric Hospital?

Whilst having access to emergency treatment for cardiopulmonary resuscitation, psychiatric wards have no capability to cannulate, give intravenous medications, or fluids. Ordering routine investigations can be delayed owing to the practicalities of sending samples to neighbouring laboratories. Mental health nursing staff may have limited experience in caring for complex physical health problems without support.

It is best practice to speak with the psychiatric team to understand what can be achieved on the ward, and what might require transfer to local acute trusts. Treating serious physical illnesses on psychiatric wards can feel isolating, overwhelming, and cause distress to other patients.

At initial review by the palliative care team, Yusuf was reluctant to engage. He understood he had cancer but didn't want to have any further treatment as he wanted to be "left alone". Yusuf hoped to return home imminently. He refused chemotherapy because he didn't "want more needles". Oncology wondered if this could be given under the MHA?

Clinical Tip Treating Physical Health under the Mental Capacity Act (MCA) and Mental Health Act (MHA)

MCA

Assessing someone's capacity is a two-stage test:

Stage one: Is there an impairment of or disturbance in the functioning of the person's mind or brain?
Stage two: Is the impairment or disturbance sufficient that the person lacks the capacity to make that particular decision?

To have capacity a person must be able to:

A. Understand the information relevant to the decision
B. Retain that information
C. Use or weigh that information up in making their decision
D. Communicate their decision

Capacity assessments are time and issue-specific (not 'Does this person have capacity regarding treatment for their cancer?', but rather 'Does this person have capacity to consent to a hemicolectomy to treat their colorectal cancer?').

If someone lacks capacity, they can be given treatment under the MCA (under restriction and/or restraint if necessary) if it is deemed necessary to prevent the person from coming to harm. Any restraint/restriction must be reasonable and proportionate to the likelihood and seriousness of harm. The MCA is not concerned with harm to others.

Decisions concerning potentially life-prolonging treatment must not be motivated by a desire to bring about the patient's death, and must start from a presumption in favour of prolonging life.[11]

Repeatedly restraining someone to give them chemotherapy may not be deemed proportionate if the likelihood of symptomatic or life expectancy improvement is small. Decisions made under the MCA must consider a patient's best interests and be least restrictive.

MHA

The MHA can be used to treat physical illness only when it is 'part of, or ancillary to, treatment for mental disorder (e.g. treating wounds which are self-inflicted as a result of mental disorder)'.[12] An overdose could be medically treated under the MHA if part of a wider treatment of mental disorder, although practically these cases are complex and often involve legal teams.

Following exploration of Yusuf's capacity to make decisions regarding receiving chemotherapy it was felt that he had capacity to refuse this. After discussion with the mental health liaison team, it was agreed that giving chemotherapy under the MHA was not appropriate.

Yusuf requested to self-discharge from hospital, where he believed his neighbours had followed him. He reported being in considerable abdominal pain. He had not requested any analgesia which had been prescribed 'as required'. After discussion, he agreed to take 5 mg oramorph which helped. Subsequently regular analgesia was prescribed, with laxatives, and antiemetics to prevent side effects.

Yusuf's mental state improved and the MHLT 'rescinded' the section three. He was agreeable to staying in hospital for a few more days to arrange a new bed for home. The palliative team continued to review Yusuf, but he remained reluctant to speak with them and could be dismissive, often saying he wants to 'go home to die'. The palliative care clinicians noticed that they often left Yusuf until the end of their ward

Expert Comment Refusal of Treatment

The palliative team need to be alert to careful exploration to ensure Yusuf is not acting out his internal world in this treatment refusal—a world that embodies deep feelings of unworthiness, neglect, un-verbalized notions of suicide, or never having mattered to anyone or been in receipt of someone's affection.

round, sometimes missing him out altogether. Yusuf explained to the palliative care nurse that he doesn't like seeing them and can 'eff and blind' at them because it is a 'constant reminder' that he is dying.

Expert Comment Psychodynamic Principles

Palliative care is highly relational in its approach. It can be difficult to establish relationships with people with SMI who may not readily attach. The following psychodynamic principles start to explain the psychology of this interaction:

Transference: the qualities a patient projects onto a clinician based on their previous experiences of relationships, e.g. Yusuf may see a female palliative nurse as overbearing because of his relationship with his mother.

Countertransference: the feeling a clinician has about their patient, based on historical, or current experiences, e.g. the palliative care doctor becomes increasingly paternalistic towards the reluctant to engage Yusuf owing to his personal experience with his teenage son.

Projective identification: a patient unconsciously projects feelings they hold onto others, e.g. Yusuf feels the ward staff want to kill him representing an internal wish to no longer be alive.

Clinical Tip Risk Assessment

It is important to ask a patient with SMI about whether they are having thoughts of ending their life or harming themselves, including towards the end of life. It is essential to consider access to end of life medications. Suicidal ideation should be discussed with a mental health professional for additional support and care planning.

Suicide risk in palliative care appears low[13]; including for those cared for at home[14] and in hospices.[15] It may be because deteriorating physical health makes suicide practically difficult, or there is a fundamentally different psychological response with a lessened propensity to act. It is also possible suicide is difficult to determine as cause of death.

As Yusuf's discharge approached, the team were concerned that he had access to large quantities of opioid and other sedating medications. Although he had started to engage with the hospital palliative care team, there was a feeling that once the community palliative care team took over his care Yusuf would quickly disengage. Yusuf chose hospice as his preferred place of death, but hospice managers were reluctant to accept someone with SMI who had been on a recent section and questioned where his mental health support would come from if he was admitted. As a result of these complexities, as Yusuf deteriorated physically, he ended up being admitted to an acute hospital once again where he died the following day.

Expert Comment Planning for Death in Severe Mental Illness

As death approaches, people with SMI may be cared for in acute hospitals because of the complexity of needs and the practical fragmentation of resources between mental health, primary care, and palliative care. When psychiatric and palliative care systems are organized in mutually exclusive ways this may undermine the notion of palliative care, particularly alleviation of suffering.

Actively dying and becoming unconsciousness is a time of great dependence and vulnerability. As consciousness loosens historical traumatic experiences can surface. The psychological care environment when someone is dying always needs to be considered carefully in SMI. This may include attending to sensory stimuli, 'being with' when there may be times of hallucinations or delirium, or 'leaving alone' when presence is too intrusive or frightening.

Expert Comment Mental Health Act in the Acute Hospital

Often a patient on a section of the MHA in an acute hospital will require a 1:1 RMN (Registered Mental Health Nurse) with them. They can be an invaluable source of support and information regarding the patient's mental state. Such patients should be known to the local mental health liaison team (MHLT), who will determine the frequency of their review.

Expert Comment Advance Care Planning in Severe Mental Illness

Advance care planning discussions can bypass people with SMI as there may be a fear of provoking psychological instability and may involve complex capacity discussions. Working collaboratively with involved mental health teams can improve such conversations. Someone with SMI may feel uncomfortable contemplating any mental, spiritual, or social suffering, given their historical traumatic experiences.

Discussion

This case typifies the journey a patient with SMI takes through the physical healthcare system, including late presentation, poor prognosis, diagnostic overshadowing, and navigation of the seemingly labyrinthine community psychiatric supports. The point whereby those with both physical and mental illnesses interact with acute medical services can be bewildering for patients and clinicians alike and may incorporate both MHA and MCA. By employing communication skills and having a basic understanding of the psychodynamic principles described within this case, the palliative care clinician will have a better chance of engaging with their patient, improving outcomes.

Evidence is limited regarding consensus approaches to delivering palliative care to those with SMI. Qualitative evidence available points to the need to adopt multidisciplinary and multi-professional care, alongside a need for extensive staff training.[16] These patients are not receiving the palliative care they should be, with both more research, and collective clinical experience being required to further shape and improve care.

A Final Word from the Expert

This case helps deepen understanding of how to identify and attend to a person's mental vulnerability at the interplay between physical and psychiatric symptoms, alongside other sources of psychological suffering over time. Practitioners need to remain curious regarding dependence and uncertainty as death approaches, whilst considering communication, and psychological skills as distinct entities. Clinicians must be able to identify and attend directly to overwhelming fear and anxiety states that are unspoken whilst coordinating palliative care where someone's psychiatric needs are complex, unpredictable, and require dynamic assessment of informed consent. Building trust over time is of fundamental significance where a person's processing of perceptual information or their beliefs about their physical illness may obstruct acceptance of care. Times of psychiatric crisis can be better predicated if there is collaboration with colleagues in mental health and clinical problems are shared.

There is also a need to grow the expertise of mental health practitioners in the identification and understanding of prognosis of physical life-limiting illness to enable them to better support someone who is dying. To achieve this an interface between relevant multidisciplinary teams (MDTs) is needed. Sometimes an individual's mental health needs will be greater than their physical health needs as dying approaches and vice-versa, emphasizing that a blended approach is necessary to best alleviate symptoms.

References

1. McGrath J, Saha S, Chant D, Welham J. Schizophrenia: a concise overview of incidence, prevalence, and mortality. *Epidemiol Rev* 2008; 30(1): 67–76.
2. Wiersma D. Needs of people with severe mental illness. *Acta Psychiatrica Scandinavica* 2006; 113: 115–119.
3. Thornicroft G. Physical health disparities and mental illness: the scandal of premature mortality. *Br J Psychiatry* 2011; 199(6): 441–442.
4. Laursen TM, Munk-Olsen T, Vestergaard M. Life expectancy and cardiovascular mortality in persons with schizophrenia. *Curr Opin Psychiatry* 2012; 25(2): 83–88.

5. Grassi L, Riba M. Cancer and severe mental illness: bi-directional problems and potential solutions. *Psycho-oncology* 2020; 29(10): 1445–1451.
6. Himelhoch S, Lehman A, Kreyenbuhl J, Daumit G, Brown C, Dixon L. Prevalence of chronic obstructive pulmonary disease among those with serious mental illness. *Am J Psychiatry* 2004; 161(12): 2317–2319.
7. Correll CU, Solmi M, Veronese N, et al. Prevalence, incidence and mortality from cardiovascular disease in patients with pooled and specific severe mental illness: a large-scale meta-analysis of 3,211,768 patients and 113,383,368 controls. *World Psychiatry* 2017; 16(2): 163–180.
8. Cai L, Huang J. Schizophrenia and risk of dementia: a meta-analysis study. *Neuropsychiatr Dis Treat* 2018; 14: 2047.
9. Walton H. Fish's Outline of Psychiatry. Edited by Max Hamilton. Bristol: John Wright & Sons, 1978.
10. Oyebode F. Sims' Symptoms in the Mind: An Introduction To Descriptive Psychopathology. London: *Elsevier Health Sciences*, 2008.
11. General Medical Council. Treatment and Care Towards The End Of Life: Good Practice In Decision Making. London: General Medical Council, 2010.
12. Great Britain. Welsh Office, Great Britain. Department of Health. Code of practice: Mental Health Act 1983. The Stationery Office, 1999.
13. Dormer NR, McCaul KA, Kristjanson LJ. Risk of suicide in cancer patients in Western Australia, 1981–2002. *Med J Aust* 2008; 188(3): 140–143.
14. Ripamonti C, Filiberti A, Totis A, De Conno F, Tamburini M. Suicide among patients with cancer cared for at home by palliative-care teams. *Lancet* 1999; 354(9193): 1877–1878.
15. Grzybowska P, Finlay I. The incidence of suicide in palliative care patients. *Palliat Med* 1997: 11(4): 313–316.
16. Edwards D, Anstey S, Coffey M, Gill P, Mann M, Meudell A, Hannigan B. End of life care for people with severe mental illness: Mixed methods systematic review and thematic synthesis (the MENLOC study). *Palliat Med* 2021; 35(10): 1747–1760.

CASE

28 Symptom Management in Organ Failure

Stephanie Lister-Flynn and Stephanie Ainley

Expert: Emma Murphy

Case history

Fred, a 74-year-old man with type II diabetes mellitus, hypertension, congestive cardiac failure, had end-stage kidney disease (ESKD) secondary to diabetes. He was on renal replacement therapy (RRT), with a dialysis vintage of 8 years, was anuric, and dialysed three times a week via a brachial arteriovenous fistula. He was referred to the community palliative care team (CPCT) due to frailty, increasing symptom burden, deterioration despite dialysis, and to commence advance care planning (ACP) discussions.

Expert Comment Identifying Symptoms

In patients with ESKD, symptoms are often under-recognized and undertreated by their healthcare teams. It is important to assess symptoms proactively alongside dialysis and the use of a valid symptom measurement can help identify symptoms that may otherwise be unrecognized. There are measures in use within renal settings that have been adapted and validated for patients with renal disease. In the UK, the Palliative Outcome Scale Symptom module (POS-S Renal) (see www.pos-pal.org) has been validated in ESKD and assesses a range of the most common physical and psychological symptoms experienced by patients with renal disease.[1] Incorporating symptom management guidelines with valid symptom measures into routine clinical practice in advanced renal disease is key to improving care and person-centred outcomes.

Expert Comment Dialysis Treatment Control Strategies

Consideration of dialysis regimen may help with the management of symptoms alongside pharmacological and non-pharmacological strategies. Physical symptoms unique to dialysis may include pain caused by vascular access, fatigue due to inadequate dialysis prescription and inadequate dry weight, poor appetite, muscle cramps, pruritus, and restless legs due to uraemia. Working alongside renal teams to understand which physical symptoms could be improved with the modification of dialysis regimen is key to improving patients' health related quality of life.

It is important to understand and communicate the evidence on survival for patients with ESKD in whom dialysis has yet to be initiated and for patients considering dialysis withdrawal. Whilst there is clear evidence that those over the age of 75 years treated with RRT can expect to live longer than patients managed conservatively without dialysis, this survival advantage diminishes when patients have higher comorbidity and poor functional status.[2]

On review, one of Fred's main symptoms was uraemic pruritus, affecting his sleep and leading to low mood. Initially he trialled menthol cream and antihistamines with minimal effect. Gabapentin 100 mg (post dialysis) caused daytime drowsiness, but he tolerated pregabalin 25 mg (post dialysis) with minimal side effects, leading to improved pruritus and sleep quality.

Learning Point and Evidence Base Uraemic Pruritus

Uraemic pruritus is a common symptom in ESKD both in dialysed patients and those managed conservatively (see Figure 28.1). It is associated with a poor quality of life including low mood and sleep disturbance.[3] It can be localized or generalized, intermittent or constant, and tends to be worse at night.

Management will depend on the individual patient's circumstances but should involve general measures such as prescribing regular emollients. Dry skin is common in patients with ESKD and while it is not believed to be the sole cause for pruritus, it may exacerbate it.

For localized pruritus, capsaicin cream 0.025–0.075% can be tried. It can cause a burning sensation at the site of application which may affect tolerability.

At present gabapentinoids are the only treatment with good evidence of effect for uraemic pruritus. This was shown in the meta-analysis 'Interventions for itch in people with advanced chronic kidney disease', which found that gabapentinoids had the most evidence of any intervention, both in effect size and number of studies.[4]

Based on this and earlier systematic reviews, gabapentin and pregabalin can be trialled for generalized pruritus. They require low starting doses based on renal function and close monitoring for side effects, particularly drowsiness. Both medications are removed by dialysis, so for this group of patients it is recommended to give doses post-haemodialysis.[5]

UVB phototherapy may also be considered, with some randomized controlled trials (RCT) showing evidence of effect, although this is not supported by more recent trials.[6] Treatment involves multiple sessions per week over a few months, which may not be practical for patients with poor mobility or a short prognosis.

Although antihistamines are often prescribed for uraemic pruritus, there is little evidence that they provide benefit. An exception to this may be doxepin, which is a tricyclic antidepressant with antihistamine activity and showed some effect in a single small RCT.[7]

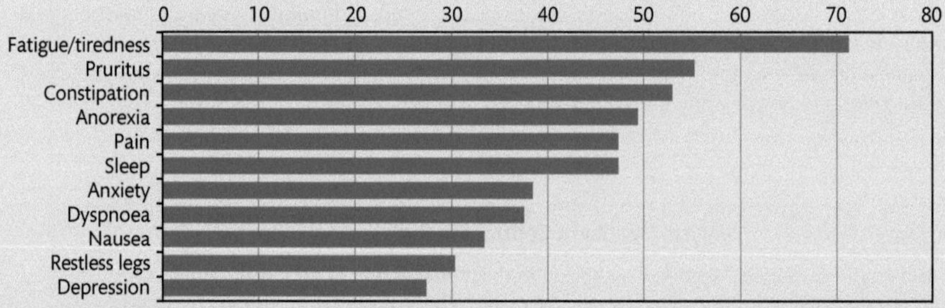

Figure 28.1 Graph to show the weighted prevalence of symptoms (%) in ESKD from systematic review

Reproduced with permission from Murtagh FE, Addington-Hall J, Higginson IJ. The prevalence of symptoms in end-stage renal disease: a systematic review. *Adv Chronic Kidney Dis* 2007; 14, 82–99.

Clinical Tip Anxiety and Depression

Renal failure also has significant psychiatric comorbidity (see Figure 28.1). In ESKD prevalence rates are found to be 12-52% for anxiety and 5–58% for depression, significantly higher than general population rates.[8] The more intensive the RRT regimen, the higher the rates of depression. In addition, there appears to be an established link between depression and negative outcomes, such as increased mortality and hospitalization.[9] It is therefore vital that patients are screened for anxiety and depression throughout their renal disease trajectory, using validated screening scales, to guide intervention.[9]

Fred also reported generalized bilateral neuropathic leg pain, likely secondary to diabetic neuropathy. Due to the large area of pain and generalized nature, it was felt to be unsuitable for capsaicin cream. Attempts to increase his pregabalin dose led to increased drowsiness and he agreed to a trial of oxycodone immediate release 1–2 mg 4 hourly prn. This had some effect on his pain, but Fred found the 4-hourly dosing burdensome, so the oxycodone was switched to a buprenorphine 5 microgram/hour patch with good effect.

Learning Point Pain (Opioids)

Studies suggest that at least half of dialysis patients experience pain (47–67%) (Figure 28.1), with a similar prevalence in those with ESKD being managed conservatively without dialysis.[8, 10, 11] In the last weeks of life, pain is reported more commonly by ESKD patients compared to patients dying from advanced cancer.[12] Pain is often multifactorial, commonly related to neuropathy, vascular disease, restless legs, bone pain, chest pain, muscle soreness, headaches, fistulae, and haemodialysis complications.[10, 12]

Pain is often underrecognized and undertreated in this patient population for a variety of reasons, including a lack of focus on symptom management early in the disease trajectory, uncertainty in pain assessment, and fear of opioid toxicity.[10] The evidence base for potential of toxicity in severe renal impairment is limited, and due to potential impact on both renal and hepatic clearance, reduced protein binding and increased central nervous system (CNS) sensitivity, opioid prescribing should always be at low doses and titrated cautiously.[5]

In severe renal impairment strong opioids with no clinically relevant active metabolites are preferred, e.g., alfentanil, buprenorphine, fentanyl, and methadone.[5] Morphine and diamorphine should be avoided in severe renal impairment due to accumulation and adverse effects; oxycodone is often used pragmatically in mild-moderate impairment in practice but should be used cautiously in severe renal impairment.[5] At the end of life, fentanyl is generally advised. Alfentanil is often used in continuous subcutaneous infusions due to familiarity and volume but is less useful as a breakthrough option due to short half-life. In RRT, drug choices tend to be similar as above, with the four drugs listed above felt to be generally safe and other opioids needing closer monitoring.[5]

Learning Point Pain (Neuropathic)

Pain in ESKD is often neuropathic in origin, so adjuvant analgesics should be considered alongside opioids. Neuropathies are common features in advanced kidney disease, and studies suggest that almost a third of patients report 'numbness/tingling in hands or feet'.[10, 12]

Tricyclic antidepressants including amitriptyline and nortriptyline can be considered for neuropathic pain, but cautious dosing should be used and avoided in cardiac comorbidity.[5] Dose adjustments are not required for dialysis.[5] Anticonvulsants including gabapentin and pregabalin are also used for neuropathic pain; however, all should be used with caution and at low doses due to possible accumulation. As previously stated, due to dialysis clearance, for these patients it is advised to administer gabapentin and pregabalin doses soon after dialysis.

Fred also experienced leg oedema and skin breakdown; in agreement with his renal team, his furosemide dose was increased with good effect. Advance care planning (ACP) conversations started, as Fred wanted to explore the possibility of stopping dialysis due to the impact on his quality of life. It was agreed the CPCT would liaise with his renal team and follow up on these discussions in two weeks' time.

Expert Comment Nausea

Nausea is common in ESKD and antiemetic choice should be based on the suspected underlying cause. It is recommended that all antiemetics should be commenced at a lower than usual dose and titrated slowly.[5] Haloperidol is recommended first-line for nausea secondary to uraemia. For nausea at end of life, either low-dose haloperidol or levomepromazine may be effective, although levomepromazine in particular can cause drowsiness.

Expert Comment Advance Care Planning

Patients with chronic kidney disease (CKD) prefer to have ACP discussions earlier in the disease trajectory.[13] However, these conversations are often challenging, and evidence suggests that nephrologists tend not to engage in ACP with patients.[14] Factors that contribute to low adoption of ACP include unpredictable trajectories, prognostic uncertainty, and lack of time by treating teams.[15] The illness trajectory experienced by dialysis patients may be similar to other chronic diseases, characterized by frequent hospital admissions and acute declines in the last year of life. ACP discussions should therefore be integrated proactively early in the course of illness, alongside active dialysis treatment, as well as reactive discussions when patients are deteriorating despite dialysis.

Clinical Tip Advance Care Planning

Whilst palliative care consultations are associated with improved rate and extent of ACP in patients with CKD, the technological focus of dialysis treatment can be challenging to change as end of life nears.[16] Integrating palliative care and supportive care upstream in the illness trajectory is key to ensure that patients with ESKD receive the care that is consistent with their values, goals, and preferences.[17] Proactive symptom dialysis rounds and joint renal and palliative outpatient clinics can help identify patients who have been on dialysis but have a poor prognosis and are increasingly less well or symptomatic, or finding it harder to tolerate dialysis and dialysis withdrawal is being considered.

Two months later, Fred decided to stop dialysis and was admitted to his local hospice for end of life care, 5 days after dialysis ceased. He was nauseous secondary to uraemia (serum urea 70 mmol/L) and was commenced on a syringe pump of haloperidol, titrated to 3 mg without significant benefit. This was switched to levomepromazine 6.25 mg over 24 hours via a syringe pump with good effect. He continued to experience leg pain due to a combination of neuropathic pain and increasing peripheral oedema. This was controlled with alfentanil titrated up to 2 mg over 24 hours in his syringe pump. Fred continued to deteriorate with reduced consciousness and died peacefully 6 days after hospice admission and 11 days after his last dialysis session.

Expert Comment Dialysis Withdrawal

More than 4,000 prevalent dialysis patients die each year in the UK. In older patients on RRT, it is common for dialysis to be withdrawn before death and dialysis withdrawal is reported as the third most common cause of death in these patients.[18] Patients on RRT will experience variability in symptoms and survival following dialysis withdrawal, influenced by their comorbid illnesses and renal failure. The average time from dialysis withdrawal to death is approximately 10 days, however, patients may live longer with residual renal function and dogmatic prognostication can cause patient and family distress.[19]

Clinical Tip Dialysis Withdrawal

Symptoms are common and the 'painless uraemic death' is not an accurate description, as most dialysis withdrawal occurs in the context of debilitating pre-existing comorbidities in an elderly frail population. In the last days of life, additional symptoms include myoclonus and pruritis from uraemia, dyspnoea, and oedema from fluid overload, muscle pain due to immobility and poor tissue perfusion. In order to anticipate symptoms and survival following dialysis withdrawal, we must first ask the question 'what is my patient dying from?'.

Future Advances

CKD is highly prevalent and represents a significant disease burden globally: a recent systematic analysis ranked it the twelfth leading cause of death globally.[20] As the prevalence of CKD increases, so too do life-limiting complications, including cardiorenal and hepatorenal syndrome. This prevalence does not appear to be declining as is the pattern with other chronic diseases, meaning increasing reliance on RRT. A future focus on early identification and treatment of risk factors for CKD, including monitoring or cessation of the multitude of causative medications, would go some way to reducing the overall burden of this condition. However, given CKD remains prevalent and will do so for many frail and comorbid patients, a focus on early palliative intervention should be prioritized. A future aim would be to make links with nephrology teams, identifying patients at risk of deteriorating whilst under their care, creating opportunities to meet patients upstream in their illness trajectory to create integrated and early palliative care interventions.

A Final Word from the Expert

This case is a good example of the symptoms, illness trajectories and decision making that a person may experience with end-stage kidney failure (ESKF) on dialysis. Dialysis patients with multiple coexisting diseases are now the norm rather than the exception, with an increasing awareness among nephrology teams of the complexity of their palliative and supportive care needs. As outlined in this case, there are challenges to providing palliative care to this population, including, unpredictable illness trajectories, prognosis, and symptoms. Consideration of the current evidence on identification, assessment and management of their palliative and supportive care needs will help deliver high quality care to patients with end-stage kidney disease.

References

1. Murphy EL, Murtagh FE, Carey I, Sheerin NS. Understanding symptoms in patients with advanced chronic kidney disease managed without dialysis: use of a short patient-completed assessment tool. *Nephron Clin Pract* 2009; 111(1): c74–80.
2. Foote C, Kotwal S, Gallagher M, et al. Survival outcomes of supportive care versus dialysis therapies for elderly patients with end-stage kidney disease: a systematic review and meta-analysis. *Nephrology (Carlton)* 2016; 21: 241–253.
3. Pisoni RL, Wikström B, Elder SJ, et al. Pruritus in haemodialysis patients: international results from the Dialysis Outcomes and Practice Patterns Study (DOPPS), *Nephrol Dial Transplant* 2006; 21(12): 3495–3505.
4. Hercz D, Jiang SH, Webster AC. Interventions for itch in people with advanced chronic kidney disease. Cochrane Database Syst Rev 2020; 12: CD011393.
5. Wilcock A, Howard P, Charlesworth S (eds). *Palliative Care Formulary*, 7th ed. London: Pharmaceutical Press, 2020.
6. Ko MJ, Yang JY, Wu HY, et al. Narrowband ultraviolet B phototherapy for patients with refractory uraemic pruritus: a randomized controlled trial. *Br J Dermatol* 2011; 165(3): 633–639.
7. Pour-Reza-Gholi F, Nasrollahi A, Firouzan A, Nasli Esfahani E, Farrokhi F. Low-dose doxepin for treatment of pruritus in patients on hemodialysis. *Iran J Kidney Dis* 2007; 1(1): 34–37.
8. Murtagh FE, Addington-Hall J, Higginson IJ. The prevalence of symptoms in end-stage renal disease: a systematic review. *Adv Chronic Kidney Dis* 2007; 14: 82–99.
9. Goh ZS, Griva K. Anxiety and depression in patients with end-stage renal disease: impact and management challenges—a narrative review. *Int J Nephrol Renovasc Dis* 2018; 11: 93–102.
10. Chambers EJ, Germain M, Brown E (eds). *Supportive Care for the Renal Patient*. Oxford: Oxford University Press; 2004.

11. Davison SN. Pain in haemodialysis patients: prevalence, etiology, severity and analgesic use. *Am J Kidney Dis* 2003; 42: 1239–1247.
12. Murtagh FE, Addington-Hall J, Edmonds PM, et al. Symptoms in the month before death for stage 5 chronic kidney disease patients managed without dialysis. *J Pain Symptom Manage* 2010; 40(3): 342–352.
13. Davison SN. End-of-life care preferences and needs: perceptions of patients with chronic kidney disease. *Clin J Am Soc Nephrol* 2010; 5(2): 195–204.
14. Tamura MK, Montez-Rath ME, Hall YN, Katz R, O'Hare AM. Advance directives and end-of-life care among nursing home residents receiving maintenance dialysis. *Clin J Am Soc Nephrol* 2017; 12 (3): 435–442.
15. O'Hare AM, Szarka J, McFarland LV, et al. Provider perspectives on advance care planning for patients with kidney disease: whose job is it anyway? *Clin J Am Soc Nephrol* 2016; 11 (5): 855–866.
16. Abdel-Rahman EM, Metzger M, Blackhall L, et al. Association between palliative care consultation and advance palliative care rates: a descriptive cohort study in patients at various stages in the continuum of chronic kidney disease. *J Palliat Med* 2021; 24(4): 536–544.
17. Sudore RL, Lum HD, You JJ, et al. Defining advance care planning for adults: a consensus definition from a multidisciplinary delphi panel. *J Pain Symptom Manage* 2017; 53(5): 821–832.e1.
18. Steenkamp R, Rao A, Fraser S. UK Renal Registry 18th Annual Report Nephron 2016; 132(suppl1):111–144 (December 2015) Chapter 5: Survival and Causes of Death in UK Adult Patients on Renal Replacement Therapy in 2014: National and Centre-specific Analyses
19. Holley JL. Palliative care in end-stage renal disease: illness trajectories, communication, and hospice use. *Adv Chronic Kidney Dis* 2007; 14: 402–408.
20. Bikbov et al. Global, regional, and national burden of chronic kidney disease, 1990–2017: a systematic analysis for the Global Burden of Disease Study 2017. *Lancet* 2020; 395: 709–733.

SECTION 5

Challenging physiology/physical conditions

CASE

29 Rigidity

Constantina Pitsillides

Expert: Lou Wiblin

Case history

Michael, a 74-year-old man, presented to his general practitioner (GP) in December 2019, complaining of stiff legs and difficulty walking. He had a history of ischaemic heart disease and had attended a local falls clinic the previous year. The GP noticed that he shuffled when he walked. After early review from a neurologist, he was diagnosed with Parkinson's disease (PD) and commenced on co-careldopa, 25/100 mg three times daily, at 9am, 1pm, and 5pm.

The onset of the COVID-19 pandemic resulted in social restrictions that limited follow-up. During this time, Michael had telephone follow-ups with his GP as face-to-face clinics were avoided where possible. He was compliant with his medications but had limited family support and lived alone. His one son lived abroad and supportive neighbours helped with food shopping. The PD specialist nurse was also providing telephone follow-up during this time. She had been increasingly concerned as voice changes (low in pitch, growly in nature and difficult to understand) had become apparent, but Michael had told the specialist nurse, 'I'm champion', and, 'I'm grand'. There was the growing concern that he was beginning to show early signs of cognitive impairment and his neighbours contacted his son, who in turn telephoned the GP practice.

Michael was reviewed by his GP in early 2021 when he complained about blurred vision when reading and neck pain. He had suffered multiple falls and was intermittently using a wheelchair, which he had purchased on the internet. The GP was struck by Michael's unsteadiness, staring expression, and difficulty to initiate walking with his feet 'sticking' to the floor. As he rose quickly from his chair in the GP room, he unbalanced and fell backwards, caught by the GP. The rather shaken GP asked for an urgent neurology review.

The neurologist found Michael had a surprised expression with overactive frontalis (furrowed forehead) and reduced vertical eye movements, so looking up and down was difficult. Michael complained his double vision was worse during the eye examination. His voice was indistinct and documented as 'gravelly' by the neurologist. His neck was very rigid compared to his arms and legs. He had very little caution and threw himself backwards into a chair, nearly tipping it backwards. A Montreal Cognitive Assessment (MoCA) cognitive test showed significant cognitive impairment of 16/30, scoring worst in verbal fluency and visuospatial function. Micheal was subsequently diagnosed with Progressive Supranuclear Palsy (PSP); the photo (Figure 29.1) shows the typical facial features of this condition.

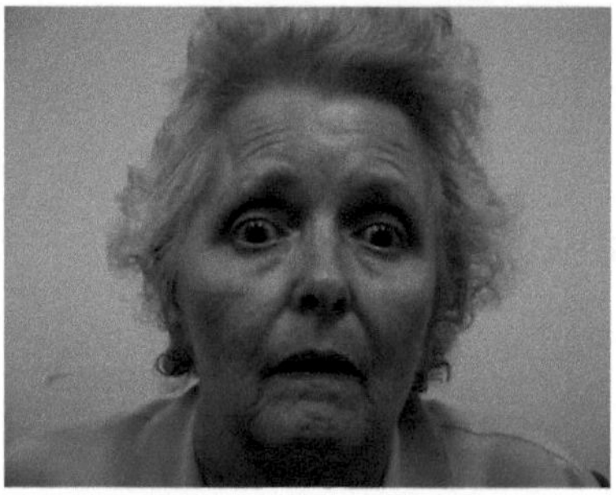

Figure 29.1 Facial characteristics seen in PSP.

Learning Point Progressive Supranuclear Palsy

PSP is a progressive movement disorder which occurs sporadically. There is often a delay in the diagnosis of PSP and often patients are diagnosed later in their disease course. They may initially present to memory clinics due to their cognitive issues or ophthalmologists due to blurred vision secondary to the restricted vertical gaze. If the syndrome is not recognized and referral to neurology is delayed, this hinders the correct diagnosis being made. It is often misdiagnosed as PD initially.[1,2] There are several different subtypes of PSP. The poorest survival is seen in PSP-Richardson's type, which is the 'classic' PSP and is associated with a rapid decline.[3]

Learning Point How Progressive Supranuclear Palsy is Diagnosed

PSP is a clinical diagnosis with the use of investigations (such as blood tests and brain imaging) to rule out potential mimics.[1] Rowe et al. described how PSP and PD present differently and having an awareness of this can aid with diagnosis. Patients with PSP often present with rigidity affecting the trunk and neck with symmetrical limb signs (with no tremor) and have a greater tendency to falls in the first year. Due to restricted vertical eye movements in PSP (which can be elicited by examination), patients will walk with their head in an up-and-forward position. In PSP, cognitive and personality changes often feature and voice changes are often noticeable.[1] Key milestones showing evidence of disease progression include the onset of falls (often the first sign experienced), change in speech, and admissions to hospital.[2]

Expert Comment Diagnosing Progressive Supranuclear Palsy

PSP-Richardson's type, which is the 'classic' PSP, has features of cognitive impairment, prominent vertical gaze palsy and axial rigidity. PSP-Parkinson's Predominant (PSP-P) appears more like idiopathic PD initially with features such as vertical gaze palsy emerging later in the disease process. Should falls, rapid cognitive and mobility impairment, personality change, and visual problems arise, rapid assessment and consideration of PSP (rather than PD) should take place. Be mindful of the speed that change has taken place. Patients may describe a stiff neck and double vision and there are often falls within the first three years of diagnosis. Patients may present in a wheelchair which is reflective of a rapid decline in function. Be mindful of patients who feel like their feet are stuck to the floor and present with a 'magnetic gait'. Voice changes with a low, growling quality and early swallowing dysfunction are further clues to a possible underlying PSP diagnosis. It is important to recognize features suggestive of a frontal lobe degenerative syndrome (as seen in PSP). This includes repeating phrases such as, 'I'm champion', (called catch phrasing) or echolalia where patients repeat all or part of what has been said by the last person speaking.

Learning Tip Rigidity and Falls—Using Levodopa in Progressive Supranuclear Palsy for Rigidity

Axial rigidity is a feature of PSP. Falls are common and are characteristically backward. Patients may comment that they feel they are being pulled backwards and have a profound loss of balance on the pull test (examiners should ensure they are steady and have another person to support them before testing this, especially in larger patients). Falls often occur because of impaired turning or pivoting. Truncal rigidity in extension (with a tendency to backwards lean) can impair the patient from maintaining a seated position.[4] Patients may also mobilize without hesitation, further contributing to the risk of falls. This is manifested when patients rush to stand, pick up a fallen object and so forth, rapidly losing balance. This is connected to a lack of inhibition and is seen in frontal lobe dysfunction.

Michael had limited response to the initiation of levodopa. Patients with PSP often respond poorly to levodopa in comparison to PD.[1] Responses to levodopa tend to occur early in the disease course and benefits may only last a few months.[4] Approximately 30% of patients with PSP report mild benefits with levodopa and until a high dose has been used, it is not possible to conclude a lack of response.[1] Although levodopa can be used alongside an additional dopaminergic medication such as amantadine, the use of other dopaminergic medications aside from levodopa have shown minimal or no benefit in PSP.[4]

Dopamine agonists can also be trialled when patients are struggling with pain, often affecting legs, arms, and back. Caution should be used when patients have significant cognitive impairment as dopamine agonists can aggravate this. For patients who have PSP, pain responds in 25% of patients when dopaminergic medications are trialled.[3]

Clinical Tip Use and Side Effects of Levodopa

Patients with PSP are less likely to experience the common side effects of levodopa and doses can be escalated faster than would be used in PD. Levodopa doses can be escalated to up to 1000 mg/day. Response to levodopa is assessed by change noticed over 2-3 months, if there is no benefit, the levodopa can be down titrated and stopped over 4-6 weeks.[1]

If during the levodopa tapering the patient shows a worsening in their condition, the levodopa should be maintained at this dosage. Further attempts at down titration can be tried at a later date.[4]

Expert Comment

In PSP higher doses of levodopa may be needed to achieve a treatment response compared to early PD. A proportion of PSP will not have any response, and some will lose their levodopa response after over time. Levodopa needs to be increased carefully with mindful consideration of the impact this can have on cognitive function. There is no evidence for dopamine agonists or MAO inhibitors in PSP. Consider a diagnosis of PSP in patients who have had a poor medication response, have early gait initiation failure or early frontal cognitive changes.

It was clear that Michael needed support at home and was assigned a social worker. Carers were also organized to come to the house four times a day. Due to Michael's cognitive impairment, he often locked the door and intermittently did not allow carers into his home. Michael, who had always been quiet and respectful, often patted the carers inappropriately, called them, 'my gorgeous girls', and commented on their dress and person. His son reported he was disinhibited during conversations and described him as, 'having no filter', which was very different to his previous behaviour, though he remained friendly and was not aggressive.

Expert Comment

If disinhibition leads to aggressive behaviour and frequent falls through being unable to understand poor balance and mobility, there can be significant carer strain and falls with injuries are very common. Medications such as cognitive enhancers have been used off-licence to try and manage this, as have agents like trazadone especially if there is patient distress, but frontal disinhibition can be very challenging. Psychiatry liaison support can be invaluable. Low dose benzodiazepines have been used

Learning Point

Involuntary eyelid closure in PSP is often seen and causes functional blindness as patients struggle to life their eyelids. This is called apraxia of eyelid opening. Botulinum toxin can selectively weaken muscles of eyelid closure to improve this.[1]

Expert Comment

Apraxia of eyelid opening is a dystonic issue. Other eye symptoms in PSP include dry eyes from reduced blinking. Diplopia (double vision) from poor vertical eye movement may benefit from prism lens in some cases. This is often interpreted as an eye problem early in disease and patients are investigated for cataract and glaucoma before eye movement issues are identified..

in this group if behaviours are resulting in significant injury or aggression; clonazepam is also helpful in poor sleep in Parkinsonian disorders but may worsen unsteadiness. Antipsychotics almost without exception worsen motor parkinsonism and should be started only with careful discussion with the patient's neurology team. Haloperidol and traditional antipsychotics should be strictly avoided.

Learning Point Use of Montreal Cognitive Assessment for Cognitive Impairment

Patients with PSP often suffer from cognitive and personality changes and there is a close association with frontotemporal dementias.[1] In patients with PSP, cognitive change is an important feature with early changes being noticeable. Cognitive changes in PSP can be identified and monitored using the MoCA and is more sensitive than using the more commonly known Mini-Mental State Examination (MMSE) at detecting cognitive impairment in PSP.[5]

Michael's son had visited from France and found his father (more) confused and drowsy. He was admitted to hospital and was diagnosed with aspiration pneumonia. He was reviewed by the speech and language therapy team (SALT) who advised he needed thickened fluids, but aspiration would continue to be a risk. A best interests meeting was called to discuss a percutaneous endoscopic gastrostomy (PEG), as Michael's impaired cognition meant he was unable to give valid consent to the procedure. He improved markedly with a course of antibiotics. This improvement coupled with his carer's report that meals were long, laborious, and caused anxiety for Michael due to the time it took for him to eat a meal, led to the multidisciplinary team (MDT) decision to insert a PEG. The ability to provide nutrition with reduced stress to the patient and his carers improved his quality of life and he took puddings and cups of his favourite coffee with some thickener for pleasure. The risk of aspiration was accepted and balanced against Michael's quality of life (QoL).

Learning Point

Aspiration and weight loss due to dysphagia is common in PSP. Early input from SALT is essential and they can provide guidance on diet and safer eating. Consideration of alternative routes of feeding such as a PEG tube should also be discussed with appropriate patients which can help prevent weight loss and ensure adequate nutrition.[1]

Expert Comment

When considering a PEG in PSP, the individual needs of a patient must be considered, including, if the patient is strong enough to have the PEG and if it is burdensome for them. Some patients with frontal lobe syndromes have utilization behaviours where they compulsively pull at clothing, catheters, etc. A PEG in this group is challenging and injury can occur when the PEG is pulled out. In a patient who is very weak and frail, enteral feeding will not prolong their life; this should be recognized and communicated when having discussions with patients and those important to them about the expectations of what a PEG can provide.

Learning Point Palliative Care Involvement

Identifying when input from palliative care (PC) is appropriate can be challenging as there is often a variable trajectory with limited pharmacological benefit to help with the distressing symptoms patients with PSP may experience. There is a need for PC to help with commonly occurring symptoms such as secretions and pain and early optimization of symptom control can help with improving QoL.[3]

Michael was placed in a nursing home after he became unable to transfer around his house and his maximal package of social care was insufficient for his needs. His son was able to 'see' placements with him using Zoom, which comforted him.

After 6 months settled in the new placement, Michael was doubly incontinent and required a hoist for washing and transfers. He had very little speech but smiled when spoken to and gave a thumbs up when happy (this is very common in PSP). He developed several chest infections and was taken to hospital, each time becoming very agitated and distressed at the new environment. Despite PEG feeding, he continued to lose weight. His GP, nursing home carer and neurology team had a virtual meeting with Michael's son and advance care planning (ACP) was initiated. It was decided to treat him at his nursing home for any further infections and, if he did not improve to keep him comfortable in his home environment. A month later, Michael died comfortably at his care home after developing a further chest infection. He had anticipatory medications in place but only required PRN medications for secretions.

Expert Comment Palliative Care

Care is needed when prescribing anticipatory medicines, particularly when managing nausea. Haloperidol can cause severe worsening of parkinsonism (otherwise known as extrapyramidal effects). Cyclizine is often used but can cause side effects (such as confusion) due to its anticholinergic properties. Levomepromazine is the antiemetic drug of choice here.

Discussion

In summary, this is a case of a patient with PSP who was initially misdiagnosed as having PD and was given their diagnosis later in the disease course. He experienced rigidity and had a poor response to dopamine agonists. He had many falls and developed cognitive impairment which made providing care more difficult. The MDT was fundamental to provide good care and the use of technology allowed his son to remain present in his father's care despite being abroad. Palliative care input for symptom control is important for patients who have a diagnosis of a movement disorder despite their variable trajectory.

A Final Word from the Expert

This case is typical of a patient receiving a diagnosis of idiopathic PD then having a re-diagnosis when early symptoms of frontal dysexecutive problems and behaviour change, poor treatment response with gait freezing and vertical gaze limitation develop. It is important to look for these features in patients who progress more rapidly than expected, attending the ED multiple times for falls or coming to clinic with a wheelchair after only a few months from diagnosis. PSP is a highly difficult condition to manage especially when considering carer strain. Patients are at greatest risk when they are still very mobile yet disinhibited and unable to control their impulses to move around, rapidly putting themselves at risk of injury due to falling. In addition, the postural instability and tendency to fall backward add to the significant challenges of keeping this group of patients safe 24 hours a day. This should be appreciated.

PSP leads to early communication challenges both through dysarthria secondary to parkinsonism and cognitive decline, so early signposting and discussion regarding future planning should be considered. Research has identified that there are low numbers of patients with movement disorders with ACP in place.[3] ACP is imperative in patients with PSP, but its unpredictable trajectory can make this difficult. Anyone who has the skillset to do so and a good relationship with the patient (and those important to them) can support ACP decisions. In most neurodegenerative conditions like PSP, multiple system atrophy (MSA) and motor neurone disease (MND), death usually comes after a period of decline with weight loss (even with a PEG in situ), recurrent infections, and a tendency to become more somnolent. Aspiration pneumonia is generally the cause of death.

References

1. Rowe J, Holland N, Rittman T. Progressive supranuclear palsy: diagnosis and management. *Pract Neurol* 2021; 21: 376–383.
2. Wiblin l, Durcan R, Galna B, Lee M, Burn D. Clinical milestones preceding the diagnosis of multiple system atrophy and progressive supranuclear palsy: a retrospective cohort study. *J Mov Disord* 2019; 12(3):177–83.
3. Wiblin L, Lee M, Burn D. Palliative care and its emerging role in multiple system atrophy and progressive supranuclear palsy. *Parkinsonism Relat Disord* 2017; 34: 7–14.
4. Bluett B, Pantelyat A, Litvan I, et al. Best practices in the clinical management of progressive supranuclear palsy and corticobasal syndrome: a consensus statement of the CurePSP centers of care. *Front Neurol* 2021; 12: 1123.
5. Fiorenzato E, Weis L, Falup-Pecurariu C, et al. Montreal Cognitive Assessment (MoCA) and Mini-Mental State Examination (MMSE) performance in progressive supranuclear palsy and multiple system atrophy. *J Neural Transm* 2016; 123(12): 1435–1442.

CASE 30 Sialorrhoea

Kirsty Douglas

Expert: Rachel Burman

Case History

Sandy, a 60-year-old retired electrician, was diagnosed with motor neurone disease (MND) 18 months ago after a lengthy period of investigation for clumsiness and falls. He used a wheelchair, relied on his husband Craig for care and received nutrition and medication via a percutaneous gastrostomy tube. His speech was effortful, quiet, and dysarthric. He was referred to the palliative care clinic as he had developed problems with drooling of saliva, which was distressing and causing excoriation around his mouth.

Learning Point Sialorrhoea

Sialorrhoea is the accumulation and unintentional loss of saliva from the mouth. It occurs due to overproduction or reduced clearance of saliva.

It is common in neurological conditions, including Parkinson's disease, stroke, and MND. In these conditions, reduced coordination or strength of bulbar and facial muscles causes a reduction in swallowing function and frequency, impaired saliva control and poor lip seal, leading to reduced salivary clearance.[1]

Sialorrhoea affects up to 50% of MND patients, and 20% of those affected report moderate to severe symptoms.[2–4] It becomes increasingly common as the disease progresses and can be challenging to manage. A recent observational survey suggested almost half of those with sialorrhoea had uncontrolled symptoms,[5] and only a quarter reported 'very effective' treatment.[4]

Sandy described 'constant watery saliva', which he struggled to swallow and cleared with tissues. As his arms had weakened, he found it harder to raise tissues to his mouth and was more reliant on others for help. Saliva escaped from the corner of his mouth and caused skin breakdown and discomfort. He found this embarrassing and no longer felt comfortable leaving the house. Night-times were more difficult, and his sleep was interrupted. At times he described feeling like he was choking and struggling for breath, which was 'terrifying'. His cough was weak and he had required hospital admissions with aspiration pneumonia.

Learning Point Motor Neurone Disease

Motor neurone disease (MND) is a progressive neurodegenerative disorder affecting the motor neurons in the anterior horn of the spinal cord, brainstem, and motor cortex.[1–6] The classic form (amyotrophic lateral sclerosis) presents with mixed upper and lower motor neurone features. Often focal at onset, progression is inevitable but individual.[7] Weakness worsens and becomes widespread, affecting the limbs, bulbar and respiratory muscles, causing progressive paralysis alongside impairment of speech, swallowing, and respiratory function. The usual cause of death is respiratory failure, often associated with infection.[7]

Bulbar symptoms are relatively uncommon at onset (occurring in 20%) and are associated with poorer prognosis.[6] In the later stages of MND, most patients have bulbar involvement leading to problems with communication, sialorrhoea, and dysphagia.

Other symptoms include pain, spasticity, fatigue, dyspnoea, anxiety, and depression.[7] Cognitive and behavioural changes occur in around 20%, and may reduce quality of life, and complicate planning and decision-making.[8]

Patients, and their families, face considerable challenges throughout the course of the illness: there is often a delay to diagnosis, symptoms are varied and tend to worsen over time, the disease is punctuated by serial losses of function, and although progression and death are inevitable, timings are uncertain.

There are no curative treatments, and the prognosis is usually short, averaging 2–3 years.[8] Riluzole is the only disease-modifying drug available but only slows the rate of decline by a few months.[9] Nocturnal non-invasive ventilation (NIV) improves 1-year survival, and maintains quality of life, in those with respiratory failure and without severe bulbar dysfunction.[10]

Care is mainly supportive and should be delivered by an experienced multidisciplinary team (MDT).[11] MDT care is associated with improved quality of life, symptom control, and survival.[7] The role of palliative care specialists within the team is increasingly recognized: potentially helping with symptom control, psychosocial support, complex communication and decision-making, and end of life care.[7, 8, 11]

Learning Point Saliva–Production and Function

The salivary glands produce between 1–1.5 litres of saliva daily.[12] Although there are hundreds of minor glands, the three major pairs (parotid, submandibular, and sublingual) produce 90% of this volume.[12] Saliva has several physiological functions and is essential for digestion, oral health, and speech.

Saliva production is under autonomic control, increasing in response to parasympathetic input, mediated by the neurotransmitter acetylcholine. In health, we swallow saliva approximately once a minute to prevent excessive accumulation.[1]

Clinical Tip Assessing Oral Secretions

It is crucial to assess what type of secretions the patient is experiencing. This case focuses on the management of thin watery 'serous' saliva. Thick, tenacious 'mucoid' secretions require a different approach, with trials of mucolytic agents and saline nebulizers. Evaluation should also include the severity, timing, and overall impact of sialorrhoea, and if relevant, the effect on the patient's ability to use NIV.

Learning Point Physical Consequences of Sialorrhoea

Chronic sialorrhoea causes a variety of physical problems. Anterior spillage of saliva results in chapping and maceration of skin around the mouth due to constant exposure to moisture. As well as being uncomfortable, this can cause an offensive smell and problems with secondary infection. Pooling of saliva exacerbates speech difficulties making communication harder. Sleep may be disturbed, worsening fatigue, and impacting on patients and carers. Posterior spillage increases the risk of aspiration pneumonia with significant distress and adverse implications in terms of hospitalization and survival. Importantly, uncontrolled sialorrhoea is associated with poorer tolerance of NIV, which is one of the few interventions that has been evidenced to improve survival and maintain quality of life in MND.[10]

Learning Point Psychosocial Consequences of Sialorrhoea

Patients describe embarrassment and may withdraw from social interaction, becoming isolated. Eating and talking become difficult, removing pleasure from otherwise sociable activities. Relationships may change as loved ones increasingly adopt caring roles and patients become more dependent. Some partners and family members may struggle to maintain intimacy and affection. Self-esteem may suffer, and social stigmatization can magnify isolation and impair quality of life.

Some people experience choking episodes which can be frightening, heightening underlying anxieties and fears. Some are scared they will die feeling 'as if they are drowning'.

Of course, sialorrhoea doesn't occur in isolation in MND. It accompanies serial losses of function which alter roles, living and working arrangements, and dictate increasing reliance on care and medical interventions. These rapid, significant changes permeate all aspects of life and carry their own psychosocial burden.

Sandy had tried several treatment options without success. A trial of a hyoscine hydrobromide patch caused itchy skin irritation despite patch rotation and topical steroids. Atropine eye drops, administered sublingually four times a day by his husband, were ineffective. Sandy found amitriptyline solution, via his gastrostomy tube, unpleasantly sedating, with only slight improvement in symptoms.

Clinical Tip Non-pharmacological Measures

Simple adjustments to correct forward neck flexion, including supportive chairs, chin supports, and soft neck collars, may help if posture is contributing to the problem. Good oral hygiene is important. Early referral to speech and language therapy is essential to optimize swallowing and lip seal.[1]

Portable suction units can be considered for those with sialorrhoea refractory to pharmacological treatment, particularly if there is pooling of saliva.[1] Patients, or their carers, should be trained to use suction safely.

Evidence Base Treatment Principles

The aim of treatment is to improve symptoms and quality of life. Difficulties occur due to systemic side effects of medications and lack of evidence base to guide choices. Studies are limited by small numbers, lack of blinding, and lack of validated outcome measures.[4] Some evidence is extrapolated from paediatric populations. Treatment decisions are mostly based on expert opinion. A 'trial-and-error' approach is adopted, working stepwise through options including conservative measures, anticholinergic medications, and intrasalivary gland botulinum toxin injections.[1, 11]

A 2022 Cochrane review explored treatment of sialorrhoea in MND and identified four randomized control trial (RCTs), concluding that there is low-certainty or moderate-certainty evidence for the use of botulinum toxin B injections to salivary glands and moderate-certainty evidence for the use of oral dextromethorphan with quinidine (DMQ) for the treatment of sialorrhoea in MND.[3]

Clinical Tip Anticholinergic Medications

Anticholinergic drugs are first-line medications.[11] They act on the salivary glands to decrease saliva production by blocking parasympathetic stimulation. However, nearly a third of treated patients don't respond, and their use is limited by side effects (urinary retention, constipation, visual disturbance, confusion, agitation, sedation, and postural dizziness).[13, 14]

Care must be taken to avoid causing an unpleasantly dry mouth or overly thick respiratory secretions, which may be more distressing than the primary problem. General advice is to start at a low dose and gradually up-titrate as tolerated.

Hyoscine Hydrobromide

Hyoscine hydrobromide is used off-licence, commonly by the transdermal route. Scopoderm® patches comprise a reservoir containing 1.5 mg hyoscine hydrobromide.[15] The patch is changed every three days and, on average, 1 mg hyoscine is absorbed in this time.[15]

The main advantages are simplicity of dosing and application, and maintenance of steady-state. However, patches are not always tolerated: one multicentre observational study reported that a third of patients discontinued them due to side effects.[14] Skin reactions are common but can be reduced by rotating sites and using topical steroid if required.[1] Hyoscine hydrobromide should be avoided in patients with, or at risk of, cognitive impairment due to central anticholinergic side effects.

Amitriptyline

Amitriptyline is available as an oral solution, or as tablets that can be crushed and dispersed in water. These can be given by mouth or feeding tube. Expert opinion recommends gradual up-titration, with effective doses in the range 10–50 mg.[1] Amitriptyline is cheap and familiar to prescribers but may be poorly tolerated due to systemic effects.[5]

Atropine Eye Drops

Atropine has a high bioavailability, rapid onset, and short duration of action.[15] 1% atropine eye drops are used off-licence and are dropped under or onto the tongue. The Palliative Care Formulary (PCF) recommends 4 drops every 4 hours as required.[15] Drop sizes, and thus doses, vary with the applicator and technique, and safe administration may require assistance from a family member or carer.

Although some clinicians have hypothesized that atropine acts topically when given in this way, with reduced systemic absorption and risk of anticholinergic side effects, this is not currently substantiated by evidence or pharmacological theory.[17] Atropine may be a good option if sialorrhoea is related to meals, as drops can be administered before eating or when the problem arises.[1]

Glycopyrronium Bromide

Glycopyrronium oral solution is used off-licence. Different brands are not interchangeable as concentrations vary. The PCF recommends a starting dose of 200 micrograms every 8 hours which can be increased every few days to a maximum of 2 mg three times daily.[1, 13, 15] The dose is measured and administered via a graduated syringe and given orally or via NG or PEG tube. Since this process requires manual dexterity, carers may be required for administration.

There are case reports of successful use of subcutaneous (continuous and intermittent), nebulized, and inhaled glycopyrronium.[1]

Its main advantage is a reduced central side effect burden.

Expert Comment

There is no evidence-based guidance to inform choices between anticholinergic options, resulting in significant variation in practice. Decisions should be patient-centred and consider route of administration, cognition, and potential beneficial side effects. Glycopyrronium is preferred in those with cognitive impairment or frailty as it has limited ability to cross the blood-brain barrier reducing central nervous system effects.[11]

Expert Comment

Clear instructions are important to avoid accidental overdose, and to limit use to specific circumstances, e.g. meals, social occasions, clinic visits.

Further treatment options were considered, including a trial of glycopyrronium bromide, intrasalivary gland botulinum toxin injections or radiotherapy. 'Fed up with side effects' from medication trials, Sandy chose to try botulinum toxin treatment. Bilateral parotid and submandibular gland injections were performed under ultrasound guidance. He reported a reduction in sialorrhoea, and opted to have a repeat procedure four months later.

Clinical Tip Botulinum Toxin

Injection of botulinum toxin into salivary glands reduces saliva production by inhibiting release of acetylcholine at the parasympathetic nerve terminal. Injections are administered in the outpatient clinic. The dose is divided between parotid and submandibular glands, which are identified by landmark technique or ultrasound guidance.[1, 18] Treatment responses are seen within a week and last 3-6 months.[18] Repeated injections may be required.

NICE approved the Xeomin® preparation of botulinum A for chronic sialorrhoea in neurological conditions in 2019.[19] At present, it is a second-line option in NICE guidance for MND and Parkinson's disease and should be 'considered if first-line treatment is ineffective, not tolerated, or contraindicated'.[11, 17] Some experts advocate its earlier use. However, access is inconsistent, with marked geographical variation in availability and service provision.

Clinical Tip Radiotherapy

Radiotherapy is not often used. Xerostomia is a common side effect of radiotherapy for head and neck cancers. As a result, it has been explored as a treatment for sialorrhoea, and observational studies suggest it is safe and effective.[20] Treatment effects last for months to years. The optimal treatment schedule is yet to be established; commonly used regimens target bilateral submandibular and caudal portions of the parotid glands. A recent review recommended 12 Gy in 2 fractions or 20 Gy in 4 fractions with treatments twice a week.[20]

Expert Comment

The recommended dose for sialorrhoea is one Scopoderm® patch every 72 hours. If needed, the dose can be increased to two patches or decreased by cutting the patch in half.[16]

Expert Comment

The sedative side effect of amitriptyline may be beneficial for some but may force others to discontinue it.

Clinical Tip Oral Dextromethorphan with Quinidine (DMQ)

DMQ is used to treat pseudobulbar affect (unprovoked and uncontrollable episodes of laughing and/or crying). As reported in the Cochrane review, a phase 2, randomized, placebo-controlled cross-over study of 20 mg dextromethorphan hydrobromide and 10 mg quinidine sulphate found that DMQ may produce a participant-reported improvement in sialorrhoea.[3] Side effects were most commonly constipation, diarrhoea, nausea, and dizziness, with no difference between the DMQ and placebo groups.

Expert Comment

One key benefit of botulinum injection is that treatment is targeted, avoiding systemic effects. There is a risk of xerostomia, which reverses slowly as it takes time for the toxin to wear off. There have been cases of worsening dysphagia following submandibular injection in MND patients[18]; it is not known whether this is a causal relationship or secondary to disease progression. As a precaution, some centres no longer offer submandibular injections to MND patients with preserved oral intake.[18]

Future Advances

New models of integrated multidisciplinary working improve outcomes in MND.[7] Early access to timely help is crucial for these patients. Holistic oral assessment should be part of routine care, and some centres advocate early referral to, or discussion with, maxillofacial colleagues for assessment of dentition, temporomandibular joint spasm, and botulinum injections. Further research is required to inform optimal timing of botulinum injections in the disease trajectory.

Learning Point

Both sialorrhoea and enteral feeding are risk factors for aspiration pneumonia. It is important to review feeding at the time of deterioration, and it is common practice to discontinue enteral feeding when someone is dying.

After several months, Sandy deteriorated significantly—he was febrile, breathless, and drowsy: a further aspiration pneumonia was suspected. In line with his wishes, a symptomatic approach was taken, with a view to supporting his last days of life at home. His PEG feed was discontinued, and subcutaneous medications via a syringe pump were used to manage breathlessness, anxiety, and respiratory secretions.

A Final Word from the Expert

Sandy's case explores a common yet challenging presentation to palliative medicine, highlighting the importance of actively managing sialorrhoea to reduce its physical and psychosocial consequences. This is, arguably, particularly important for those who use NIV since uncontrolled sialorrhoea reduces NIV tolerance, potentially reducing life expectancy and quality of life. Currently, management involves a trial-and-error approach working stepwise through options with the individual patient, and their family, at the centre of all decisions.

References

1. McGeachan AJ, Mcdermott CJ. Management of oral secretions in neurological disease. *Pract Neurol* 2017; 17(2): 96–103.
2. Bradley WG, Anderson F, Bromberg M, et al. Current management of ALS. *Neurology* 2001; 57(3): 500–504.
3. James E, Ellis C, Brassington R, Sathasivam S, Young CA. Treatment for sialorrhea (excessive saliva) in people with motor neuron disease/amyoptrophic lateral sclerosis. Cochrane Database Syst Rev 2012; 5(5): CD006981.
4. McGeachan AJ, Hobson E v., Shaw PJ, McDermott CJ. Developing an outcome measure for excessive saliva management in MND and an evaluation of saliva burden in Sheffield. *Amyotroph Lateral Scler Frontotemporal Degener* 2015; 16(1–2): 108–113.
5. Hobson E v., McGeachan A, Al-Chalabi A, et al. Management of sialorrhoea in MND: a survey of current UK practice. *Amyotroph Lateral Scler Frontotemporal Degener* 2013; 14(7–8): 521–527.
6. McDermott CJ, Shaw PJ. Diagnosis and management of motor neurone disease. *BMJ* 2008; 336(7645): 658–662.
7. Oliver DJ. Palliative care in motor neurone disease: where are we now? *Palliat Care* 2019; 12: 117822421881391.
8. Oliver D. Palliative care for patients with MND: current challenges. *Degener Neurol Neuromuscul Dis* 2016; 6: 65–72.
9. Miller RG, Mitchell JD, Moore DH. Riluzole for amyotrophic lateral sclerosis ALS/MND. *Cochrane Database Syst Rev* 2012; 2: CD001447.

10. Bourke SC, Tomlinson M, Williams TL, Bullock RE, Shaw PJ, Gibson GJ. Effects of NIV on survival and quality of life in patients with ALS: a randomised controlled trial. *Lancet Neurol* 2006; 5(2): 140–147.
11. National Institute for Health and Care Excellence. Motor neurone disease: assessment and management. NICE Guideline (NG42). 2016. Available at: https://www.nice.org.uk/guidance/ng42
12. Hockstein NG, Samadi DS, Gendron K, Handler SD. Sialorrhea: a management challenge. *Am Fam Physician* 2004; 69(11): 2628–2634.
13. Banfi P, Ticozzi N, Lax A, Guidugli GA, Nicolini A, Silani V. A review of options for treating sialorrhea in ALS. *Respir Care* 2015; 60(3): 446–454.
14. McGeachan AJ, Hobson E v., Al-Chalabi A, et al. A multicentre evaluation of oropharyngeal secretion management practices in ALS. *Amyotroph Lateral Scler Frontotemporal Degener* 2017; 18(1–2): 1–9.
15. Wilcock A, Howard P, Charlesworth S. *Palliative Care Formulary*, 7th ed. London: Pharmaceutical Press, 2020.
16. NHS Scotland. Hyoscine hydrobromide 1.5mg transdermal patch for respiratory secretions (Scopoderm®). Scottish Palliative Care Guidelines. 2020. Available at: https://www.palliativecareguidelines.scot.nhs.uk/media/83345/hyoscine-hydrobromide-scopoderm-pil-2020-10.pdf
17. National Institute for Health and Care Excellence (NICE). Parkinson's disease in adults: diagnosis and management (NG71). 2017. Available at: https://www.nice.org.uk/guidance/ng71
18. Harbottle J, Carlin H, Payne-Doris T, Tedd HMI, de Soyza A, Messer B. Developing an intrasalivary gland botox service for patients receiving long-term NIV at home: a single-centre experience. *BMJ Open Respir Res* 2022; 9(1): e001188.
19. National Institute for Health and Care Excellence. Xeomin (botulinum neurotoxin type A) for treating chronic sialorrhoea; Technology appraisal guidance [TA605]. 2019. Available at: https://www.nice.org.uk/guidance/ta605
20. Hawkey NM, Zaorsky NG, Galloway TJ. The role of radiation therapy in the management of sialorrhea: a systematic review. *Laryngoscope* 2016; 126(1): 80–85.

CASE

31 Frailty and Multiple Long-Term Conditions

Felicity Dewhurst

Expert: Caroline Nicholson

Case history

Florence (Flo) was an 82-year-old woman who lived alone. She rarely left the house except for frequent hospital appointments with her cardiologist, nephrologist, and respiratory physician for her respective diagnoses of heart failure, chronic kidney disease, and chronic obstructive pulmonary disease. She had a historic diagnosis of hypertension, for which she took multiple medications. Flo's clinic letters to her general practitioner included 'frailty' and 'multiple long-term conditions (MLTC)' in her problem list.

Flo was referred to geriatric services due to falls, necessitating review by her GP, emergency department visits, and hospital admissions. At the clinic visit, she was screened for frailty, her 'frailty syndromes' were described and she underwent a comprehensive geriatric assessment (CGA).

Evidence Base Definitions of Frailty and Multiple Long-Term Conditions (MLTC)

Frailty

Frailty is defined as age-related decline across multiple systems, increasing vulnerability to health stressors.[1]

MLTC

The term MLTC as opposed to multimorbidity and comorbidity is preferred by patients and the public. The National Institute for Health and Care Research and the World Health Organization, support the use of the Academy of Medical Sciences definition: The coexistence of two or more chronic conditions, each one of which is either; a physical non-communicable disease, an infectious disease, or a mental health condition of long duration.[2] Complex MLTC is also an accepted concept. There is variation in how this is defined. Definitions include three or four long-term conditions or multiple affected body systems and/or significant functional limitation.[3]

Expert Comment The Associations of Frailty and Multiple Long-Term Conditions

Both Frailty and MLTC increase your susceptibility to deteriorate and die at any point.[4]

Age

In an era of unprecedented global ageing, death is now an event of older age. By 2040, most deaths (54%) will be amongst people aged ≥ 85 years.[5] The prevalence of MLTC increases with age and is now the norm in later life.[3] Frailty is also common amongst older adults: Approximately 11% of people >65 years and 25–50% of those >85 years are frail.[6]

In older people, physical illness has a greater social, functional, and psychological effect.[7] There is an increasing need for geriatric, palliative and primary care, and community services. These services must work together to ensure continuity and coordination of care.

Socioeconomic and Ethnic Inequity

Living with and dying of MLTC is even more common if people are from poor socioeconomic backgrounds or ethnic minority groups. In these communities, the prevalence of MLTC is comparable to their more affluent counterparts who are one to three decades older and life expectancy is reduced by up to 15 years due to the rapid accumulation of conditions, disability, and frailty. Despite this, care provision generally and palliative care specifically is particularly poor.

Learning Point Why are Frailty and Multiple Long-Term Conditions such a Big Problem for Society and Healthcare in General and Palliative Care Specifically?

Frailty

In palliative care, frailty may be endemic across all age groups.[8–10] There is evidence that frail older people commonly experience high levels of untreated symptoms and poorly recognized and managed dying.[6] Frailty has received increased consideration in recent palliative care literature, but appropriate models of palliative care (regardless of diagnosis) need ongoing consideration.[4,11] The Clinical Frailty Scale has been used as a way of measuring and promoting the use of the concept of frailty.

MLTC

MLTC are one of the biggest problems facing the health service.[12,13] Prevalence is increasing significantly, resulting in high levels of morbidity and disability associated with poor quality of life, increased health and social care service use, and subsequently mortality. The burden of MLTC is often greater than the sum of their parts, particularly where patients are nearing the end of their lives.[3]

Clinical Tip What are the Benefits of Recognizing Frailty?

The purpose of identifying frailty varies depending on where a patient is on their illness trajectory. Attempts at reversal are often appropriate in the early stages; however, coordinated end of life care is important in the latter stages but however identification of dying is often missed.

Identifying frailty improves prognostication and decision-making, particularly in the setting of critical illness or interventions that may cause significant injury (e.g. chemotherapy and surgery).

Knowledge gained from identifying and grading frailty can help engage with patients and their families in order to produce individualized goal-centred plans of care.[6]

Grading and Acting Upon Frailty

A positive screen for frailty should prompt a comprehensive geriatric assessment (CGA), 'a multidimensional, interdisciplinary diagnostic process to determine the medical, psychological, and functional capabilities of in order to develop a coordinated and integrated plan for care'[14] (Figure 31.1).

Clinical Tip Frailty and Multiple Long-Term Conditions are not the Same Thing, but they are Interwoven

NICE guidance recommends that when patients are frail, identification, and appropriate management of associated MLTC is paramount. Conversely, frailty is one way of describing functional limitation amongst people with MLTC.[3]

Expert Comment Goals of Care

It is fundamental that a comprehensive assessment goes beyond a purely medical review. Goals of care and what matters most to the person should be central. The CGA is a tool most often used to assess frail patients considering functional, practical, and social need; palliative care reviews often include spiritual and psychological issues. There is merit in bringing these together.

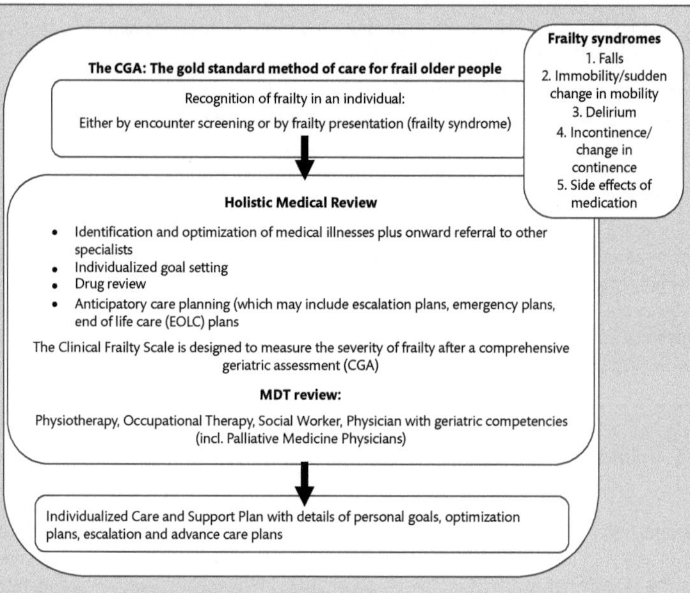

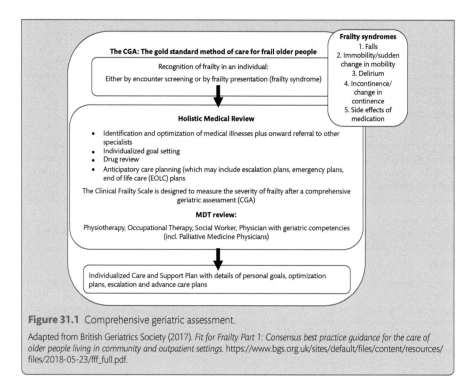

Figure 31.1 Comprehensive geriatric assessment.

Adapted from British Geriatrics Society (2017). *Fit for Frailty Part 1: Consensus best practice guidance for the care of older people living in community and outpatient settings.* https://www.bgs.org.uk/sites/default/files/content/resources/files/2018-05-23/fff_full.pdf.

Flo's CFS was 6. Following her CGA she was noted to have postural hypotension. As she had not had angina for 'years', her amlodipine and isosorbide mononitrate were stopped.

Expert Comment Falls, Hypotension, and Heart Failure

In older adults, a systolic BP of below 110 mmHg is associated with falls.

Recommendations for de-prescribing include stopping nitrates, calcium channel blockers, and other vasodilators. If there is no evidence of congestion, reduce diuretics.[14, 15]

Angiotensin-converting enzyme inhibitors and beta blockers have a survival benefit in systolic cardiac failure and should be maintained if possible if patients have systolic dysfunction.

However, most cardiac failure in older people is diastolic (preserved left ventricular function). Angiotensin-converting enzyme inhibitors and beta blockers have little survival benefit in diastolic failure and may be discontinued.

Involve occupational and physiotherapists for environmental assessment, equipment, and walking aids.

Flo had recently been bereaved. Her husband of 64 years had died 6 months previously following a diagnosis of dementia. She was his main carer and following his death, described herself as 'lacking purpose and lonely'. She now lived alone in a four-bedroom house; her two children both lived within the UK but were geographically distant.

Expert Comment Palliative Care Services Need to Change

More people will die of frailty and MLTC than of cancer (severe frailty results in a five times increased risk of mortality over one year). However, palliative care services remain focused on the needs of those with cancer and single diseases.[4] The need for palliative care services to change to accommodate frail patients and those with MLTC is increasingly recognized as is the lack of a clearly transferrable model of care.[4]

Evidence Base How do the Factors Described Above Make the Patient More Vulnerable?

The frailty fulcrum is a useful way of considering frailty and explaining the concept to patients and relatives. Frailty is a dynamic process, and in advanced frailty, deterioration is more common than improvement (Figure 31.2).

The reduced reserve of patients with frailty results in a relatively large impact or unbalancing of the fulcrum because of small insults.[16] The fulcrum can be rebalanced through increased resilience across the domains. There are numerous factors which make Flo more vulnerable. She is socially withdrawn following her husband's death (bereavement of a long-term spouse is associated with poorer health outcomes), she has MLTC, and has had recent acute health events.

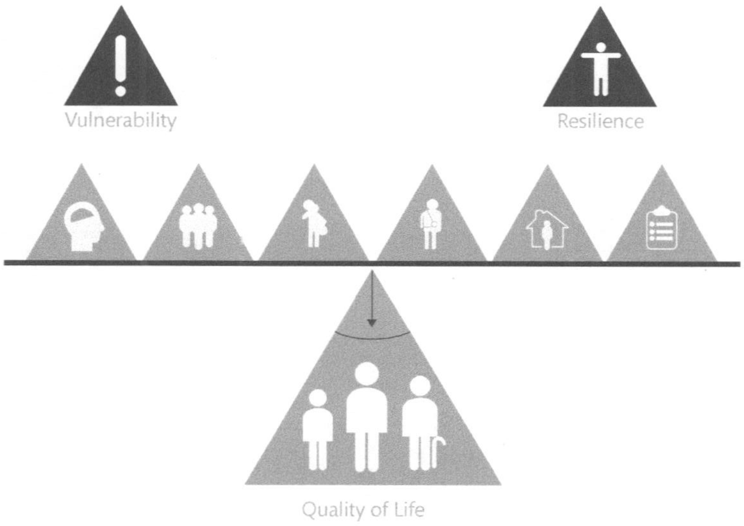

Integrated Assessment

Domain	Areas to Consider
Social Environment	• Main carer & carer network • Next of kin & wider family • Friends & community • Preferred methods of interaction
Physical Environment	• Think from the skin outwards • Clothing & footwear • Main daily living areas • Beyond the doorstep & transport
Systems of Care	• Health & social care integration • Sharing information & care records • Respite & carer support • Funding & benefits
Psychological Status	• Recognised conditions or symptoms • Motivation & confidence • Emotional well-being • Spiritual & cultural fulfilment
Multimorbidity	• Treatment burden of multiple long term conditions • Physical & mental health • Vision, hearing, dentition, continence • Strength & mobility
Acute Health Events	• Frailty syndromes: delirum, falls, immobility, incontinence, medication side effects • Planned acute care (e.g. surgery)

Figure 31.2 Frailty fulcrum.

Reproduced from the Frailty Toolkit (2020). *Frailty Fulcrum Animation*. https://www.frailtytoolkit.org/frailty-fulcrum-animation/.

Following Flo's CGA, she was reviewed by occupational and physiotherapists and a social worker. Equipment was prescribed for her house, and she was given a walking aid. The social worker arranged for a care package and for Flo to attend a weekly day centre.

Six months later, Flo complained of increasing breathlessness. A CT scan resulted in a radiological diagnosis of metastatic lung cancer. Her oncologist decided that due to her 'level of frailty and multiple long-term conditions' she was not suitable for active oncological treatment and advised she should be flagged on the GP palliative care register.

Learning Point Is This An Appropriate Time to Refer to Palliative Care Services or Should This Have Been Considered Before Now?

The scale of the problem of frailty and MLTC and the question of how to provide appropriate end-of-life care is massive and an international priority.[6, 8, 11] End of life care provision in care homes and the community needs to double by 2040.[11] Fewer older patients and those with a non-cancer diagnosis access palliative care. A recent quantitative review described the significant unmet physical, psychological, and social needs of patients with frailty, particularly at the end of life.[6] As a result, many people like Flo will only get referred to palliative care when a malignant diagnosis is made.

Flo was looking to plan for the future and as part of this, she asked, 'How long have I got and where and how might I die?'

Evidence Base Prognosis

Frailty

Frailty as measured by CFS can predict patient outcomes: the higher the level of frailty the shorter a patient's prognosis. Severe frailty results in a five times increased risk of mortality over one year. The CFS has been validated as an adverse outcome predictor in hospitalized older people. However, because of the multifactorial nature of problems presented by the frailty state, and although literature supports the fact that prognosis is poor, the exact timescales can vary widely, making appropriate future management difficult and highlighting the importance of individual indicators of decline.[7, 9, 17, 18]

Frailty and Heart Failure

Frailty is common in chronic heart failure and is associated with adverse outcomes including death. Frailty can be used to predict mortality in heart failure patients both in the hospital and the community setting.[18]

Frailty and COPD

Frailty level captures the deterioration of multiple systems in COPD and provides an overview of impairments, identifying individuals at increased risk of mortality.[19]

Frailty with Malignancy

Frailty can be used to predict mortality in patients with solid organ and haematological malignancy.[20] It can also predict survival following oncological treatments including chemo/radiotherapy and surgery.[21]

Evidence Base What Palliative Management Strategies Could and Should be Considered?

Following an interdisciplinary palliative care intervention in advanced heart failure patients showed consistently greater benefits in quality of life, anxiety, depression, and spiritual well-being compared with usual care alone. Early input from palliative care should be increasingly considered in patients with non-malignant disease, MLTC, and frailty.[22]

Learning Point The Key Factors for Palliative Care for Patients with Frailty

Consideration of the five Ms of geriatric medicine are required: Mobility, Mind, Medications, Multicomplexity, and Matters Most.[23]

Expert Comment What Palliative Management Strategies Could and Should be Considered?

Patients with frailty and MLTC often receive poor end of life care. Many of the services available to these patients are reactive. More proactive care is required. Frequent reflection with the older person and their family on where they are in their life course is important, consequently the right care can be offered at the right time.[4]

There is a need to change policy and palliative care provision to provide more equitable services based on the opinion of patients, relatives, and care givers. Older people express a need for care continuity and assistance to navigate services.[6]

New models of care are required with the potential to provide a single point of care provision without compromising specialist multidisciplinary team input. There is a moral and clinical imperative for palliative care services to contribute to the support of patients with frailty and MLTC as they near the end of their lives. Remodelling of palliative care services should ensure we focus more on need than diagnosis and prognosis. Age-attuned palliative care has been one suggested solution.[4] This model of care provision aims to balance continuity of care with ongoing adaptation to loss. Hospices and community palliative care services could work with surrounding services to produce mutually advantageous relationships, reducing hospital visits and admissions. Specialist clinicians could provide remote support, advice, and guidance. Palliative care services in all settings need to be more integrated and proactive to better meet need. Hospices could act as hubs in the local community, providing multidisciplinary team assessment to improve holistic symptom control, rehabilitation, identification and optimization of medical illnesses including discussion with other specialists, individualized goal setting, drug review and de-prescribing, signposting to local services, and advance care planning.[4, 6]

Flo was visited weekly by her district nurses, and they noticed a weekly deterioration in her general condition. She had problematic pain and nausea and was referred to the community specialist palliative care team. At the time of the initial review, they felt that Flo was dying and arranged for her to be admitted to the hospice for end of life care. Flo died in the hospice two days following admission, having only received specialist palliative care input for a total of one week.

A Final Word from the Expert

People with Frailty have the same symptomatic problems as those conventionally seen by palliative care services. However, their problems are underreported and undertreated. Older people often have much more capability and resilience than health and social care providers recognize and societies appreciate.[4] They want to remain active and connected with society and as such communities need to change to become more compassionate, recognizing the value and contribution of older people and playing an increasingly significant role in the health and social care of their older members. Community engagement, e.g. compassionate communities (see Case 43) at this stage can influence complex issues such as well-being and social isolation, key challenges for people in late older age. There are potential savings (both financial and personal) through the provision of good palliative care to frail older people with MLTC. Advance care planning, appropriate prognostication and the delivery of realistic medicine could reduce hospitalizations and outpatient appointment visits whilst improving care satisfaction and improving well-being and quality of life.

Providing appropriate palliative care for people with MLTC and frailty may be the key to improving palliative care equity. Due to their associations with socioeconomic deprivation and ethnically diverse communities palliative care provision for these communities would also improve.

References

1. Clegg A, Young J, Iliffe S, Rikkert M, Rockwood K. Frailty in elderly people. *Lancet* 2013; 381(9868): 752–762.
2. MacMahon S, The Academy of Medical Sciences. Multimorbidity: a priority for global health research. *Acad Med Sci*. 2018. Available at: https://acmedsci.ac.uk/file-download/82222577

3. National Institute for Health Research. NIHR Strategic Framework for Multiple Long-Term Conditions (Multimorbidity) MLTC-M Research. 2020. Available at: https://www.nihr.ac.uk/documents/research-on-multiple-long-term-conditions-multimorbidity-mltc-m/24639?pr =
4. Nicholson C, Richardson H. Age-attuned hospice care: an opportunity to better end of life care for older people. 2018. Available at: http://www.stchristophers.org.uk
5. Etkind SN, Bone AE, Gomes B, et al. How many people will need palliative care in 2040? Past trends, future projections and implications for services. *BMC Med* 2017; 15(1): 1–10.
6. Stow D, Spiers G, Matthews FE, Hanratty B. What is the evidence that people with frailty have needs for palliative care at the end of life? A systematic review and narrative synthesis. *Palliat Med* 2019; 33(4): 399–414.
7. Bone AE, Gomes B, Etkind SN, et al. What is the impact of population ageing on the future provision of end-of-life care? Population-based projections of place of death. *Palliat Med* 2018; 32(2): 329–336.
8. Hamaker M, van den Bos F, Rostoft S. Frailty and palliative care. *BMJ Support Palliat Care* 2020; 10: 262–264.
9. Harwood RH, Enguell H. End-of-life care for frail older people. *BMJ Palliat Care*. 2019 Nov 15. Available at: http://spcare.bmj.com/content/early/2019/11/14/bmjspcare-2019-001953.abstract
10. Nicholson C, Gordon AL, Tinker A. Changing the way 'we' view and talk about frailty. *Age Ageing* 2017; 46(3): 349–351.
11. Bone AE, Morgan M, Maddocks M, et al. Developing a model of short-term integrated palliative and supportive care for frail older people in community settings: perspectives of older people, carers and other key stakeholders. *Age Ageing* 2016; 45(6): 863–873.
12. Pearson-Stuttard J, Ezzati M, Gregg E. Multimorbidity-a defining challenge for health systems. *Lancet Public Health* 2019; 4(12): e599–600.
13. Marmot M, Allen J, Boyce T, Goldblatt P, Morrison J. *Health Equity in England: The Marmot Review 10 Years On*. 2020. Available at: https://www.instituteofhealthequity.org/resources-reports/marmot-review-10-years-on/the-marmot-review-10-years-on-full-report.pdf
14. British Geriatric Society. Fit for Frailty Part 1 Consensus best practice guidance for the care of older people living in community and outpatient settings. 2017;1–22. Available at: http://www.bgs.org.uk/campaigns/fff/fff_full.pdf
15. Darowski A, Dwight J, Reynolds J. Medicines and falls in hospital. 2011; 1–4. Available at: https://www.bgs.org.uk/sites/default/files/content/attachment/2018-05-22/Falls_drug_guide.pdf
16. Moody D. The Frailty Fulcrum. 2016. Available at: https://www.england.nhs.uk/blog/dawn-moody/
17. Vernon MJ. NHS RightCare Frailty Toolkit. 2019;(June). Available at: https://www.england.nhs.uk/rightcare/wp-content/uploads/sites/40/2019/07/frailty-toolkit-june-2019-v1.pdf
18. Jha SR, Ha HSK, Hickman LD, et al. Frailty in advanced heart failure: a systematic review. *Heart Fail Rev* 2015; 20(5): 553–560.
19. Gale NS, Albarrati AM, Munnery MM, et al. Frailty: a global measure of the multisystem impact of COPD. *Chron Respir Dis* 2018; 15(4): 347–355.
20. Welford J, Rafferty R, Hunt K, et al. The Clinical Frailty Scale can indicate prognosis and care requirements on discharge in oncology and haemato-oncology inpatients: A cohort study. *Eur J Cancer Care* 2022; 31(6): e13752. https://doi.org/10.1111/ecc.13752
21. Ethun CG, Bilen MA, Jani AB, Maithel SK, Ogan K, Master VA. Frailty and cancer: Implications for oncology surgery, medical oncology, and radiation oncology. *CA Cancer J Clin* 2017; 67(5): 362–377.
22. Rogers JG, Patel CB, Mentz RJ, et al. Palliative care in heart failure: the PAL-HF randomized, controlled clinical trial. *J Am Coll Cardiol* 2017; 70(3): 331–341.
23. Molnar F, Frank CC. Optimizing geriatric care with the GERIATRIC 5Ms. *Can Fam Physician* 2019; 65(1): 39.

CASE

32 Diabetes Management at the End of Life

Jaspal Kaur Mann

Expert: Alastair Lumb

Case history

Harry, a 44-year-old man, with a background of adenocarcinoma of the distal sigmoid colon, was admitted to a tertiary oncology centre for symptom control with severe, worsening abdominal pain and distension. Imaging revealed widespread disease progression with pleural effusions, extension of lung metastases, multiple enlarging liver metastases, and extensive peritoneal disease. A large abdominopelvic collection was noted, containing gas and fluid, secondary to suspected stent perforation of the distal colonic wall. He had no further systemic anticancer treatment options.

He had been diagnosed with type 1 diabetes aged 16 years and was under the care of his General Practitioner. Glycosylated haemoglobin (HbA1c) was within target limits. His mother (who lived abroad in his country of origin) also had type 1 diabetes. At the time of admission, he had stopped both his basal (Lantus®/insulin glargine) and bolus (Humalog®/insulin lispro) insulin injections. He had not eaten for 36 hours and had deliberately omitted his insulin due to low blood glucose readings (between 5 to 6 mmol/L). Admission bloods revealed a blood glucose of 6 mmol/L, severely deranged liver function with raised white cells, inflammatory markers, and urea. A venous blood gas (VBG) showed normal pH, low bicarbonate, and a base deficit indicative of metabolic acidosis with respiratory compensation.

Lantus® was restarted after Harry's wife and mother raised concerns that he may develop diabetic ketoacidosis (DKA). However, he subsequently developed hypoglycaemic episodes and the Lantus® was again stopped by the medical team.

Learning Point Epidemiology of Type 1 Diabetes and Cancer

Just under 4 million people in the UK have a diagnosis of diabetes, of which approximately 8% have type 1 diabetes. It is the commonest form of diabetes found in children,[1] but can be diagnosed at any stage of life. Management of type 1 diabetes involves lifelong treatment with exogenous insulin guided by glucose monitoring. Glycaemic targets are set to reduce the risk of developing long-term micro- and macrovascular complications. Relatively few deaths are attributable to diabetes directly, most are due to cardiovascular disease (e.g. ischaemic heart disease, chronic kidney disease, heart failure) or cancer. There is also growing epidemiological evidence of an association between diabetes and an increased risk of cancers,[2, 3] particularly those of the breast, lung, colon, prostate, and pancreas.[4]

Expert Comment Treatment Regimens for Type 1 Diabetes

The majority of people with type 1 diabetes manage their condition using multiple daily injections of insulin. Insulin is administered to try to mimic physiological insulin secretion. Long-acting basal insulins are injected once or twice daily, and rapid-acting bolus insulin injected with food. Some people use insulin pumps, where basal insulin is provided by a continuous infusion of rapid-acting insulin, which can be varied through the day.

Expert Comment

People with type 1 diabetes self-manage their condition with support from a specialist healthcare team. They routinely make detailed decisions about medication dosing, with bolus insulin doses adjusted according to a range of factors such as blood glucose, activity, and the carbohydrate content of food. People with type 1 diabetes should be viewed as experts in the management of their condition, and their opinion sought about treatment changes where possible.

Clinical Tip Diabetic Ketoacidosis

DKA is an acute metabolic crisis, most often seen in people with type 1 diabetes, and caused by absolute insulin deficiency. It usually develops rapidly when insulin is omitted for whatever reason (over hours to days) and can also be associated with intercurrent illness. There are specific diagnostic criteria.[5] It should be considered as a differential in all unwell patients with type 1 diabetes.[6]

Expert Comment Ketone Measurement

Ketones can be measured in urine, capillary samples, and whole blood. Guidelines on DKA management in adults recommend capillary ketone measurement which provides quick, precise, and quantitative ketone assessment.[5] Urinary ketone measurements are non-invasive but less useful as they are not specific for the ketones which develop in DKA and may not represent current clinical status.[7] Ketones can also be elevated by starvation, which may cause confusion at the end of life as oral intake diminishes.

The Oncology team recognized that Harry was rapidly approaching the end of life. He was referred to the Hospital Palliative Care Team (HPCT) for symptom control and psychological support for his wife and young family. He was commenced on a morphine and levomepromazine syringe driver for moderate to severe pain, nausea, and vomiting. He appeared very jaundiced, frail, and cachectic, managing only monosyllabic responses on questioning. Episodes of confusion were also reported.

Harry's mother was unable to travel to the United Kingdom, but his wife and children were granted urgent access for visiting. His family raised concerns that he was not on insulin treatment, with a particular concern about the risk of DKA. A VBG excluded a metabolic acidosis and urinalysis excluded ketones. Blood glucose readings monitored 6-hourly from admission were stable (between 5.3 and 8.5 mmol/L). In response to the family's concerns, the HPCT prescribed a significantly reduced dose of Lantus® insulin to be given immediately, and then regularly once daily in the morning. Treatment for hypoglycaemia was also prescribed in case it was required.

Overnight, blood glucose dropped to below 4 mmol/L. Treatment was given with an oral glucose gel and subsequently 10% IV dextrose, with advice to hold insulin in the morning. Blood glucose pre-breakfast was 4.2 mmol/L. Following senior HPCT review, insulin was again stopped. Over the next 24 hours, further episodes of hypoglycaemia were noted and treated with IV glucose via a peripherally inserted central catheter or PICC line which was in situ. His family remained concerned about the risk of DKA but VBG monitoring was reassuring. The HPCT recognized that death was imminent, and he sadly died a few hours later.

Evidence Base End of Life Guidance for Diabetes Care, 4th Edition. Trend Diabetes Endorsed by Diabetes UK

A few countries, such as Australia[1] and the UK[8] have specific guidance regarding the management of diabetes at the end of life. Prior to the development of this guidance, there was a lack of consensus regarding best practice,[9, 10] with inconsistencies in quality standards and management. This could lead to inconsistent advice from Diabetes and Palliative Care teams.

In order to achieve high-quality diabetes care at the end of life, recommendations are based on illness stage and prognosis:

- Proactive, regular review and rationalization of glucose-lowering therapies and other medications (e.g. statins) with joint decision-making involving patient and carers
- Avoidance of metabolic emergencies, e.g. hypoglycaemic episodes, persistent symptomatic hyperglycaemia and DKA in type 1 diabetes
- Early recognition of illness stage and potential for deterioration, with discussion of advanced care planning
- Supporting the patient and carers in self-management as long as possible
- Effective symptom control at the end of life
- Care of patients with diabetes not influencing patient, carer, or healthcare professional (HCP) preference for preferred place of care (PPC) or preferred place of death (PPOD)

Clinical Tip Recommended Management for Type 1 Diabetes at the End of Life

People with type 1 diabetes usually require daily insulin to avoid DKA, even when not eating or drinking. At the end of life, UK guidance[8] recommends switching to a simplified treatment regime, with once-daily long-acting basal analogue insulin (e.g. Lantus®/Glargine or Tresiba®/Degludec). This type of insulin gives a stable level of insulin with a relatively low risk of hypoglycaemia (Figure 32.1).

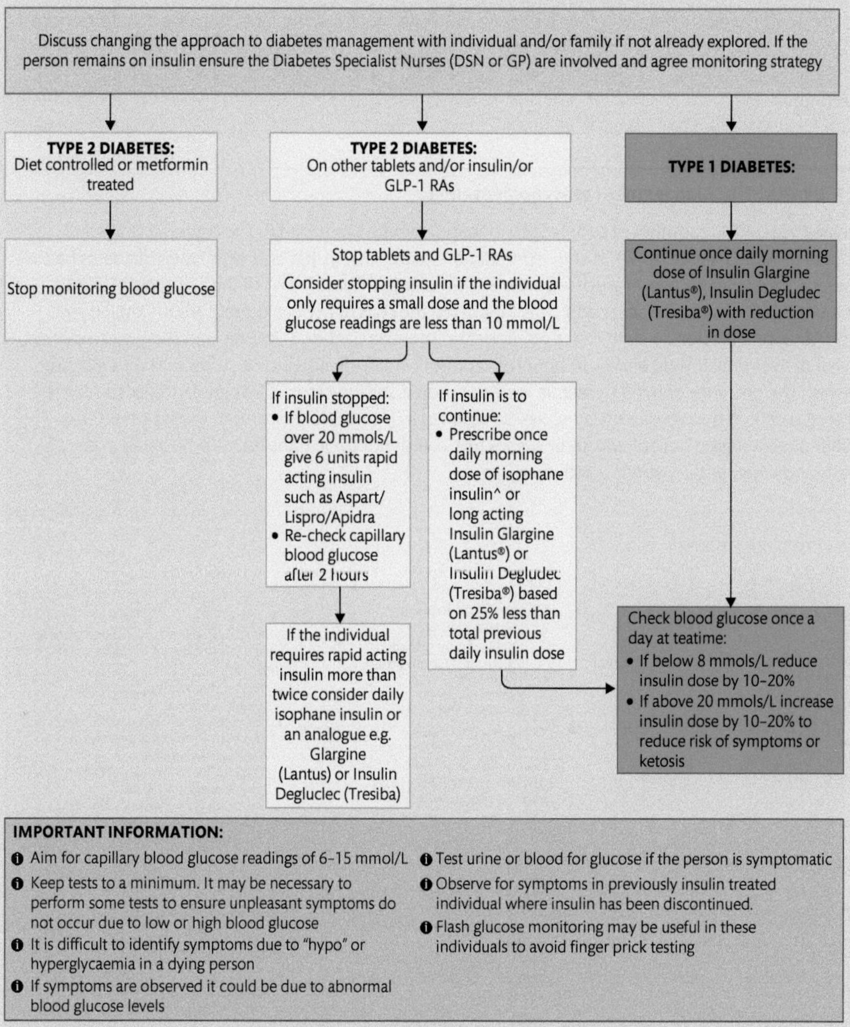

Figure 32.1 Algorithm for diabetes management in the last days of life.

Reproduced with permission from Trend Diabetes & Diabetes UK.

Learning Point Blood Glucose Targets and Monitoring at the End of Life

Blood glucose levels can influence symptom severity (e.g. fatigue, pain) and overall quality of life, but no published data or prospective studies exist for ideal blood glucose or Hba1c ranges at the end of life.[4,8] An individualized approach is required, considering illness stage, prognosis, the presence of hypoglycaemia, nutritional status, and the wishes of people with diabetes and their carers. A capillary blood glucose range of 6–15 mmol/L is recommended,[8] to avoid hypo- and hyperglycaemia and any associated symptoms. Monitoring frequency can potentially be reduced to once daily. In this case, blood glucose monitoring was continued four times a day due to concerns about stopping basal insulin in a person with type 1 diabetes.

Expert Comment Continuous Glucose Monitoring (CGM)

CGM involves a sensor under the skin which measures interstitial glucose readings, and its use has increased significantly over recent years. It offers a less invasive way to obtain frequent glucose readings, with insertion of a single sensor providing readings for around 7–14 days. Sensor readings

Expert Comment The Impact of Treatment De-escalation

At the end of life, the focus of treatment shifts from tight glucose management and avoidance of long-term complications to more relaxed blood glucose targets and an overall holistic approach.[11] This de-escalation of treatment can be challenging for patients and carers. Careful explanation and reassurance are required to ensure people do not feel as though diabetes management is being overlooked or HCPs are 'giving up' on them.

include information about whether glucose is currently steady, rising, or falling. Most systems have alarms that can alert to high or low glucose readings and hence support treatment adjustments. If readings are outside a target range, then confirmation with a fingerstick reading is usually recommended.

Clinical Tip Management of Hypoglycaemia

Hypoglycaemia is common in people with diabetes admitted to hospital. The National Diabetes Inpatient Audit (NaDIA) in 2019, showed that more than 1 in 4 in-patients with type 1 diabetes had experienced at least 1 blood glucose below 3.0 mmol/L in the last 7 days of their hospital stay.[12] In the setting of advanced disease and type 1 diabetes, the risks of hypoglycaemia are multiplied by a combination of factors: weight loss, poor appetite, anorexia-cachexia, nausea, vomiting, gastroparesis, renal or liver impairment and poor symptom control (which affects glucose stores and thus glucose levels). The presence of hypoglycaemia is a poor prognostic indicator.[1] Clear guidance exists for the management of hypoglycaemic episodes, as outlined in Figure 32.2.[8] However, management may differ depending on patient and carer wishes (e.g. a wish not to be transferred to hospital), place of care, and whether the patient is actively dying.

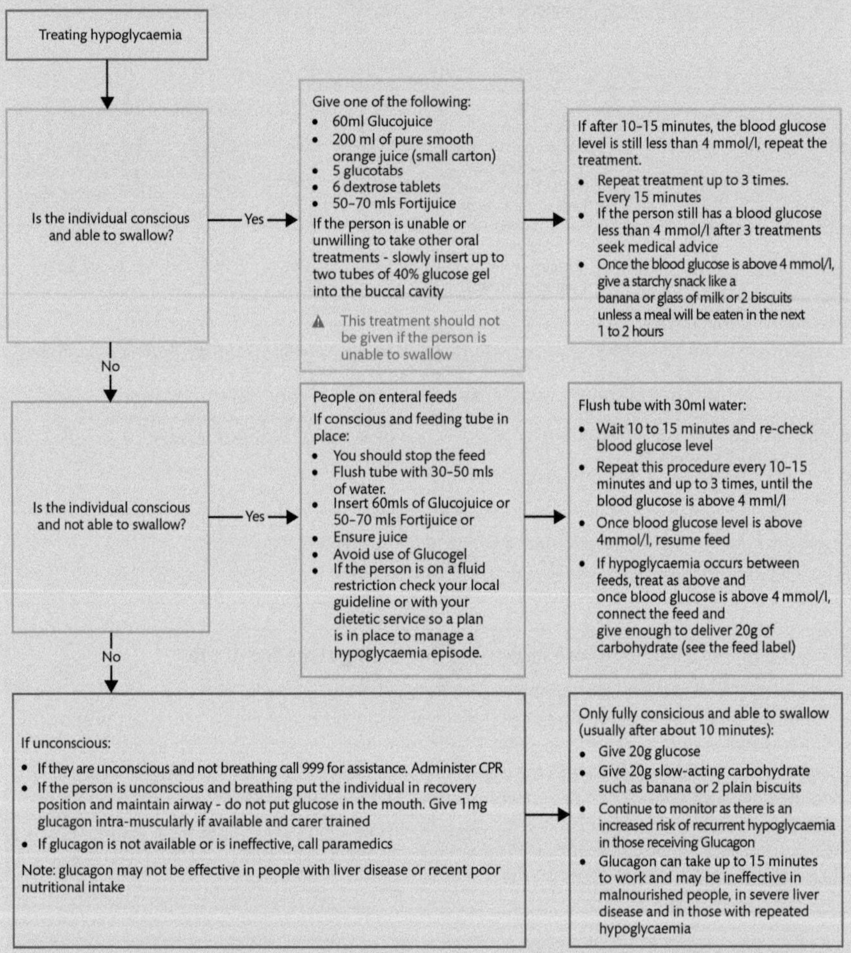

Figure 32.2 Algorithm for treating hypoglycaemia.

Reproduced with permission from Trend Diabetes & Diabetes UK.

Expert Comment Recurrent Hypoglycaemia

While it is unusual to need to stop insulin treatment at the end of life in type 1 diabetes, there were a number of factors that contributed to hypoglycaemia, including anorexia-cachexia secondary to cancer, nausea, vomiting, impaired gastrointestinal function due to bowel perforation and the dying process. We would usually expect withdrawal of exogenous insulin to precipitate DKA, but in this case saw blood glucose measurements below 6 mmol/L, which is the recommended lower limit for glucose[8] in the last few days of life. The re-introduction of insulin caused recurrent hypoglycaemia, demonstrating that it wasn't required. Insulin was therefore withdrawn, with monitoring to ensure this did not result in DKA and hence further distress.

Expert Comment Insulin Treatment and Renal Impairment

It is possible that this patient's renal function had deteriorated further after blood tests were stopped. The kidney is responsible for between 30% and 80% of insulin removal, so a decline in renal function is associated with an increase in insulin half-life and a decrease in insulin requirement.[13] The actual dose reduction will need to be individualized and guided by monitoring but a 50% reduction may offer similar glycaemia with a reduced risk of hypoglycaemia.

Discussion

Guidelines advise continuation of basal insulin in patients with type 1 diabetes at the EOL, but individual circumstances have to be considered. In this case, Harry himself had made the decision to stop his basal insulin. Insulin omission carries a risk of DKA, and his family were concerned about this, but metabolic testing was reassuring. Accepting his expertise in diabetes self-management, it would have been important to assess whether he had the capacity to make the decision to stop insulin treatment. A combination of delirium, lethargy, pain, and distress could have impacted his decision-making capacity, although no concerns were raised at the time of admission. Insulin may also have been deliberately withheld as a means of hastening death.

Harry was cared for in a tertiary oncology hospital with a PICC line in situ, allowing blood samples to be taken and intravenous medication administered. Where IV access is an issue, the patient is at home or IV medications or fluids cannot be given (such as some inpatient palliative care units), management, and treatment escalation decisions should be discussed with patients and carers, ideally early on and as part of an advance care plan (ACP). Early ACP may have addressed some of the issues raised by Harry's case, in particular action plans for DKA, and symptomatic hyperglycaemia and hypoglycaemia. Good communication is vital in any therapeutic relationship but absolutely essential where management decisions deviate from usual practice.

Harry had not informed his mother of his decision to omit insulin or the reasons for it. She was afraid that his diabetes was being either ignored or mismanaged, and her fears would also have been compounded by her own distress and grief of having an imminently dying son who she was unable to visit. Regular monitoring of glucose and VBG results aided discussion with the family, providing reassurance and acceptance of clinical management. They also helped to distinguish whether his symptoms and clinical status were due to the dying process or diabetes.[14]

People with type 1 diabetes, and their carers, can struggle to accept a switch in focus from tight glycaemic management. In palliative care, non-essential drugs are often rationalized or used for off label indications, in up to one-third of prescriptions.[15] While some insulin is usually essential for people with type 1 diabetes, the doses required for tight glycaemic targets are no longer required. Guidelines support reducing the frequency of blood glucose monitoring and other invasive testing as a patient approaches the end of life, to reduce patient burden and avoid unnecessary tests. CGM may be useful in this context, providing useful information about glucose levels without significant burden. It is important to note that the idea of what constitutes burden in this context should be guided by patients and carers, rather than HCPs.

This was a complex case involving a young person with aggressive metastatic cancer, and type 1 diabetes, where it was appropriate to stop insulin in the last few days of life. Although UK and Australian guidelines[1, 8] recommend continuing insulin for people with type 1 diabetes, both guidelines recognize instances when stopping insulin is appropriate (such as frequent, persistent hypoglycaemic episodes). This case offers such an example and should encourage medical and nursing teams to be familiar with diabetes end of life guidelines for consistent, holistic care, and to exercise an individualized approach, depending on the clinical presentation and other circumstances.

Future Advances

The bulk of the caseload in palliative care currently involves patients with cancer, followed by organ failures, such as cardiac and renal failure, which are often secondary complications of diabetes. It is therefore inevitable in palliative care we will manage patients with type 1 diabetes. The use of wearable technologies and other technological developments will also increase and it is important HCPs have some familiarity with these and are able to access specialist advice and support. Discussion of alternatives to wearable technologies with close liaison and advice from the diabetes teams is helpful, especially where newer technologies may be unfamiliar to staff. Management of devices or metabolic emergencies should not negatively impact patient or carer choice regarding place of care and death.

A Final Word from the Expert

The case described here illustrates the complexity of diabetes management at the end of life. Standard glucose targets are aimed at reducing the risk of longer-term complications associated with diabetes, and hence become less relevant as the end of life approaches. In the final stages of life, guidance suggests the focus of treatment should be on reducing both the burden of diabetes management and the risk of symptoms arising from low or high glucose levels. Hypoglycaemia is a particular risk at this stage, as factors which increase the occurrence of low glucose such as anorexia-cachexia, impaired liver and renal function, and weight loss are all common at the end of life. A simplification of diabetes treatment is usually suggested, and there are guidelines in place to support this. Insulin should usually be continued in a reduced dose for people with type 1 diabetes. Advance care planning discussions can be extremely helpful, allowing people with diabetes and their carers to understand the reasons for the change in focus and agree an approach to diabetes management. Wearable diabetes technologies, such as continuous glucose monitors, are increasingly used to support treatment decisions. These can offer valuable information with limited burden, but palliative care staff may require additional training to support their use.

References

1. Dunning TM, Peter. Revised guidelines for deciding Palliative and End of Life Care with People with Diabetes Australia: Australian Disease Management Association (ADMA) 2019. Available at: https://adma.org.au/download/revised-guidelines-for-deciding-palliative-and-end-of-life-care-with-people-with-diabetes/.
2. Giovannucci E, Harlan DM, Archer MC, et al. Diabetes and cancer: a consensus report. *Diabetes Care* 2010; 33(7): 1674–1685.
3. Jacob P, Chowdhury T. Management of diabetes in patients with cancer. *QJM* 2015; 108(6): 443–448.

4. Hershey DS. Importance of glycemic control in cancer patients with diabetes: treatment through end of life. *Asia-Pac J Oncol Nurs* 2017; 4(4): 313–318.
5. Dhatariya KK; Joint British Diabetes Societies for Inpatient Care. The management of diabetic ketoacidosis in adults—an updated guideline from the Joint British Diabetes Society for Inpatient Care. *Diabet Med* 2022; 39(6): e14788.
6. Muneer M, Akbar I. Acute metabolic emergencies in diabetes: DKA, HHS and EDKA. *Adv Exp Med Biol* 2021; 1307: 85–114.
7. Brewster S, Curtis L, Poole R. Urine versus blood ketones. *Practical Diabetes* 2017; 34(1): 13–15.
8. Diabetes UK and Trend Diabetes. *End of Life Guidance for Diabetes Care 2021*, 4th ed. Available at: https://diabetes-resources-production.s3.eu-west-1.amazonaws.com/resources-s3/public/2021-11/EoL_TREND_FINAL2_0.pdf
9. James J. Dying well with diabetes. *Ann Palliat Med* 2019; 8(2): 178–189.
10. Ford-Dunn S, Smith A, Quin J. Management of diabetes during the last days of life: attitudes of consultant diabetologists and consultant palliative care physicians in the UK. *Palliat Med* 2006; 20(3): 197–203.
11. King E, Haboubi H, Evans D, Baker I, Bain S, Stephens J. The management of diabetes in terminal illness related to cancer. *QJM* 2012; 105(1): 3–9.
12. NHS Digital. The National Diabetes Inpatient Audit (NaDIA) 2019 2019. Available at: https://files.digital.nhs.uk/F6/49FA05/NaDIA%202019%20-%20Full%20Report%20v1.1.pdf
13. Hahr A and Molitch M. Management of diabetes mellitus in patients with chronic kidney disease. *Clin Diabetes Endocrinol* 2015; 1: 2.
14. Quinn K, Hudson P, Dunning T. Diabetes management in patients receiving palliative care. *Aus Nurs Midwifery J* 2006; 13(8): 29.
15. Hagemann V, Bausewein C, Remi C. Drug use beyond the licence in palliative care: a systematic review and narrative synthesis. *Palliat Med* 2019; 33(6): 650–662.

CASE

33 Malignant Spinal Cord Compression

Mairi Finlay and Oliver Jackson

Expert: Mark Teo

Case history

Chris, a 55-year-old man, presented to the emergency department with a 6-month history of progressive thoracic back pain that had significantly worsened over the preceding week, accompanied by right leg weakness and paraesthesia. He was able to mobilize independently with no urinary or bowel symptoms. In recent months, Chris had noticed weight loss of a stone, a persistent cough, and episodes of coughing up blood.

Neurological examination revealed loss of power throughout the entire right leg (Medical Research Council (MRC) score 4 + /5) and altered sensation to light touch in dermatomes L3–S2. Perineal sensation and anal tone were intact. Gait was normal with appropriate speed and no ataxia.

Chris had no significant past medical history and worked as a joiner. He was an ex-smoker with a 20-year pack history. He had a World Health Organization (WHO) performance status of 1.

The clinical impression was a high suspicion of malignant spinal cord compression. Chris was commenced on 16 mg oral dexamethasone with proton-pump inhibitor (PPI) cover, and urgent whole spine MRI requested. He was prescribed 5 mg immediate release oral morphine QDS, with 2 mg immediate release oral morphine PRN for breakthrough pain.

Learning Point Diagnosis of Malignant Spinal Cord Compression

A full neurological examination is essential for all patients with suspected MSCC to correlate clinical examination findings with radiological imaging and ensure the correct site(s) treated.

It is important to have a high level of suspicion for MSCC in patients with known cancer and those with high risk factors for cancer. Clinical predictors for MSCC include presence of neurological signs, cervical or thoracic back pain, known vertebral metastases, and known metastatic disease, with an MSCC risk of 8% for no risk factors up to 81% for more than three risk factors.[1] Unless contraindicated, a loading dose of 16 mg oral dexamethasone should be given immediately on suspicion of MSCC. The caveat is for suspected new haematological cancers (e.g. plasmacytoma, lymphoma), as the high steroid doses would make subsequent tissue diagnosis difficult, hence an urgent biopsy and/or surgical decompression is needed.

An urgent MRI of the whole spine should be obtained within 24 hours[2] as multilevel MSCC is common and will influence treatment options. CT imaging may be a pragmatic alternative if MRI is contraindicated. If emergency surgical intervention is planned, overnight imaging should be considered. For suspected MSCC such as cancer patients with neuropathic back pain but no neurological signs, urgent imaging should be performed within seven days.[2]

Clinical Tip Dexamethasone Prescribing

Ensure that dexamethasone is prescribed in the morning as prescribing later in the day increases the risk of insomnia and disturbed sleep.

Learning Point Managing Steroid Side Effects

Dexamethasone is a corticosteroid with potent glucocorticoid activity. Adverse effects include steroid-induced hyperglycaemia, deterioration of existing diabetes mellitus, and increased risks of gastrointestinal bleeding, infection and psychiatric disturbances (e.g. agitation, paranoia). When initiating prescriptions, there must be a clear plan for dose reduction or dose review date.

All patients should be issued a steroid alert card. In a meta-analysis,[3] adrenal insufficiency has been reported with short steroid courses less than a month (absolute risk 1.4%) and low doses of less than 1 mg oral dexamethasone equivalent (absolute risk 2.4%). This risk increases to over 11% for steroid courses over one month and over 21.5 % for doses greater than 8 mg oral dexamethasone.

A gastroprotective agent, typically an oral proton-pump inhibitor, should be routinely coprescribed for the duration of the course of high-dose steroids. Regular capillary blood glucose monitoring is needed to identify patients who develop steroid-induced hyperglycaemia (consider prescribing a sulphonylurea with a target blood glucose between 6–15 mmol/l). For patients with pre-existing diabetes, more frequent monitoring may be required with support from the Diabetes Specialist Team.[4]

Longer-term adverse effects of corticosteroids include proximal myopathy, cushingoid appearance, and skin changes. To minimize these effects, dexamethasone therapy should be reduced over 5–7 days once definitive MSCC treatment has started. If neurological function deteriorates during dose reduction, it may be necessary to increase dexamethasone in the short term. When neither surgery or radiotherapy are indicated, dexamethasone should be gradually reduced with the eventual aim to discontinue; some patients may require long-term low-dose dexamethasone, e.g. if neurological function worsens during dose reduction.[2]

Clinical Tip Pain Management in Malignant Spinal Cord Compression

Pain from MSCC is often severe and patients may experience escalating pain prior to diagnosis. The pain management strategy will depend on the patient's current analgesia regimen. Access to short-acting opioid analgesia for breakthrough pain is important for all patients. Some may also benefit from regular paracetamol and/or non-steroidal anti-inflammatories (NSAIDs); be especially cautious of prescribing dual NSAIDs alongside high-dose steroids, in view of gastrointestinal bleeding risk.[2] Individualized risk versus benefit assessment is needed to optimize analgesia, especially if inadequate pain management is preventing diagnostic imaging or radiotherapy treatment.

Treatment with radiotherapy can improve pain control but may take over 2 weeks to see the full effect. Over this period, the overall analgesia requirements may reduce. Pain control should be reviewed regularly with analgesia doses titrated accordingly.

Patients with breast cancer, prostate cancer or myeloma who develop MSCC may benefit from treatment with bisphosphonates or RANK ligand inhibitors (denosumab) to reduce pain and the risk of further bone complications. This should be discussed with the treating cancer team.[2]

An MRI revealed extensive extradural spinal metastases (Figure 33.1) with multi-level MSCC at C5/C6 from mixed degenerative and malignant compression, with pathological collapse of T1, and early MSCC around T6/T7 due to extradural soft tissue. A staging CT imaging demonstrated a right lower lobe primary lung cancer with malignant effusion, mediastinal and hilar lymphadenopathy, and widespread bone metastases. The intrathoracic disease was suitable for biopsy.

Chris's case was discussed with the on-call spinal surgical team to explore if surgical management would be suitable. In view of the spinal column being stable, the extensive vertebral metastases, and multilevel cord compression, surgery was felt to be inappropriate.

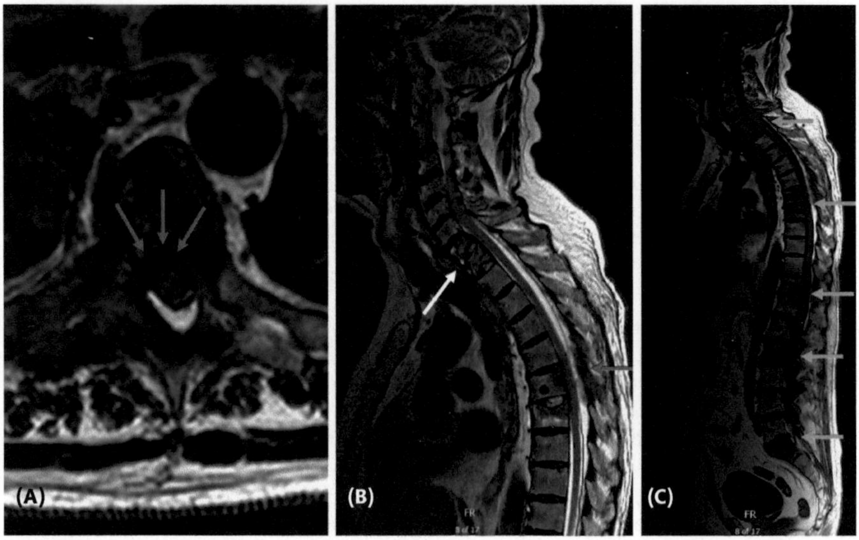

Figure 33.1 MRI imaging of the whole spine demonstrating: i) on T2-weighted sequences effacement of CSF anteriorly secondary to large volume right sided vertebral body soft tissue at T6 and T7 from metastatic disease (Figure 33.1A and 33.1B arrowed red); ii) mixed degenerative and malignant compressive myelopathy in the cervical spine (Figure 33.1B arrowed white); and on T1-weighted sequences, extensive multilevel extradural spinal metastases (Figure 33.1C arrowed blue).

Learning Point Surgical Management of Malignant Spinal Cord Compression

The objectives of surgery in MSCC are spinal decompression to restore neurological function, halt further neurological deterioration, and to maintain spinal stability. Surgical suitability is based on a variety of factors, including comorbidities, frailty, number of sites of disease, the speed and severity of the onset of neurological symptoms, and cancer prognosis. Suitable patients should have surgery before they lose the ability to walk; in patients with a good prognosis, those with residual motor or sensory function should be offered surgery with the aim of restoring function.

Surgical intervention often includes posterior decompressive laminectomy, with or without internal fixation or bone grafting. En-bloc radical excision of metastases should only be attempted in rare cases (isolated thyroid or renal cell metastases after complete staging). Definitive treatment should be started within 24 hours of diagnosis if possible.

Evidence Base Decompressive Surgical Resection in Malignant Spinal Cord Compression

There has been one randomized control trial and one systematic review assessing surgical decompression and stabilization followed by radiotherapy versus radiotherapy only.[5, 6] These demonstrated significantly better ambulatory recovery with surgery compared to radiotherapy (64% vs. 29%, respectively), longer median duration of retaining walking function (122 days vs. 13 days, respectively), and pain relief (88% of patients vs. 74%, respectively). Surgical complication rates of 29% (range 5–65%) and 30-day postoperative mortality of 5% (range 0–22%) have been reported. Median overall survival for all cancer types were better with surgery (17 months) versus radiotherapy (3 months), likely due to improved ambulatory function following surgery (potentially influenced by patient selection bias).

Chris was referred to the regional clinical oncology team for radiotherapy. He received a single fraction of radiotherapy treating from C4 to T7 vertebrae (Figure 33.2). Chris tolerated radiotherapy well, noting side effects of mild self-limiting fatigue and odynophagia, which was managed with oxetacaine suspension. A flare of his thoracic back pain was managed with oral morphine suspension 5 mg PRN, alongside regular paracetamol, and codeine.

Learning Point Radiotherapy Treatment Pathway/Techniques/Side Effects

Radiotherapy fractionation regimens vary but is commonly a single 8 Gy fraction.[7] Higher radiotherapy dose regimens, e.g. 30 Gy in ten daily fractions, are associated with better local control but are more resource and time intensive; prolonged control may be irrelevant for patients with poor prognosis.

Treatment involves a planning CT scan for target localization and radiotherapy dose-planning. To ensure patient set-up reproducibility, appropriate patient positioning and immobilization devices such as radiotherapy masks may be required. For urgent MSCC treatments, often a single rectangular radiotherapy field, or an opposing pair of fields are applied (Figure 33.2) with delivery of a single radiotherapy fraction taking 10–15 minutes. With a single fraction of radiotherapy, planning and treatment is often delivered in a single day. The anticancer response to radiotherapy typically takes 10–14 days from treatment.

Palliative radiotherapy side effects are dose-dependent and occur 24–48 hours after treatment, with peak severity under two weeks from treatment and resolving by 2–4 weeks. Fatigue and mild skin dermatitis are common, with other side effects typically mild relating to the treatment site and adjacent organs (e.g. cervical/upper thoracic spine—mucositis of the oesophagus; lower lumbosacral spine—diarrhoea from large bowel enteritis). Ten per cent of patients may develop a flare of pre-existing pain occurring 24–48 hours after treatment. This pain flare is self-resolving within a week and is managed with breakthrough analgesia.

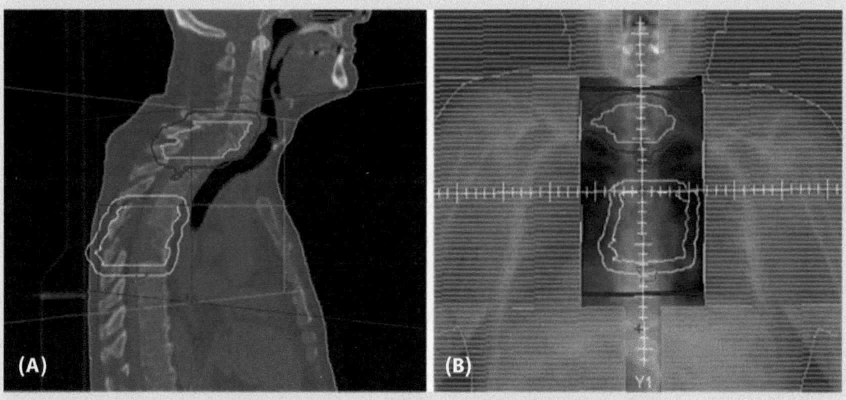

Figure 33.2 Radiotherapy virtual simulator planning. Figure 33.2A shows Mr Brown's two target areas of MSCC delineated (light and dark blue areas) with a parallel opposed field arrangement with the posterior radiation field edge in red, and the anterior field in pale blue. Figure 33.2B shows the anterior field 'Beam's eye view' on the planning CT digital reconstructed radiograph.

Learning Point Suitability for Radiotherapy

It is important to consider if radiotherapy is suitable for each patient at the time of referral. To deliver radiotherapy safely, patients must be able to lie supine and still for 10–15 minutes. This may preclude treatment for patients with uncontrolled pain, delirium or cognitive impairment, and clinically unstable patients. For clinically unstable patients, it is often not suitable to transfer between hospitals for treatment.

It is essential to recognize those that will not benefit from radiotherapy, either because their prognosis is too poor (i.e. less than a few weeks) or where there is no scope for functional recovery (e.g. complete motor loss for over 24 hours with no response to high-dose steroids). For the latter group, radiotherapy can still be considered for pain control.

Clinical Tip Other Options for Treatment of Malignant Spinal Cord Compression

Whilst most treatment for MSCC is either surgery or radiotherapy, systemic therapies may be appropriate in select scenarios. In untreated prostate cancer, gonadotropin-releasing hormone antagonists, e.g. degarelix can have a very rapid effect on testosterone-driven tumour cells and is usually given synchronously with radiotherapy. Emergency primary chemotherapy may be considered in chemo-sensitive cancers, such as small cell lung cancers, lymphomas, or plasmacytomas, especially if there is a curative treatment intent involving radical radiotherapy doses.

Expert Comment Radiotherapy

Radiotherapy remains the mainstay treatment for MSCC in patients unsuitable for surgery. A meta-analysis has demonstrated that single-fraction radiotherapy (8–10 Gy in one fraction) compared to multifraction regimens has equivalent ambulatory motor response, risk of bladder dysfunction, and overall survival.[7] Multifraction radiotherapy is considered for patients with good prognosis where longer local control from a higher dose may be preferred.

For a radiation myelopathy risk of <1%, the maximum lifetime dose tolerance for the spinal cord and cauda equina are 50 Gy and 60 Gy in equivalent dose in 2 Gy fractions, respectively. Decisions to re-irradiate the same spinal level is thus dependent on prior radiotherapy dose received, duration of disease control from last treatment, and patient prognosis (radiation induced myelopathy typically occurs more than 6 months after radiation treatment). Stereotactic ablative radiotherapy (SABR) for spinal metastases have reported greater local cancer control and symptom control than conventional radiotherapy, but due to the longer radiotherapy treatment planning time required, has no routine role in the emergency treatment of MSCC.

Two weeks following treatment, neurological examination showed persistent but stable weakness of his right leg. Chris remained independently mobile and developed no further neurological deficits. The pleural effusion was sampled for histology and cancer molecular profiling, and Chris was referred to the medical oncology team for consideration of palliative systemic therapies.

Learning Point Spinal Instability and Mobilization

Scoring systems, such as Spinal Instability Neoplastic Score (SINS),[8] are useful to predict the likelihood of spinal instability to identify the patients most likely to benefit from referral for surgical stabilization. For patients with stable SINS or surgically stabilized spines, graduated mobilization should be encouraged with careful monitoring for any worsening pain or neurology.

For patients with unstable SINS who are unsuitable for surgery, cervical collars and/or spinal bracing should be considered for both pain control and protecting the spinal cord, but these are often poorly tolerated by patients. Patient involvement in deciding the extent of spinal immobilization and the level of mobility allowed is needed taking into account the risk of neurological deterioration versus quality-of-life considerations and the overall poor prognosis of MSCC.[2, 9]

Learning Point Palliative Rehabilitation and Psychological Impact

Multidisciplinary care is core to the management of MSCC, including expert nursing care and early involvement from physiotherapy and occupational therapy. Palliative rehabilitation focuses on specific, short-term patient-chosen goals, often with a focus on quality of life. Functional status varies widely following MSCC and rehabilitation needs to be adaptive to the individual patient. MSCC can have profound physical, psychological, and social effects on patients, families, and carers. Rehabilitation plays an important role in enabling patients to adapt to new disabilities, achieve short-term goals, and plan longer-term goals that are important to them.[2, 10]

Clinical Tip Bladder and Bowel Dysfunction

Proactive management of bladder and bowel disturbance is vital for symptom control and to prevent other complications. Specific interventions will vary depending on the degree of spinal cord injury so early assessment of bladder and bowel function is essential. Discussion with patients and carers is essential to understand the patient's priorities and how interventions (e.g. bowel routine, catheterization) can best be adapted to their circumstances including prognosis.[9, 11]

Expert Comment Rehabilitation

Published data on rehabilitation outcomes in MSCC patients are limited and retrospective in nature. A Canadian retrospective population registry study of following inpatient rehabilitation[12] found that MSCC patients had equivalent functional outcome scores to non-malignant spinal cord injury (SCI) patients with 75% of MSCC patients achieving their rehabilitation goals. In this study, the median inpatient rehabilitation stay was about 30 days with a median survival of 9.5 months. Despite a diagnosis of incurable cancer, rehabilitation in MSCC patients remains beneficial but will need to be patient goals specific and balanced against their likely prognosis. Early physiotherapy and occupational therapy assessments should be carried out within 24–48 hours of admission for MSCC inpatients.[9]

Expert Comment Prognostication

With an overall one-year survival of 20% following MSCC,[13] prognostication is critical to guide decision-making on the aggressiveness of MSCC treatment (e.g. surgery, higher radiotherapy doses) and potential for rehabilitation. Several clinical scoring systems have been reported, with the Revised Tokuhashi score the most widely used, yet this only has an overall predictive value of 66% and may have lower accuracy in different cancers.[14] A systematic review identified additional clinical prognostic factors such as age, ambulatory status, and duration of motor neurology prior to radiotherapy, as well as cancer-specific prognostic factors such as tumour histopathology, hormone receptor expression status, and oncogenic driver mutations.[15]

However, most of these scoring systems were prior to the advent of immunotherapy and molecular targeted therapies which have led to survival times in the order of years in select cancers. With evolving targeted cancer treatments, a patient's cancer molecular profile is increasingly relevant in managing MSCC.

A Final Word from the Expert

This case is a common example of a new first presentation of metastatic cancer with MSCC. These patients are often younger with a prolonged history of back pain and due to their younger age, malignancy is not suspected. The priority is for urgent diagnosis and cancer staging to determine the extent of malignant disease and suitable sites for histological sampling (including adequate biopsies for cancer molecular profiling for targeted therapies). This information alongside assessment of patient fitness for oncological treatments will guide the optimum management of their MSCC, whether surgical (better functional outcomes) or non-surgical/radiotherapy (less invasive treatment allowing earlier commencement of systemic anticancer treatment). Acute oncology advice is needed to aid prognostication (especially potential anticancer treatments), determine rehabilitation potential, and holistic care needs. A good functional outcome will dictate patient quality of life and the feasibility to offer life-prolonging oncological treatment.

References

1. Lu C, Gonzalez RG, Jolesz FA, Wen PY, Talcott JA. Suspected spinal cord compression in cancer patients: a multidisciplinary risk assessment. *J Support Oncol* 2005; 3(4): 305–12.
2. National Institute for Health and Care Excellence (NICE). Spinal metastases and metastatic spinal cord compression. NICE guideline (NG234) 2023 [6 September 2023. Available at: https://www.nice.org.uk/guidance/ng234]
3. Broersen LH, Pereira AM, Jorgensen JO, Dekkers OM. Adrenal insufficiency in corticosteroids use: systematic review and meta-analysis. *J Clin Endocrinol Metab* 2015; 100(6): 2171–80.
4. Joint British Diabetes Societies for Inpatient Care. Management of Hyperglycaemia and Steroid (Glucocorticoid) Therapy. 2021. Available at: https://diabetestimes.co.uk/wp-content/uploads/2021/06/JBDS-08-Steroids-and-DM-Guideline-FINAL-28.05.21-1.pdf
5. Kim JM, Losina E, Bono CM, et al. Clinical outcome of metastatic spinal cord compression treated with surgical excision +/− radiation versus radiation therapy alone: a systematic review of literature. *Spine (Phila Pa 1976)* 2012; 37(1): 78–84.
6. Patchell RA, Tibbs PA, Regine WF, et al. Direct decompressive surgical resection in the treatment of spinal cord compression caused by metastatic cancer: a randomised trial. *Lancet* 2005; 366(9486): 643–8.
7. Donovan EK, Sienna J, Mitera G, Kumar-Tyagi N, Parpia S, Swaminath A. Single versus multifraction radiotherapy for spinal cord compression: A systematic review and meta-analysis. *Radiother Oncol* 2019; 134: 55–66.

8. Fisher CG, DiPaola CP, Ryken TC, et al. A novel classification system for spinal instability in neoplastic disease: an evidence-based approach and expert consensus from the Spine Oncology Study Group. *Spine (Phila Pa 1976)* 2010; 35(22): E1221–9.
9. Guidelines and Audit Implementation Network (GAIN). Guidelines for the rehabilitation of patients with metastatic spinal cord compression (MSCC)2014 8/2/2022. Available at: https://www.rqia.org.uk/
10. Manson J, Warnock C, Crowther L. Patient's experiences of being discharged home from hospital following a diagnosis of malignant spinal cord compression. *Support Care Cancer* 2017; 25(6): 1829–36.
11. Multidisciplinary Association of Spinal Cord Injured Professionals. Guidelines for Management of Neurogenic Bowel Dysfunction in Individuals with Central Neurological Conditions. Available at: https://www.mascip.co.uk/wp-content/uploads/2015/02/CV653N-Neurogenic-Guidelines-Sept-2012.pdf2012
12. Fortin CD, Voth J, Jaglal SB, Craven BC. Inpatient rehabilitation outcomes in patients with malignant spinal cord compression compared to other non-traumatic spinal cord injury: a population based study. *J Spinal Cord Med* 2015; 38(6): 754–64.
13. Hoskin PJ, Hopkins K, Misra V, et al. Effect of single-fraction vs multifraction radiotherapy on ambulatory status among patients with spinal canal compression from metastatic cancer: the SCORAD randomized clinical trial. *JAMA* 2019; 322(21): 2084–94.
14. Quraishi NA, Manoharan SR, Arealis G, et al. Accuracy of the revised Tokuhashi score in predicting survival in patients with metastatic spinal cord compression (MSCC). *Eur Spine J* 2013; 22 Suppl 1: S21–6.
15. Luksanapruksa P, Buchowski JM, Hotchkiss W, Tongsai S, Wilartratsami S, Chotivichit A. Prognostic factors in patients with spinal metastasis: a systematic review and meta-analysis. *Spine J* 2017; 17(5): 689–708.

CASE 34 Seizures

Geoffrey Wells

Expert: Jane Neerkin

Case history

Peter was a 77-year-old man, who presented with new onset confusion. His wife described a 5-day history of headache and mild nausea, with Peter acting in a strange and confused way. She called an ambulance and upon arrival the paramedics found him to be experiencing word-finding difficulties.

Peter was a retired accountant and had remained active during his retirement playing badminton regularly. In the previous 8 weeks he had begun to find it difficult to maintain his usual standard of play and had missed several games due to tiredness. His wife noticed he had become increasingly short-tempered.

His past medical history includes benign prostatic hypertrophy, hypertension, and type-2 diabetes (diet controlled).

On review in the emergency department, Peter had expressive dysphasia and became increasingly frustrated when asked questions. Fifteen minutes after arrival, he suddenly developed a fixed gaze, his head turned to the right and his right arm flexed. After twenty seconds all four limbs began to shake violently. The attending team instigated emergency management following an ABCDE approach, and the seizure was terminated following the administration of 4 mg intravenous lorazepam.

Learning Point **Causes of Seizures in Patients with Brain Tumours**

Even when a patient with a known brain tumour presents with worsening of their seizures or different types of seizures, rule out other causes.

Tumour itself	
Treatment related	Chemotherapy or radiotherapy
Infection	Direct: CNS infection Indirect: Systemic infection lowering seizure threshold
Metabolic	Low sodium, magnesium, calcium or glucose
Vascular	Concomitant venous thrombosis
Paraneoplastic	e.g. limbic encephalitis

Learning Point Correlation of Symptoms with Brain Tumour Site

Site of brain tumour	Symptom/Signs	Type of seizure
Frontal Lobe	Hemiparesis/paralysis of a limb or side Perseverance (repetition of thought) Difficulty focussing on tasks Disinhibition, mood swings, irritability Aphasia, language difficulty Problem solving issues	Ipsilateral head and eye movements Difficulty speaking Explosive screams/laughter Abnormal body posturing Repetitive movements
Temporal Lobe	Receptive and/or expressive aphasia Face blindness Aggressive behaviour Short- and long-term memory issues Difficulty naming objects	Auras Deja-vu Impending feeling of doom Unusual smell Auditory (e.g. buzzing) Complex partial seizures Fixed stare Posturing Speaking gibberish Generalized tonic clonic
Parietal Lobe	Neglect of body parts Poor hand-eye coordination Difficulty with literacy, numeracy, naming things Difficulty distinguishing left from right	Uncommon. Sensory disturbances—feeling of heat, numbness, weakness, dizziness, hallucinations, distortions of space
Occipital lobe	Altered/blurred vision, blind spots, Visual hallucinations Difficulty reading and writing	Rare Flashing bright lights or other visual changes
Cerebellum	Coordination Tremors Vertigo Slurred speech Difficulty walking	Infratentorial tumours do not cause seizures
Brain stem	Changes in breathing Vertigo—balance issues and nausea Difficulty swallowing	

Learning Point Benzodiazepine Choice in the Management of Seizures

Acute management

Choice of benzodiazepine	Dose and route of administration	Other points to consider
Lorazepam	4 mg IV	**Hospital and hospice setting** Diluted 1:1 with 0.9% NaCl or WFI. Given as a bolus over 2 minutes. Can be repeated ONCE after 10-20 minutes if seizures persist[1, 2]

Midazolam	10 mg buccal/SC/IM 10 mg IV	**Hospital, hospice, and home setting** Given as STAT dose if administered buccal, SC, or IM (IM midazolam as effective as IV lorazepam). Buccal midazolam administered as oromucosal solution (prefilled oral syringe) into the buccal space (between gums and cheek) **Hospital setting** Given as a bolus over 2 minutes. Midazolam dose (by any route) can be repeated ONCE after 10 minutes if seizures persist
Diazepam	10 mg PR 2 mg IV	**Hospital or home setting** **Hospital setting.** Intravenous emulsion preferred (e.g. Diazemuls) Diazepam (by either route) can be repeated ONCE after 10 minutes if seizures persist. Note that diazepam is irritant and **must not** be administered SC or via CSCI.
Chronic management *Due to development of tolerance, chronic management of seizures with benzodiazepines should be reserved for seizures refractory to other treatments*		
Clobazam	10–30 mg PO once at night (some prescribe in divided doses)	Can be increased by 20–30 mg every 5–7 days to a maximum dose of 60 mg/24h (doses >30 mg should be divided)
Clonazepam	0.5–1 mg PO once at night	Can be increased by 0.5 mg every 3–5 days up to a maximum of 4 mg/24 hrs. Doses above 2 mg/24hrs should be divided
In the imminently dying patient		
Midazolam	Midazolam remains the benzodiazepine of choice in the imminently dying. Acute management of seizures remains the same. Maintain with 10–60 mg/24 h via CSCI doses. Note that if seizures persist despite 60 mg midazolam/24 hrs then treatment with **phenobarbital*** is recommended.	
Phenobarbital	100–200 mg IM STAT (loading dose) followed by 100 mg/24hrs via CSCI	Patients commencing phenobarbital will need to be in either a hospital or hospice setting. STAT loading dose can be repeated after 20 minutes if seizures persist. CSCI dose can be titrated to 400 mg/24 hrs Alternatively loading dose can also be diluted in 100 ml normal saline and administered by slow subcutaneous injection over 20–30 mins

Investigation Results

Blood profile: Unremarkable

CT head: Left frontal lobe mass. Appearance highly suggestive of a primary brain tumour.

MRI head: Solitary mass measuring 6.2 × 3.5 × 4.8 cm with surrounding vasogenic oedema confined to the left frontal lobe. Appearance highly suggestive of a primary brain tumour (Figure 34.1)

CT Chest Abdomen Pelvis: No evidence of malignancy seen.

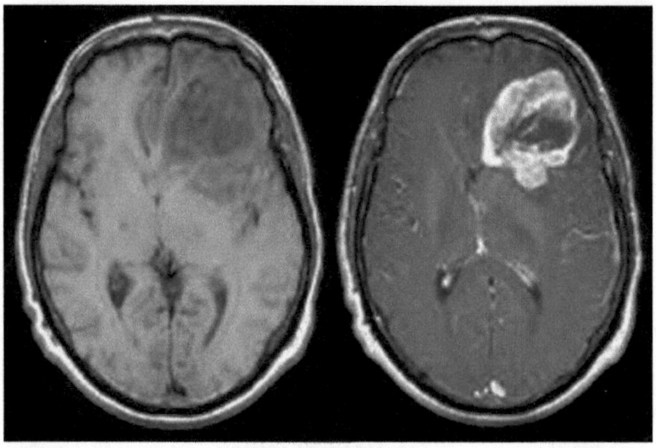

Figure 34.1 MRI demonstrating solitary left frontal lobe mass.

Reproduced with permission from David C Preston ©2006.

Initial Treatment Plan

Peter was discussed with the neurosurgical team, who advised commencing dexamethasone 16 mg daily to reduce vasogenic oedema, and levetiracetam 500 mg BD to prevent further seizures.

Clinical Tip Corticosteroids in Patients with Brain Tumours

Glucocorticoids (dexamethasone) are used to reduce tumour-related oedema and radiation-induced encephalopathy in patients with brain tumours.

Dexamethasone has a long half-life and low mineralocorticoid activity, which makes it beneficial to use in this patient group; however, there is limited evidence to guide dosage in management of tumoural oedema.[3] A randomized controlled trial comparing dexamethasone 8 mg/d vs. 16 mg/d, and 4 mg/d vs. 16 mg/d, concluded that 4 mg/d resulted in the same degree of improvement as 16 mg/d after 1 week of treatment in patients with no signs of impending herniation and lower incidence of side effects.[4] However, patients can become tolerant to steroids with the return of symptoms on maintenance doses meaning higher doses will be required.

Side Effects of Steroids

Glucocorticoids have many side effects which can accumulate over time. Side effects such as osteoporosis and cataract formation can still occur even after steroids have been stopped.

Common side effects of Steroids	Less common side effects
Proximal myopathy—up to 10% of patients may develop this, usually 2–3 months after commencing the steroids[5]	Infections—prolonged high dose steroid use can lead to the immune system becoming suppressed which can lead to an increased risk of acquiring opportunistic infections
GI bleeding—this is seen in practice rather than a clinical correlation in trials[6]	Psychosis—florid psychosis is not very common, although if the patient has pre-existing psychiatric problems, they are at increased risk
Osteoporosis—this has become more common as prognosis has improved. As patients are more likely to develop osteoporosis, uncontrolled seizures can lead to increased risk of fractures	Pancreatitis
Insomnia	Small bowel perforation
Behavioural changes	Hiccups

Common side effects of Steroids	Less common side effects
Glucose intolerance/Steroid-induced diabetes	
Cushingoid appearance including striae, bruising	
Glaucoma and cataracts	
Hypertension	
Avascular necrosis	

Interaction of Drugs and Steroids

Certain drugs that are liver enzyme inducers can increase the metabolism of dexamethasone by up to 50%. Phenytoin, carbamazepine, and phenobarbital are those more routinely used in patients with underlying gliomas and in these cases higher doses of steroids may be required.

Expert Commentary Choice of Antiepileptic Drug

The choice of AED should be based on seizure type whilst also trying to minimize the side effects a patient may experience. Newer drugs are no more efficacious than older drugs (such as phenytoin, carbamazepine, or phenobarbital)[7]; however, they have less drug-drug interactions and less side effects. Phenytoin, for example, is a potent enzyme inducer, resulting in an increased rate of metabolism and clearance of certain drugs, including dexamethasone.[8]

There is no specific evidence-based guidance available for which AED should be used for patients with brain-tumour-related epilepsy. A 2016 metanalysis recommended levetiracetam as the preferred drug in brain-tumour-related epilepsy, particularly when looking to avoid drug interactions.[9]

Where more than one antiepileptic is required, it is important to use drugs with a different mechanism of action. Early neurology advice is recommended for all patients with complex seizure management.

First line	Levetiracetam, lamotrigine, sodium valproate
Second line	As above, carbamazepine, lacosamide, clobazam
For rapid effect to treat seizure clusters whilst titrating antiepileptics	Clobazam
Sodium channel blockers	Carbamazepine, lamotrigine, lacosamide, sodium valproate (weak)
Calcium channel blockers	Sodium valproate (weak)
NMDA glutamate receptor antagonist	Sodium valproate (weak)
Inhibition of vesicle release	Levetiracetam
Augmented $GABA_A$ receptor activation	Benzodiazepines, phenobarbital
Altered GABA reuptake and breakdown	Sodium valproate (weak)

Neuro-oncology multidisciplinary team meeting (MDM) outcome: Australia-modified Karnofsky Performance Scale (AKPS) 80%. Likely primary brain tumour, appropriate for tumour de-bulking surgery and histological testing.

Peter consented to surgery and was transferred to the local neurosurgical unit. He did not experience any further seizure activity and his dysphasia responded well to the steroids.

Histology: High-grade glioma, WHO grade IV (Glioblastoma Multiforme), isocitrate dehydrogenase (IDH)-wild type.

Peter made a good postoperative recovery. With physiotherapy and occupational therapy support he was discharged home the following week with an AKPS of 70%. He was taking levetiracetam 500 mg BD and 4 mg dexamethasone daily, with a plan to reduce dexamethasone by half every 5 days to 1 mg then stop.

Expert Commentary Weaning Steroids

Prolonged use of glucocorticoids can lead to negative feedback on the hypothalamic-pituitary-adrenal (HPA) axis resulting in reduction in the endogenous production of glucocorticoids. Patients taking 5 mg prednisolone (0.75 mg dexamethasone) for longer than 4 weeks are at risk of HPA axis suppression, which may lead to an adrenal crisis if physiologically stressed, for example, during acute illness. These patients will need to have their steroids carefully weaned.

Patients at increased risk of an adrenal crisis include those that have repeated short courses of oral steroids and those with shorter courses of steroids who have also had intraarticular injections of steroid.[10]

During withdrawal, the dose of oral corticosteroids may be rapidly reduced (by 10 mg prednisolone/1.5 mg dexamethasone every 3 days) to physiological doses (about 7.5 mg of prednisolone or 1 mg dexamethasone) and then reduced more slowly thereafter (by 5 mg prednisolone/0.5 mg dexamethasone) every 5 days.[11] However, if symptoms of raised intracranial pressure recur, the patient should resume the dose that previously achieved symptomatic control.

He was referred to a neuro-oncologist to discuss further treatment options.

Peter and his wife met with the oncologist; they were informed that the tumour was aggressive, and that his prognosis was likely to be less than one year. He consented to palliative chemo-radiotherapy with the aim of improving prognosis and quality of life and a community palliative care team (CPCT) referral.

Change in Condition

Approximately 3 months into treatment, Peter's wife called the CPCT for advice as she had noticed he was becoming increasingly fatigued, irritable, and was experiencing episodes of shaking in his right arm. The team advised increasing the levetiracetam to 750 mg BD, ensured his GP was made aware of the medication change, and arranged repeat head imaging via his oncologist. This showed new lesions in both frontal lobes with surrounding vasogenic oedema.

Peter was reviewed 1 week later by his oncologist. His AKPS was 40%. The oncologist explained that the tumour had progressed on the scan despite treatment and no further treatment was available. Dexamethasone was restarted at 8 mg daily to reduce vasogenic oedema and see if his overall condition would improve.

Despite steroid treatment, Peter began to experience nausea. He was reviewed at home by the CPCT who commenced cyclizine. His random blood glucose had risen to 16 mmol/l and the decision was made to wean the steroids given they were no longer providing symptomatic benefit.

Expert Commentary

Seizure threshold describes a balance that exists between excitatory and inhibitory signals in the brain. The exact threshold to provoke a seizure will vary from person to person. There are certain drugs that can lower the seizure threshold: In patients with pre-existing epilepsy, they should be used with caution or avoided altogether.

The classes and types of drugs commonly used in palliative care:

Class of drug	Names
Antiemetics (antipsychotics)	Levomepromazine Haloperidol
Psychiatric medication	SSRIs TCAs SNRIs
Antimicrobials	Cephalosporins (fourth generation) Fluoroquinolones (e.g. ciprofloxacin)

If the patient is having more seizures than usual it is important to undertake a full review of both prescribed and over-the-counter medications to identify any that may be lowering the seizure threshold.

Although his clinical condition was deteriorating, Peter remained capacitous and wished to discuss his future care; his wishes were documented in an advance care plan.

As Peter remained at risk of seizures at home, the CPCT asked the GP to prescribe buccal midazolam for seizure emergency management. His wife was shown how to administer it and advised to dial 999 if a seizure was to occur that did not respond to buccal midazolam. Peter's condition deteriorated over the next few weeks and a twice-daily package of care was arranged. He remained clear that he wished to remain at home for as long as possible.

Expert Commentary Management of Seizures in the Community

Seizures are often frightening for families and carers to witness. It is helpful to explain what they can do if a seizure occurs at home and ensure acute antiseizure medications are available. Carers and relatives can be taught how to administer buccal midazolam/PR diazepam and advised when and how to seek help. The importance of planning ahead for acute and longer-term seizure management at home should not be underestimated (e.g. the availability of injectable anticonvulsants at home for when the patient is no longer able to swallow). By writing appropriate prn and syringe driver administration charts in advance, clinicians can facilitate the commencement of anticonvulsants by subcutaneous administration to ensure seizure activity is controlled.

Peter's swallow began to deteriorate, and he missed several doses of levetiracetam resulting in twitching of his right arm. He was commenced on a continuous subcutaneous infusion (CSCI) of levetiracetam 1500 mg/24 hours. It became clear that he was reaching the last days of life with evidence of terminal agitation, and he and his wife agreed to admission to the hospice. On admission, Peter was no longer able to take oral medications. Despite the subcutaneous infusion of levetiracetam, the twitching in his right arm had worsened. Midazolam 30 mg was added into the CSCI to manage both terminal agitation and seizures. Peter remained settled over the next 7 days requiring small increases in midazolam. He died peacefully in the hospice setting.

Clinical Tip Management of Terminal Agitation in Patients at Risk of Seizures

First line: **Midazolam:** 2.5–5mg SC/IV stat and up to once every hour. Maintain with 10–60 mg/24 h via CSCI doses. Mean effective dose 15–60 mg/24 hrs (range 5–200 mg/24 hrs).[1]

Haloperidol and levomepromazine are often used in the management of terminal agitation. Like most antipsychotics they can lower the seizure threshold and should be used with caution in those patients with seizures.

Phenobarbital: Patient requires loading dose, typically 200 mg IM (undiluted) or IV (diluted with 10 ml water for injection of sodium chloride over 2 minutes). May require 1 or 2 repeat doses 30 mins apart (median loading dose 600 mg). Maintain with 800 mg/24 hrs via CSCI (use higher initial CSCI dose if the patient requires a loading dose of ≥600 mg). Typical CSCI dose 800–1,200 mg/24 hrs (range 200–3800 mg/24 hrs). This is a much higher dose than that required to manage seizures, although higher doses are required for status epilepticus.

Discussion

This case details the complexities of seizure management from initial presentation to end of life care. The ability of clinicians to manage seizures in an appropriate and timely fashion, particularly in community settings, will have an important and positive impact for the patient and their family. Whilst management in the hospital setting will likely be consistent and guideline driven across the NHS, management in hospice and community settings needs to be flexible and adaptive to factors such as clinician skill mix and medicine availability. Clinicians need to consider adapting prescribing practice when maintaining seizure control in the deteriorating patient, particularly when treating patients who can no longer swallow oral medications, or when there is a requirement to co-administer drugs for other symptoms (e.g. nausea) which may lower the seizure threshold. When seizure management becomes complex, it is important to seek the advice of the local neurologist to support management rather than manage this complexity in isolation. By drawing together details within published guidelines this case aims to provide the reader with a focused yet comprehensive resource to support the management of seizures in the palliative care population.

A Final Word from the Expert

This is a good example of the multiple challenges experienced by patients with seizures secondary to an underlying brain tumour. The higher the grade of brain tumour, the less epileptogenic they tend to be. Patients with lower grade brain tumours often require multiple antiepileptic medications to manage their seizures compared to those with more aggressive brain tumours. Patients with brain tumours can develop nausea and vomiting secondary to the tumour or chemotherapy, they can develop infections and can become agitated towards the end of life. When treating all these symptoms, it is important to avoid medication that may lower the seizure threshold. The approach to managing patients with brain tumours should always be with the multidisciplinary team and joined-up working between the hospital and community is paramount.

References

1. Wilcock A, Howard P, Charlesworth S. *Palliative Care Formulary PCF7*, 6th ed. London: Pharmaceutical Press, 2021.
2. Watson M, Armstrong P, Back I, Gannon C, Sykes N (eds). *Palliative Adult Network Guidelines*, 4th ed. Lisburn, NI: Tricord, 2016.
3. Dietrich J, Rao K, Pastorino S, Kesari S. Corticosteroids in brain cancer patients: benefits and pitfalls. *Expert Rev Clin Pharmacol* 2011; 4(2): 233–242.
4. Vecht CJ, Hovestadt A, Verbiest HB, van Vliet JJ, van Putten WL. Dose-effect relationship of dexamethasone on Karnofsky performance in metastatic brain tumors: a randomized study of doses of 4, 8, and 16 mg per day. *Neurology* 1994; 44(4): 675–680.
5. Dropcho EJ, Soong SJ. Steroid-induced weakness in patients with primary brain tumors. *Neurology* 1991; 41(8): 1235–1239.
6. Conn HO, Blitzer BL. Nonassociation of adrenocorticosteroid therapy and peptic ulcer. *N Engl J Med* 1976; 294(9): 473–479.
7. Nakken KO, Brodtkorb E. Are the new anti-epileptic drugs any better than their predecessors? *Tidsskr Nor Laegeforen* 2020; 140(17). doi: 10.4045/tidsskr.20.0657.
8. Riva R, Albani F, Contin M, Baruzzi A. Pharmacokinetic interactions between antiepileptic drugs. Clinical considerations. *Clin Pharmacokinet* 1996; 31(6): 470–493.
9. Fröscher W, Kirschstein T, Rösche J. [Anticonvulsant therapy for brain tumour-related epilepsy]. *Fortschr Neurol Psychiatr* 2014; 82(12): 678–690.
10. Erskine D, Simpson H. Exogenous steroids treatment in adults: The Society for Endocrinology. 2020. Available at: https://www.endocrinology.org/media/4091/spssfe_supporting_sec_-final_10032021-1.pdf
11. National Institute for Health and Care Excellence (NICE). Clinical knowledge summaries: corticosteroids—oral. 2020. Available at: https://cks.nice.org.uk/topics/corticosteroids-oral/

SECTION 6

Personalised palliative care

CASE

35 Goal Setting and Interdisciplinary Support and Care Planning

Rebecca Tiberini

Expert: Jonathan Martin

Case history

Lucy, a 77-year-old woman, was ten minutes from her home when she found herself overcome with a racing heart, dizziness, sweating, and a sensation of gasping for air. She was so breathless that she felt petrified that she was going to die. A concerned neighbour called an ambulance, and assisted Lucy to a nearby bench. By the time the ambulance arrived Lucy's breathing had recovered. The paramedics diagnosed a panic attack related to her known advanced chronic obstructive pulmonary disease (COPD) and assisted her home.

Six weeks later Lucy attended an appointment at the hospice interdisciplinary breathlessness clinic. The holistic assessment with the palliative care doctor and physiotherapist identified that Lucy was anxious, as it was the first time she had left her house since the panic attack. Housebound, Lucy was less active in a smaller living space. She felt increasingly breathless on exertion and more unsteady on her feet, which further discouraged her from being active. Lucy was deeply lonely and isolated from her friends and social network in her community. She felt she was a burden on her son who was now doing all of her shopping, which she had previously been managing independently. Lucy was low in mood and had lost her sense of purpose and meaning in her life.

Lucy's phase of illness was unstable and performance status on the Australian Karnofsky Performance Scale was 60%. She identified her top three problems on the IPOS (Integrated Palliative Care Outcome Scale) as: 1) breathlessness (overwhelming); 2) anxiety (most of the time); and 3) mobility (moderate). Lucy's SpO_2 was 93% on room air; she desaturated to 91% on exertion, stabilizing within 5 minutes of rest and recovery.

Meet Lucy here.[1]

> **Expert Comment Problems Versus Concerns**
>
> Research shows that as professionals, we have a tendency to focus on symptoms and 'problems' which represent something we can 'fix' or manage. This is in contrast to patients' concerns which focus on what they want to be able to do.[2] In practice, as professionals expertly zone in on patients' active problems and symptoms, and the solutions they can bring to improve these, they may inadvertently miss the opportunity to explore and understand what matters most to the patient. Without the intentional exploration of the patient's priorities, there is a risk that instead of 'person-centred' care, we are in fact providing 'professional-centred' care based around what we, as professionals, think we can influence, or what we perceive to be important to the patient.[3]
>
> The IPOS system of assessing patients' symptom burden is very helpful, but it tends to draw us down a problem-orientated rather than patient (person)-orientated path if we are not careful, which may, in turn, result in dissonance between our priorities for the patient and the patient's actual priorities.
>
> Such a lack of concordance in priorities of care can result in professionals focusing on impairments (e.g. optimizing pain control) which may be not only incongruent with patients' personal goals, but

antithetical to them (e.g. A patient's goal to return home from an inpatient admission to be with family as soon as possible, even if pain management is suboptimal) and as a consequence opportunities for palliative care to help the person find more meaning in life can be missed.

Consciously shifting the focus from 'What's the matter with you' (impairments) to 'What matters to you?' (patient priorities) serves to place the person at the centre of their care and well-being and empowers them as an equal partner in the therapeutic relationship, avoiding an unbalanced dependency on professionals.

Making 'person-centred goal-setting' the *goal* of every holistic assessment is essential to actively identify patients' priorities and aspirations and to position these as the central, unifying focus of the interdisciplinary palliative care team.

Learning Point Person-centred Goal-setting

Person-centred goal-setting involves working in partnership with patients to actively identify their priorities and aspirations and then tailoring our interdisciplinary support to best enable these.

The key starting point is establishing what is most important to each patient as a *person*. Whilst it may be a priority for a patient to have their symptoms well controlled, person-centred goal-setting is about going beyond this to explore and understand the *'so what?'*. If their symptoms were well controlled, what would they want to be able to do? What really matters to them? What would they like to be able to do that adds meaning and quality to their life? And/or death?

Evidence Base Patients' Experiences and Perceptions of Goal-Setting in Palliative Care

A mixed methods study found that all patients admitted to a hospice inpatient unit spoke of goals that were important to them. Some goals were about maintaining hope, such as living to attend a significant personal event like a birthday, some were about preparing for death whilst affirming life, such as writing a will and sorting out personal affairs, however the majority of goals were about doing simple, everyday things such as washing, showering, and dressing independently. Significantly, patients rarely articulated their personal goals to palliative care professionals as they did not perceive these to be of relevance or interest to them. This resulted in missed opportunities for the interdisciplinary team to support patients to achieve their personal goals. Incorporating person-centred goal-setting in an explicit and structured way is recommended.[4]

Clinical Tip Establishing Patients' Personal Priorities and Goals

Incorporate the following questions into every holistic assessment to enable the patient to identify and share their personal priorities and goals:

Personal Priorities	'Tell us about what matters most to you ... ?' 'What is really important to you?'
Personal Goals	'What would you like to be able to do in the next ... few weeks/ month/ short while?' 'What is important for you to achieve in the next ... few weeks/months?' 'What are your best hopes for ... this admission/the next few weeks?'

During the clinic assessment, the palliative care physiotherapist asked, 'Tell us about what matters most to you, Lucy?' She answered, 'My family and friends are the most important things in my life ... and I feel terrible because since I can't go out, my son has to do all my shopping and I never see my friends anymore. I'm so depressed, I just spend every day at home, every day is the same and my world feels so small'. The doctor then asked, 'And what would you like to achieve in the next month?' Lucy answered, 'Well I would like my breathing to be better ... ' The doctor followed with, 'And if your breathing was better, what is it that you would really like to be able to do?' Lucy responded, 'I would like to be able to walk down the road to the shop, to get a few things and see all my friends at the centre ... even if it was for just one last time'.

The interdisciplinary team had now established Lucy's personal priorities and goals and used these as the focus of their shared work.

Learning Point Goal-orientated Interdisciplinary Support and Care Planning

Interdisciplinary working involves team members of different disciplines working collaboratively with a common shared purpose to enable patients to achieve their personal goals. As such, person-centred goal-setting is not unique to one profession but the shared remit of all interdisciplinary team members.

Person-centred goal-setting enables collaborative action planning between the patient, family, their community, and the interdisciplinary team which places the patient actively at the centre of their care. It provides a unifying framework for professions within the team to contribute their unique knowledge and expertise in a coordinated and coherent approach - including symptom control, rehabilitation, psychological, social, and spiritual support - to optimize a patient's current issues with the shared common objective of enabling them to achieve their goals.

Creating interdisciplinary support and care plans with an explicit and intentional focus on patients' personal goals enables patients and families to:

- Have open and honest conversations with each other about what matters most.
- Feel listened to and valued as a person, not 'just a patient', by the professionals involved in their support and care.
- Know that their personal priorities are paramount.
- Have a more seamless experience of support and care across the interdisciplinary team.
- Find focus and meaning in life and death.
- Increase motivation and effort to achieve what is important to them.
- Develop resilience and coping, enabling reframing of goals as their illness progresses and mourning for unachievable goals as an important aspect of adapting to illness and approaching death.
- Live actively while dying (Figure 35.1).

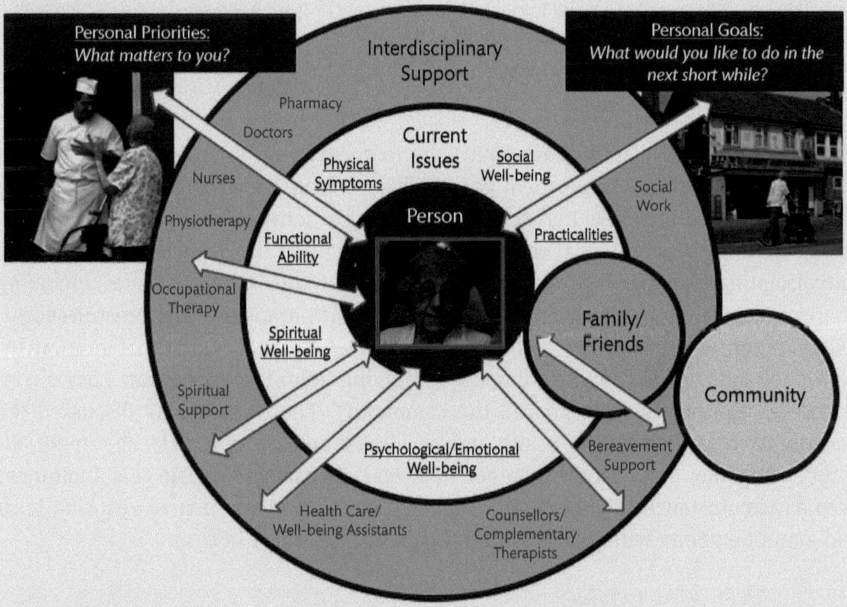

Figure 35.1 Integrating the person's goals with the context of their current issues and available support.

Clinical Tip Establishing Patients' Goals as the Central Focus for the Interdisciplinary Palliative Care Team

- Ensure all members of the interdisciplinary palliative care team understand person-centred goal-setting.
- Include identification of person-centred goals as a best practice standard for all holistic assessments.
- Incorporate questions on patients' personal priorities and goals alongside problem-orientated outcome tools such as IPOS to ensure they are identified.
- Document person-centred goals in the patient electronic records to share with interdisciplinary team and avoid duplication of patient questioning.
- Ensure interdisciplinary team meetings present each patient's personal goals. Link the professional contributions to address the patient's current issues through to how this will enable the person to achieve their goals.
- Establish a culture where person-centred goal-setting is 'everybody's business'. All members of the team make it a priority to ensure they identify or are aware of the patient's goals.
- Use outcome frameworks such as goal attainment scale (GAS)[5] or goal-setting and action planning for palliative care (G-AP PC)[6] to document and evaluate patients' goals in a structured way to evidence goal achievement, give feedback, and adapt if necessary, as a measure of personalized care and service effectiveness.
- Use person-focused outcome measures such as Life Space Assessment[7] to assess goal progress and provide positive motivation.

Expert Comment Palliative Medicine in the Interdisciplinary Team Context

The importance of interdisciplinary working reflects the different training, skills, and experiences that each profession brings. Person-centred goal-setting receives little emphasis in the palliative medicine training curriculum, which has been criticised for ignoring the 'personal and community dimensions of dying, caregiving, and bereavement'[8] and in palliative care practice a central focus on the patient as a 'person' can be peripheralized, for example in acute trusts where the emphasis is often on solving the 'problem' of the patient being in hospital.[9] As a result, particularly as doctors, we may rely on colleagues in the interdisciplinary palliative care team to help us maintain an appropriate focus on the patient, as opposed to their illness and symptoms only, when this should be central to doctors' practice in palliative medicine.

Consultation openers, such as Chochinov's 'What should I know about you as a person to help me take the best care of you that I can?',[10] help set the tone of the subsequent discussion and patients are frequently both surprised and pleased with the shift in emphasis away from the usual 'presenting complaint' conversation starting point that is so prevalent in the 'linear' and task-orientated medical model.

The palliative care team worked with Lucy to cocreate an interdisciplinary support plan to work towards her personal goal.[11] This built on Lucy's strengths and coping strategies, which included her determination to be active and the support she received from her son and local shop. The plan drew upon the diverse expertise of the interdisciplinary team to optimize the management of Lucy's current issues, including pharmacological and non-pharmacological approaches to manage her breathlessness, rehabilitation to improve her mobility and exercise tolerance, emotional support for both Lucy and her son, and an Empowered Living Volunteer to support Lucy's confidence as she pursued her goal in the community. The team openly discussed the uncertainty regarding Lucy's health and well-being and possible risks she might encounter. Together they 'parallel planned' to keep Lucy safe and enable goal attainment even as circumstances changed. This included back up plans such as ensuring Lucy had a mobile phone with her and ordering a wheelchair just in case.

Expert Comment Positive Risk-Taking—Welfare Versus Autonomy

Professionals in palliative care can be challenged by two important but competing agendas—keeping patients safe whilst enabling their pursuit of personal goals which may place them at risk. It can be helpful to keep in mind that we all take risks every day to achieve what is important to us, whether it's running across a busy road to catch a bus or fulfilling a resolution to skydive. In the context of advanced illness, where time is short, the positive benefits gained from taking risks to achieve a personal goal can outweigh the negative effects of attempting to avoid risk altogether.[12] Adopting a culture of positive risk-taking enables palliative care teams to adopt a starting point of maximizing opportunities for people and then exploring how any risks can best be mitigated. This values our patients as people, respects their autonomous/capacitous choice and importantly, enables us to support them to maintain hope and personal agency until they die.

Clinical Tip Parallel Planning

Goal-setting in palliative care, where patients' health status can change quickly, can be challenging. The uncertainty inherent in the trajectory of advanced illness means that it is frequently impossible to know if a patient's goal is realistic or achievable—this is true for both the patient and the professional team. Do not let this be a barrier to person-centred goal-setting. Proactively name the uncertainty and invite it into the conversation with the patient and their family. With this out in the open, you can then, as far as possible, plan for how to manage it together.

- Openly acknowledge that we cannot be certain what the future holds. This is upfront, honest, and frequently welcomed by patients and families who recognize the truth in this.
- Practice 'parallel planning'—the process of actively acknowledging and planning for two or more possibilities at the same time, or 'hoping for the best while planning for the worst'. This involves having 'Plan A' as the best-case scenario but also having back up 'Plans B and C' ready in case the patient's situation changes. Planning for several possibilities concurrently can help to (i) introduce and allow for anticipation of possible deterioration in a safe way, and (ii) help prevent crisis situations which place the patient at undue risk.

Through interdisciplinary rehabilitative palliative care,[13] Lucy was supported to achieve her personal goals. Four weeks later, Lucy managed to walk independently to her local shop and spend the afternoon with close friends at her community centre.

Learning Point Rehabilitative Palliative Care

Rehabilitative palliative care is a paradigm which integrates rehabilitation, enablement, self-management, and self-care into the holistic model of palliative care. It is an interdisciplinary approach in which all members of the team, including nurses, doctors, psychosocial practitioners, and allied health professionals, work collaboratively with the patient, their relatives, and carers to support them in achieving their personal goals and priorities. Rehabilitative palliative care aims to optimize people's function and well-being and to enable them to live as independently and fully as possible, with choice and autonomy, within the limitations of advancing illness. It is an approach that empowers people to adapt to their new state of being with dignity and provides an active support system to help them anticipate and cope constructively with losses resulting from deteriorating health. Rehabilitative palliative care supports people to live fully until they die.[13]

Two weeks after Lucy achieved her goal, she developed a chest infection. Her breathing significantly worsened and she struggled to manage at home. Lucy agreed to be admitted to the hospice for symptom control. The nurse consultant explored with Lucy what matters most to her now and Lucy spoke of being independent and returning home to sit out in her garden with her son. She naturally reframed her goal to something more realistic as her condition changed. The interdisciplinary team treated Lucy's chest infection, supported her to mobilize with a new walking frame, and made adaptations to enable her to be safe and independent at home. As she was much less well, the team were uncertain if Lucy would achieve her new goal, but discussed this openly with her and her son, recognizing how important it was for Lucy to maintain hope. Lucy achieved her goal to return home and have a cup of tea in her garden. She died peacefully at home with her son present the following day.

A Final Word from the Expert

Research suggests the process of setting goals and working towards them is more important than achieving them: the pursuit of goals, even if somewhat unrealistic, can help patients understand, and come to terms with, what is manageable and what is not.[5] Although patients naturally reframe and adapt their goals as health and well-being changes, it is through the process of working towards goals that they constructively adapt to progressive and accumulating losses encountered in advancing illness. Pursuit of meaningful goals supports acceptance of approaching death and impacts positively on bereavement outcomes.

It should go without saying but crucial to the success of a goal-orientated strategy is that the goals are those of the person, not the professional; as far as possible we should dance to the patient's tune. To do this, we have to ask each person what matters to them and keep this focus at the heart of both our personal and interdisciplinary practice of palliative care.

References

1. Rehabilitative Palliative Care: Enabling people to live fully until they die—YouTube. 2015. St Joseph's Hospice, Hackney. Available at: https://www.youtube.com/watch?v=eIEQOZEr3Lo
2. Baile WF, Palmer JL, Bruera E, Parker PA. Assessment of palliative care cancer patients' most important concerns. *Support Care Cancer* 2011; 19(4): 475–481.
3. Tiberini R, Turner K, Talbot-Rice H. Rehabilitation in palliative care. In: MacLeod R., Van den Block L. (eds). *Textbook of Palliative Care*. Oxford: Springer, 2019, pp. 579–607.
4. Boa S, Duncan E, Haraldsdottir E, Wyke S. Mind the gap: Patients' experiences and perceptions of goal setting in palliative care. *Progr Palliat Care* 2019; 27: 291–300.
5. Fettes L, Ashford S, Maddocks M. *Setting and Implementing Patient-set Goals in Palliative Care*. London: King's College London, 2018. Available at: https://www.kcl.ac.uk/nmpc/assets/rehab/gas-booklet-2018-final.pdf
6. Boa S. The development and evaluation of a Goal setting and Action Planning framework for use in Palliative Care (G-AP PC). Thesis, University of Stirling, 2013.
7. McCrone A, Smith A, Hooper J, Parker RA, Peters A. The life-space assessment measure of functional mobility has utility in community-based physical therapist practice in the United Kingdom. *Phys Ther* 2019; 99(12): 1719–1731.
8. Abel J, Kellehear A. Palliative curriculum re-imagined: a critical evaluation of the UK palliative medicine syllabus. *Palliat Care* 2018; 11: 1178224218780375.
9. Robinson J, Gott M, Gardiner C, Ingleton C. The 'problematisation' of palliative care in hospital: an exploratory review of international palliative care policy in five countries. *BMC Palliat Care* 2016; 15: 64.
10. Chochinov H. Dignity and the essence of medicine: the A, B, C, and D of dignity conserving care. *BMJ* 2007; 335: 184–187.
11. Care Act 2014: Strengths-based approaches. *SCIE* 2015. Available at: http://www.scie.org.uk/care-act-2014/assessment-and-eligibility/strengths-based-approach/
12. Morgan S, Williamson T. How can positive risk-taking help build dementia-friendly communities? *Joseph Rountree Foundation* 2014. Available at: https://www.jrf.org.uk/report/how-can-positive-risk-taking-help-build-dementia-friendly-communities
13. Tiberini R, Richardson H. Rehabilitative palliative care: enabling people to live fully until they die. A challenge for the 21st century. *Hospice UK* 2015. Available at: https://www.hospiceuk.org/publications-and-resources/rehabilitative-palliative-care-enabling-people-live-fully-until-they-die

CASE

36 Advance Care Planning

Georgina Osborne

Expert: Bee Wee

Case history

Marion was a 62-year-old woman. She was diagnosed with motor neurone disease (MND) six months ago. Marion still worked as an architect, but had reduced her hours due to arm weakness and painful spasm. She was otherwise asymptomatic and fully independent. Marion had a strong sense of wanting to stay in control of her situation for as long as she was able. Her hospice doctor broached what her wishes may be as her condition worsens and whether she would want to consider advance care planning (ACP). Marion didn't want to think about this yet; 'I'm trying to take this one day at a time, it's the only way I can cope'.

Clinical Tip Finding the Right Time

- People have different levels of 'readiness' to consider the implications of ACP[1]; while it is important to offer the opportunity to discuss ACP, any patient wishes to not participate should be respected.
- Unwanted pursuit of ACP can cause harm and may put up barriers to later conversations.[2, 3]
- Broaching ACP when people are receptive and accepting of their life-limiting condition[2] facilitates engagement. Exploring a person's information needs first allows ACP to develop more naturally.
- People may avoid ACP for fear of treatments becoming unavailable to them (e.g. cardiopulmonary resuscitation (CPR)) or that talking about bad outcomes will precipitate them. Others may not know what their wishes would be or want to commit beforehand. In these circumstances, agreeing that certain decisions can be made with them as more urgent situations arise (accepting they may then lack capacity) can help.
- Consider offering a patient information leaflet, signposting local ACP initiatives, or a time in future to sensitively revisit the topic.

Expert Comment

Individual factors that increase people's readiness include acceptance of their situation, previous experience, prior conversations with those they trust, feeling confident or empowered, specific concerns (e.g. of 'being a burden', or the dying process), or a desire to exercise personal autonomy. Focus on building trust and a good relationship. Explore what is important to the person now, their support networks, and specific social and spiritual care needs that they may have. Explore any key plans they have for the future. Appreciate that this may develop over multiple conversations.

Clinical Tip Resources to Start the Conversation

Many lay initiatives introducing ACP have been developed, for example 'Respecting Choices', 'Death Cafes', 'The Conversation Project', 'Go wish' and programmes offering support around will-making. There may also be programmes run through local hospices alongside consumer products such as My Directives, Best Endings, and My Living Will.

Learning Point Advance Care Planning and Emergency Care Planning

ACP explores a breadth of future care preferences when a patient has capacity for these. This contrasts with care planning that is urgently undertaken as a person's condition becomes unstable, having often lost capacity to engage. In the latter, content of decision-making usually focuses on immediate setting of care, levels of treatment, and CPR decisions though any previous ACP should inform this process.

Useful patient information guides include:

- https://advancecareplanning.org.uk/planning-ahead
- https://compassionindying.org.uk/making-decisions-and-planning-your-care/
- https://www.macmillan.org.uk/_images/no-regrets-talking-about-death-report_tcm9-311059.pdf
- For healthcare professionals (HCPs), supporting resources include:
- http://www.instituteforhumancaring.org/documents/Providers/Serious-Illness-Guide-old.pdf
- https://northerncanceralliance.nhs.uk/deciding-right/deciding-right-education-resources-for-professionals/
- http://talkcpr.wales/

Learning Point Definitions of Advance Care Planning

'ACP is a **voluntary process** of person-centred discussion between an individual and their care providers about their preferences and priorities for their **future care, while they have the mental capacity** for meaningful conversation about these. The process, which is likely to **involve several conversations over time**, must always **respect the person's wishes and emotions**. As a result, the person should experience a **greater sense of involvement** and opportunity to reflect and share what matters most to them'.[4]

In Scotland, ACP is known as anticipatory care planning. In Wales, ACP falls under the umbrella term 'Future Care Planning', which includes patients with diminished mental capacity.[5] For children and young people who lack capacity, the term ACP is used differently and is outside the scope of this case.

Expert Comment Six Universal Principles

The guide 'Universal Principles for Advance Care Planning' was published in March 2022 to provide a consistent national approach to 'what good looks like' in ACP in England.[4] This sets out six universal principles for a personalized approach, focusing on:

- the person being central to the process, including deciding who else to involve
- personalized conversations about future care, based on what matters to the person
- outcomes of the conversations being agreed through shared decision-making
- documented advance care plans being shareable
- opportunity and encouragement for the person to review and revise the plan
- ability to speak up if these principles are not being followed

Clinical Tip Who Might Benefit from Advance Care Planning Conversations?

'Any individual who wishes to plan for their future care or who may be at risk of losing their mental capacity, including:

- People facing deteriorating health due to long-term conditions or life-limiting illness, e.g. dementia, frailty, kidney, heart or liver failure, lung disease, progressive neurological conditions, incurable cancer.
- People with declining functional status, increased illness burden, or persistent symptoms.
- People facing key transitions in their healthcare needs, e.g. multiple hospital admissions, focus of treatment to more palliative intent, moving into a care home.
- People facing major surgery or high-risk treatments e.g. bone marrow transplant.
- People facing acute life-threatening conditions'.[4]

Specific tools are also available to identify such patients, such as the Gold Standards Framework Prognostic Indicator Guide and the Supportive and Palliative Care Indicators Tool (SPICT).[6]

After six months, Marion was weaker and her hospice doctor had many telephone consults supporting her and her partner Bill. They had no children and Marion had been estranged from her sister for thirty years. Marion could no longer concentrate sufficiently to work and had started having breathing problems at night. She was 'really scared about what might happen at the end'. Marion did not identify herself as religious and declined a spiritual care referral. Her hospice doctor asked if it would now be helpful to talk about the future and she agreed. 'What do I need to think about?'

Expert Comment Advance Care Planning Components

Components can vary but generally include:

1. General expressions of care wishes (e.g. advance statements)
2. Decisions made in advance that have legal force (advance directives, e.g. advance decision to refuse treatment (ADRT))
3. Nomination of surrogate decision-makers (e.g. lasting power of attorney)

Where the person lacks mental capacity, decisions made must be in their best interests, either by a legally appointed surrogate decision-maker or by the responsible clinician.

Learning Point What Can Advance Care Planning Encompass?

Advance care plans are individual, with variation in detail and scope. Discussion may include:

- Details of significant others and information-sharing permissions. Is there something the person does not want discussed (with them or others)?
- Understanding of condition, prognosis, and related information needs (person and significant others)
- General priorities and preferences. What matters most when thinking about the future?
- Social, e.g. dependents and how they may be cared for, financial concerns, interest in will-making
- Spiritual, religious, and cultural considerations
- Preferences on future treatments and care (person and significant others):
  - Preferred place of care (PPC) and death (PPOD)
  - Treatment escalation plans (TEP), CPR decisions, emergency hospital admissions, and routine outpatient attendance
  - Symptom control in community settings
  - Preferences regarding life-prolonging treatments, e.g. antibiotics
  - Disease-specific considerations, e.g. non-invasive ventilation (NIV) and withdrawal, oxygen, clinically assisted nutrition and hydration, dialysis withdrawal, blood transfusions.
  - Organ donation
- Consent for involvement of certain services, e.g. community palliative care
- Consent for shared documentation
- Review date

Learning Point Documentation—Paper Versus Electronic Palliative Care Coordination Systems (EPaCCS)

Documenting ACP decisions is a key step in sharing information across services, guiding future decision-making. Across the UK, many documents exist, each with differing content and format (paper, online, or electronically coordinated). HCPs should be familiar with and have access to documentation locally available and be aware of its strengths and limitations.

Some documents cover ACP more broadly (e.g. Planning Ahead) while others focus on emergency treatment (e.g. Recommended Summary Plan for Emergency Care and Treatment (ReSPECT)). The PEACE tool has a medicalized focus, being designed as a TEP for care home residents who may lack capacity.

EPaCCS are more accessible across services, can offer patient-facing portals and facilitate research and outcome measurement; they are however, challenging to develop and implement.

Marion was clear that what mattered most was her independence and to not prolong her life once unable to 'go outside (unaided or not) and walk my dogs'. As a result, she stopped taking riluzole (which can prolong MND's terminal phase) and stated in her advance care plan that she would not want any life-prolonging measures (e.g. antibiotics) if she became housebound. Marion agreed with a DNACPR order and referral to community palliative care. She underwent NIV assessment for symptom control but wanted to outline a withdrawal process once more unwell. Marion remained

Expert Comment Supporting Patients and Families

ACP is often emotive for people and their families, triggering differences in belief systems, experiences, and needs for hope and control. While the person remains the decision-maker, it is important to engage significant others as much as the person and they allow; hearing and addressing their concerns may alleviate current anxieties, reduce potential conflict later if best interest decisions need to be made and reduce distress in bereavement.

undecided about percutaneous endoscopic gastrostomy placement, aware that enteral nutrition may make her feel stronger but was unsure how she would engage with this, given her love of cooking and eating with friends. Marion wanted to die at home with significant others around her. Bill found these conversations very challenging, struggling with Marion's pragmatism and wanting to remain optimistic; 'I'm worried she is writing herself off'.

A year later, Marion was struggling to stay in her wheelchair for more than fifteen minutes. Beforehand, she could use this independently for a few hours and enjoy being outside. Furthermore, Marion's swallow had deteriorated, now choking on her favourite foods. She requested discussion regarding NIV withdrawal, on which she was now dependent on for more than 16 hours per day. Marion was finding her recent deterioration 'intolerable'. She talked to Bill frequently of 'wanting it all to be over', which he found very unsettling.

In the meantime, Marion became acutely unwell, feverish, and delirious, lacking capacity to make healthcare decisions. Bill was distressed and instead of calling the hospice team, called 999 wanting her to have 'full treatment'. A paramedic attended and thought Marion had aspiration pneumonia. He saw on the electronic ACP that Marion did not want antibiotic treatment but that there was no specific ADRT. He called the duty doctor for advice, and together were able to use Marion's ACP to guide decision-making and support Bill. She died at home the next day.

Clinical Tip Acknowledging Imperfection

ACP is a complex process. It can be challenging to form a plan that accurately reflects the wishes of a person and their family ahead of the situation arising. 'Goals-of-care conversations require sophisticated knowledge of prognosis, disease, associated comorbidities, and treatment outcomes' that not everyone involved has.[7] ACP cannot account for every eventuality; 'decisions near end of life are not simple, logical, or linear. They are uncertain, emotionally laden, and can change rapidly with clinical conditions'.[7] Patients may see ACP as a means of taking control of an unpredictable situation, though end of life events may not materialize as planned and can lead to conflict.[8] Successful ACP requires communication between several acute and community healthcare services, often out-of-hours. As a result, despite ACP engagement, patients may continue to receive burdensome treatments that do not match their preferences.[9]

If conducted and delivered well, ACP exemplifies 'goal-concordant care that is the foundation of palliative care',[7] reducing situations where patients die in a manner at odds with their preferences. ACP can facilitate a holistic, collaborative approach, give people a greater sense of control, improve symptom assessment, and reduce misunderstandings between HCPs and families.[2,4] For this reason, despite much imperfection, the concept of ACP is supported internationally.[10-12]

Expert Comment COVID-19 and Advance Care Planning

While the COVID-19 pandemic has brought ACP into sharp focus and provided a catalyst for HCPs less experienced in these conversations to initiate them, an over-emphasis on ACP 'completion rates' and an association with DNACPR decision-making, has been a concern for some people, their families, and HCPs.[15] ACP must not be reduced to a simple administrative task; it requires time, reflection and shifting conversational focus to 'what matters most' rather than end of life care decisions.[16]

Learning Point The Importance of Healthcare Professionals Communication and Engagement

Effectively implementing high-quality ACP, notwithstanding wider care planning, all require conversations to be ably raised. Confidence in communication skills and nuanced clinical acumen is needed, but often lacking.[2] 'HCPs often fail to initiate these discussions, possibly due to reluctance to discuss death and difficultly managing their own emotions during challenging conversations'.[13] HCPs underestimate patient and carer information needs and overestimate their understanding[14]; they often want to 'maintain hope' and may feel that ACP undermines this. Others show reluctance with ACP, perceiving it as a 'tick-box exercise'. Improved training is needed, alongside a shift in culture.

Evidence Base

Evidence supporting ACP is mixed, highlighting research challenges in evaluating such a complex intervention. For example, the ACTION project aimed to measure ACP's effect on the quality of life and symptoms of advanced cancer patients but was confounded by patients' 'readiness' to engage.[1] Finding meaningful key performance indicators and valid outcome measures is also difficult. The most consistently measured outcome is dying in PPOD, an indicator of end of life quality but contingent on many other individual and environmental factors. Study population bias also results from most ACP research originating from high-income countries, given an emphasis on autonomy and individual decision-making.[12] Few studies address cost-effectiveness.[17]

An overview of eighty systematic reviews, including over 1660 original articles, showed weak evidence that ACP can lead to improved communication at the end of life, dying in preferred place and healthcare savings.[18] Strikingly, when HCPs have a record of PPOD, people are almost twice as likely to die in the place of their choosing.[19]

For people with multiple sclerosis and Parkinson's disease, ACP contributed to reduced dying in hospital, with those initiated by GPs most likely to be effective.[20] When end of life issues were discussed with cancer outpatients, less intensive medical care near death was received and family bereavement was improved.[21] In care homes, ACP has reduced inappropriate hospital admissions and mortality.[22]

Future Advances

ACP continues to evolve with increased possibilities brought about by medical advances that sustain life while prolonging dying.[9] Advance directives originally allowed people to record an advance refusal of specific life-prolonging intervention but their limitations drove a broader ACP process, with international consensus on definition only later developed in 2017.

As a result, there remain many inconsistencies across healthcare settings in approach, terminology, communication, and understanding of ACP. Future advances in policy need to address such barriers and inequity, with new national guidance identifying key requisites for achieving good practice in ACP[4]:

- Public and professional awareness
- Clear information
- Proactive identification of those who would benefit from ACP
- Education and training
- Record keeping and information sharing
- Organizational culture
- System culture

Revised approaches to ACP have been suggested. 'Adaptive care planning' is not yet widely integrated but focuses on 'decisions made in the moment to unfolding clinical events'[8]; two parallel plans are made: one for stability/improvement, one for deterioration. Research relating to ACP effectiveness and clinical uncertainty is also underway.

A Final Word from the Expert

Marion's story provides a good example of advance care planning. It illustrates the benefit and assurance it gave Marion, when she was ready to undertake these conversations. It shows how her husband, Bill, was involved and able to hear what mattered most to her. But it also demonstrates that such conversations can be emotionally tough. Advance care planning can help the person feel more confident in maintaining some control over future decisions. Those close to them can be more reassured that they are contributing to decisions that are aligned with the person's preference. In Marion's case, Bill took comfort from knowing that he was able to fulfil her wish to die at home even though he found it challenging and stressful at times. Advance Decisions to Refuse Treatment are legally binding provided they are valid and applicable. Advance statements are not legally binding but healthcare professionals should do their best to honour these in making best interests decisions on behalf of the person who lacks capacity. The legal framework for decision-making in situations where the person lacks capacity is different across countries, and for children as opposed to adults. It is imperative that healthcare professionals understand their local legal framework and take into account the cultural context and other needs of their individual patient and those important to them.

References

1. Zwakman M, Milota MM, van der Heide A, et al. Unravelling patients' readiness in advance care planning conversations: a qualitative study as part of the ACTION Study. *Support Care Cancer* 2021; 29(6): 2917–2929.
2. Cottrell L, Economos G, Evans C, et al. A realist review of advance care planning for people with multiple sclerosis and their families. *PLoS One* 2020; 15(10): e0240815
3. Korfage IJ, Carreras G, Arnfeldt Christensen CM, et al. Advance care planning in patients with advanced cancer: a 6-country, cluster-randomised clinical trial. *PLoS Med* 2020; 17(11): e1003422.
4. NHS England and NHS Improvement. Universal Principles for Advance Care Planning. Available at: https://www.england.nhs.uk/publication/universal-principles-for-advance-care-planning/
5. Taubert M, Bounds L. Advance and future care planning: strategic approaches in Wales. *BMJ Support Palliat Care* 2022: bmjspcare-2021-003498. https://pubmed.ncbi.nlm.nih.gov/35105552/
6. The Supportive and Palliative Care Indicators Tool (SPICT). Available at: https://www.spict.org.uk
7. Sean Morrison R. Advance directives/care planning: clear, simple, and wrong. *J Palliat Med* 2020; 23(7): 878–879.
8. Johnson S, Butow P, Kerridge I, Tattersall M. Advance care planning for cancer patients: a systematic review of perceptions and experiences of patients, families, and healthcare providers. *Psychooncology* 2016; 25(4): 362–386.
9. Moody SY. 'Advance' care planning re-envisioned. *J Am Geriatr Soc* 2020; 62(2): 330–332.
10. National Palliative and End of Life Care Partnership. The Ambitions for Palliative and End of Life Care: A National Framework For Local Action 2021–2026 in England. Available at: https://www.england.nhs.uk/wp-content/uploads/2022/02/ambitions-for-palliative-and-end-of-life-care-2nd-edition.pdf
11. Lin CP, Evans CJ, Koffman J, Chen PJ, Hou MF, Harding R. Feasibility and acceptability of a culturally adapted advance care planning intervention for people living with advanced cancer and their families: a mixed methods study. *Palliat Med* 2020; 34(5): 651–666.
12. Sallnow L, Smith R, Ahmedzai SH, et al. Lancet Commission on the Value of Death. Report of the Lancet Commission on the Value of Death: bringing death back into life. *Lancet* 2022; 399(10327): 837–884.
13. Brighton LJ, Selman LE, Gough N, et al. 'Difficult conversations': evaluation of multiprofessional training. *BMJ Support Palliat Care* 2018; 8(1): 45–48.
14. Hancock K, Clayton JM, Parker SM, et al. Discrepant perceptions about end-of-life communication: a systematic review. *J Pain Symptom Manage* 2007; 34(2): 190–200.
15. Care Quality Commission. Protect, Respect, Connect—Decisions About Living And Dying Well During COVID-*19*. Available at: https://www.cqc.org.uk/publications/themed-work/protect-respect-connect-decisions-about-living-dying-well-during-covid-19

16. Abel J, Kellehear A, Millington Sanders C, Taubert M, Kingston H. Advance care planning re-imagined: a needed shift for COVID times and beyond. *Palliat Care Soc Pract* 2020; 14: 2632352420934491.
17. Dixon J, Matosevic T, Knapp M. The economic evidence for advance care planning: systematic review of evidence. *Palliat Med* 2015; 29(10): 869–884.
18. Jimenez G, Tan WS, Virk AK, Low CK, Car J, Ho AHY. Overview of systematic reviews of advance care planning: summary of evidence and global lessons. *J Pain Symptom Manage* 2018; 56(3): 436–459.
19. Macmillan analysis of Office for National Statistics, NHS England. (2015).
20. Nicholas R, Nicholas E, Hannides M, Gautam V, Friede T, Koffman J. Influence of individual, illness and environmental factors on place of death among people with neurodegenerative diseases: a retrospective, observational, comparative cohort study. *BMJ Support Palliat Care* 2021:bmjspcare-2021-003105.
21. Wright AA, Zhang B, Ray A, et al. Associations between end-of-life discussions, patient mental health, medical care near death, and caregiver bereavement adjustment. *JAMA* 2008; 300(14): 1665–1673.
22. Caplan GA, Meller A, Squires B, Chan S, Willett W. Advance care planning and hospital in the nursing home. *Age Ageing* 2006; 35(6): 581–585.

CASE

37 Pandemics and Disaster Response

Athul Manuel

Expert: Sunitha Daniel

Case history

Thomas, a 68-year-old retired carpenter, lived with his 60-year-old wife, younger son, daughter-in-law, and two grandchildren aged 8 and 5 years of age. His older son was married and lived abroad with his family. They lived in a terraced house in Kothamangalam, a town approximately 30 miles from the Oncology centre situated in Kochi, Kerala, a state in South India. He had hypertension and diabetes, which were controlled with medication.

Thomas was diagnosed with carcinoma of the lung with spinal metastasis after presenting to his doctor with a long-standing cough and a new onset of severe back pain. His pain score was 8/10 on presentation and he was started on strong opioids. Following this, his pain score improved to 3/10 but he developed some side effects to opioids. Given his disease burden, Thomas was referred for urgent palliative radiotherapy for pain control.

There had been incessant rains in the state over the days prior to Thomas's hospital appointment to start radiotherapy and his house and surrounding houses were flooded. The family managed to move to a higher ground and were subsequently moved to a relief camp at a nearby village. Thomas and his family had to leave most of their belongings, household items, clothing, and school books and equipment. Thomas was not able to carry his medical records with him; he was due to get a repeat prescription for his medication during the hospital visit for radiotherapy. Thomas's pain worsened as he ran out of strong opioids and he and his family became extremely anxious due to the delay in treatment. His son, who lived abroad, has not seen his father since the diagnosis of cancer and was unable to travel home as local airports were shut.

Learning Point

Humanitarianism is the compassionate response to the suffering and needs of others. It aims to prevent and relieve human suffering wherever it may be found, to protect life and health, and to ensure respect for all. Mass Casualty Events (MCE) involve hundreds, thousands, or even tens of thousands of victims that affect the ability of local or regional health systems to deliver services consistent with the established standards of care. There are two categories of MCE: 'big bang' single incidents with immediate or sudden impact like hurricanes, tornadoes, tsunamis, earthquakes, and terrorist attacks; and 'rising tide' incidents with prolonged impact like pandemic flu outbreaks.[1] Health services can be overwhelmed by natural disasters due to the physical destruction of facilities as well as the sheer increase in number of people with resulting acute injuries and illnesses. This can affect the care provided for the patients with chronic illnesses, the elderly, and other vulnerable populations.

Clinical Tip

Patients needing palliative care during humanitarian crisis include[2]:

1. Previously healthy individuals who are directly affected by MCE making them injured or critically ill.
2. People with pre-existing life-threatening illnesses like advanced cancer and dialysis dependant renal failure.
3. Individuals who are imminently dying, e.g. those receiving hospice care.
4. People with comorbidities whose health deteriorates due to the disaster.
5. People awaiting curative medical management with symptom control and supportive care needs.
6. Individuals who might be triaged out of curative medical care due to scarce resources.

Expert Comment

Palliative care aims to improve quality of life, provide dignity and comfort, whilst advising how to alleviate financial suffering due to illness or disability. Integration of palliative care into public healthcare systems is an essential part of universal health coverage.[3] People living in low- and middle-income countries (LMICs) are more vulnerable to needless suffering due to disasters as they have limited access to disease prevention, diagnosis, management, and social care as compared to high-income countries (HICs).[4] A number of principles apply to palliative care in any humanitarian crisis and a recommended triage category is given in Figure 37.1.[5]

Category	Colour code	Description
1. Immediate	Red	Survival possible with immediate treatment. Palliative care should be integrated with life-sustaining treatment as much as possible.
2. Expectant	Blue	Survival not possible given the care that is available. Palliative care is required.
3. Delayed	Yellow	Not in immediate danger of death, but treatment needed soon. Palliative care and/or symptom relief may nevertheless be needed immediately.
3. Minimal	Green	Will need medical care at some point, after patients with more critical conditions have been treated. Symptom relief may be needed.

Figure 37.1 Recommended triage categories in humanitarian emergencies and crises

Reproduced with permission from World Health Organization. (2018) . *Integrating palliative care and symptom relief into responses to humanitarian emergencies and crises: a WHO guide*. World Health Organization. https://apps.who.int/iris/handle/10665/274565.

Learning Point

Following a disaster, patients could either die in the first hours or days or could live for days or weeks with injuries and illness that are life-threatening. Both these groups of patients need symptom control and psychosocial support. Palliative care uses the skills from multiple disciplines to improve the quality of life of seriously ill patients and their families based on evidence-based medical treatment, robust symptom relief, and humanitarian care when there is nothing else to offer.[6] The World Health Organization (WHO) guide on integrating palliative care and symptom relief into the response to humanitarian emergencies and crises describes the types of suffering of people affected by sudden onset of MCEs and recommended steps to integrate palliative care into the humanitarian response[5] (Table 37.1).

Table 37.1 Types of suffering of people affected by sudden onset disasters, war, political conflict, or ethnic violence, and recommended steps to integrate palliative care into the humanitarian response

Type of suffering	Recommended palliative care responses to suffering
Physical suffering	
Symptoms due to acute injury or illness Symptoms due to injury-related complications and subacute or chronic illnesses	• Put in place policies clarifying that humanitarian medical assistance aims to both save lives and relieve suffering. • Develop protocols for a minimum standard of symptom assessment and treatment, and for care of expectant patients, by international and national emergency medical teams (EMTs) and local healthcare providers. • Train and equip EMTs and local healthcare providers to reach a minimum standard of symptom assessment and treatment and care of expectant patients. • Include the essential package of palliative care medicines and equipment for humanitarian emergencies and crises in all emergency health kits; ensure that oral and injectable morphine are included in all kits and are both secured and accessible in adequate quantities by EMTs and local healthcare providers. • Include in all Type 1 EMTs at least one physician and nurse with at least basic palliative care training. • Include in all Type 2 and 3 EMTs at least one physician with at least intermediate palliative care training and that all anaesthetists and anaesthesia technicians have at least basic palliative care training.
Psychological suffering	
Acute psychological effects (including acute anxiety, acute depressed mood, acute grief) Chronic psychological effects (including PTSD, chronic anxiety disorders, chronic depression, complicated grief, survivor's guilt)	• Train EMT staff members and local healthcare providers in psychological first aid (PFA). • Train and equip EMTs and local healthcare providers with protocols for psychological symptom assessment and treatment. • Include the essential package of palliative care medicines and equipment for humanitarian emergencies and crises in all emergency health kits; include oral fluoxetine, injectable diazepam, and oral and injectable haloperidol in all kits so that they are accessible in adequate quantities to EMTs and local healthcare providers.[7] • Train and equip all EMTs in palliative care. • Seek partnerships with local community and spiritual leaders for advice on cultural values and beliefs relevant to mental illness and to inform the local community about the EMTs' activities. • Recruit local mental healthcare providers who can provide culturally and linguistically appropriate care and advise foreign team members on cultural values and beliefs relevant to mental illness. • Offer training to local volunteers to provide basic mental health interventions as appropriate. • Organize support groups for patients and survivors who may wish to share experiences and challenges. • Include mental healthcare providers in humanitarian response teams that are likely to encounter many patients with mental health consequences.

Type of suffering	Recommended palliative care responses to suffering
Social suffering	
Loss of access to shelter, clothing, food, sanitation, protection from violence Extreme vulnerability (including frail older people, unaccompanied children, people with mental or physical disabilities, people living in extreme poverty)	• Ensure access to shelter, clothing appropriate to climate and culture, food, sanitation, school. • Seek to arrange protection from physical or psychological abuse. • Organize support groups for patients and survivors who may wish to share experiences and challenges.
Spiritual suffering	
Loss of sense of meaning of life Loss of faith/anger towards God	• Seek partnerships with local spiritual counsellors willing to visit patients and family members on request

Reproduced with permission from World Health Organization. (2018) . *Integrating palliative care and symptom relief into responses to humanitarian emergencies and crises: a WHO guide.* World Health Organization. https://apps.who.int/iris/handle/10665/274565. License: CC BY-NC-SA 3.0 IGO

Expert Comment

The essential package includes safe, effective, inexpensive, off-patent, and widely available medicines, simple and inexpensive equipment and basic social supports, which is aimed at preventing and relieving all types of suffering–physical, psychological, social, and spiritual. It also includes the human resources needed to apply them appropriately, effectively, and safely, and to provide psychological and spiritual support.

Expert Comment

Emergency medical teams (EMTs) are groups of health professionals (doctors, nurses, paramedics, etc.) who could come from governments, non-governmental organizations (NGO), international humanitarian organizations like Red Cross, academic institutions, and military. They provide medical aid both locally and internationally for people affected by humanitarian emergencies and crises.

The WHO has classified EMT into three types:

1. EMT Type 1 provides outpatient emergency care, including emergency care of injuries and other significant healthcare needs.
2. EMT Type 2 provides inpatient surgical emergency care including acute care, general, and obstetric surgery for trauma and other major conditions.
3. EMT Type 3 provides complex inpatient referral surgical care including intensive care. These groups involve additional specialized care teams within inpatient settings of hospitals, including palliative care clinicians.

Two days after the relocation Thomas was reviewed by a community palliative nurse, who was part of a well-established team consisting of doctors, nurses, social workers, and volunteers trained in principles of palliative care. They provide door to door care, at his new location (Figure 37.2). On evaluation he had a WHO Performance status of 2, an Edmonton symptom assessment scale (ESAS) score of 7/10 for pain and 6/10 for anxiety (mainly related to delays in treatment) plus additional symptoms of cough and insomnia. The nurse contacted Thomas's previous medical team to access his medical records, and was able to arrange for his prescriptions including his opioids to be renewed. Thomas and his family had lost most of their possessions. The volunteers in the team were able to liaise with a NGO involved in relief activities and the family were supplied with clothes, food kits, school books, and uniform for children and other household items. The team also contacted the radiotherapy department of the nearest cancer centre and arranged to start radiotherapy. The nurse continued to visit weekly for symptom assessment, to provide psychosocial support, and to monitor for any signs of post-traumatic stress disorder. She also provided the contact details of

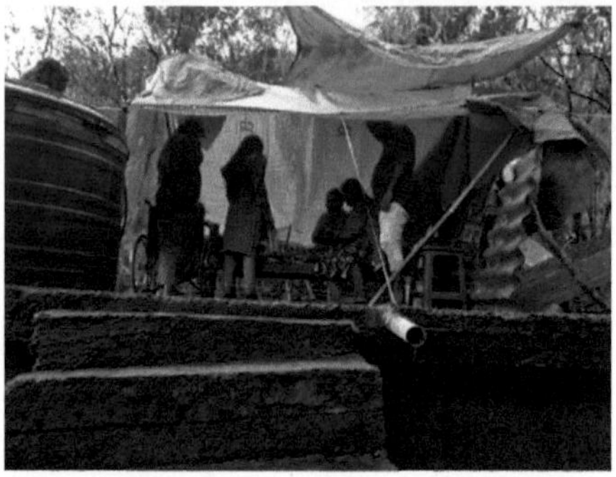

Figure 37.2 Community palliative care team visiting patient and family.

the tele helpline services providing psychological support and District Mental Health Programme, a multidisciplinary team, consisting of a psychiatrist, social worker, clinical psychologist, psychiatric nurse, and support staff that are trained to provide psychological first aid (PFA).

Expert Comment

Floods are the commonest natural disaster globally. Impacts include high rate of somatization, depression, psychological distress, anxiety, and post-traumatic stress disorder,[8,9] which can even persist up to 2 years after the disaster.[10] Support from family and friends have been shown to reduce the incidence of PTSD and depression post-flood-exposure.[11] Psychological First Aid (PFA) is compassionate, sympathetic response to anyone who is suffering and who may need support can be provided by non-professionals. It involves three steps: look (for safety, to protect people from further harm and to identify people with urgent basic needs or serious distress reactions), listen (to the needs and concerns, help to calm people), and link (address basic needs and provide information about services and support, connect people with loved ones).[12]

Learning Point

Any humanitarian crisis goes through two major phases—Response and Relief—followed by Recovery, which includes three intersecting phases of emergency relief, rehabilitation, and reconstruction.[13] The duration of each phase depends on the type of humanitarian crisis. Preparedness towards humanitarian crises must be part of community awareness, especially in terms of common incidents that pertain to the geography of a place. Community response is key in the rescue phase. Palliative care volunteers can lead the civil society response by forming community rescue camps at shelter points which prioritize care to women, children, and house-bound people. Nurses can help with wound dressings, urinary catheter changes and other minor procedures as a part of the campsite activities for ongoing care of the chronically ill patients.

Expert Comment

Volunteers are an important part of the hospice and palliative care movement in many countries in North America and Europe as well as in India and Uganda.[14] They provide support in number of ways including visiting patient in hospices, sitting with dying patients, help in day care and bereavement services, running complementary therapy and pastoral/faith-based care services.[15] Neighbourhood Network in Palliative Care (NNPC) was formed in 2001 and is community-led initiative aiming to provide home-based palliative care to all those in need in Kerala, South India.[16] It provides support with training volunteers, access to medical and nursing skills, and initial funds to start the work. Groups are managed by people from the local communities, such as farmers, teachers, and local business people, and draw on existing community resources and assets. Currently over 1,600 institutions deliver palliative care services throughout the state; and tens of thousands of volunteers have been trained.[17] These trained volunteers become the first response group during any humanitarian crisis in the state.

Expert Comment

Future research and work. There are several organizations formed to develop guidelines and training for palliative care in humanitarian settings. These include: 1) PALCHASE (Palliative Care in Humanitarian Situations & Emergencies), which is an international network of practitioners and scholars advocating for research on and practice of palliative care in humanitarian crises (https://www.pallchase.org); 2) WHO working group to develop guidelines for palliative care provision in humanitarian emergencies; 3) Research colloquium on palliative care for children in humanitarian emergencies; 4) Médecins Sans Frontières (MSF); 5) The Sphere Handbook 2018.[2]

Expert Comment

Pandemics and natural disasters can adversely impact end of life care services including detrimentally affecting service provision, service providers and service users. Adaptations need to be made in terms of location, mode of consultation, and drug prescription. Modifications to practice need to be made in response to; changes in disease trajectories, problems with accessing care, shortage of resources, lack of specific guidance, and increased pressure on healthcare workers. Awareness of isolation, dehumanization of care, and extra burdens on caregivers are also important. In the context of increasing number of natural disasters globally there is an urgent need to develop end of life care policies and practices that can be rapidly implemented natural disasters occur.[18]

Discussion

Thomas had been newly diagnosed with cancer and was receiving strong opioids for pain whilst awaiting oncological treatment. Thomas had to be relocated to a new village as his house was affected by unprecedented floods. He and his family lost all their possessions as well as medications, which resulted in worsening of physical and psychological symptoms. The palliative care team made a significant difference to Thomas's situation by evaluating his symptoms and addressing all his needs including the supply of prescriptions and relief and rehabilitation kits. They were also able to refer to available oncology centres for further continuation of treatment.

A Final Word from the Expert

This case is a good example of a patient with palliative care needs, with a recent life changing diagnosis. He had to face a once in a lifetime natural calamity with the loss of all his possessions. The case demonstrated how his palliative care needs worsened during the crisis due to problems with access to medications and treatment and how this can worsen the suffering and distress of patient. An already established palliative care network with strong roots in the community was able to appropriately care for the patient and his family, providing symptom control and needed psychosocial care.

References

1. Wilkinson A. The potential role for palliative care in mass casualty events. *J Palliat Care Med* 2012; 2: e112.
2. Nouvet E, Sivaram M, Bezanson K, et al. Palliative care in humanitarian crises: a review of the literature. *Journal of International Humanitarian Action* 2018; 3(1): 5.
3. Knaul FM, Bhadelia A, Rodriguez NM, Arreola-Ornelas H, Zimmermann C. The Lancet Commission on Palliative Care and Pain Relief—findings, recommendations, and future directions. *Lancet Glob Health* 2018; 6: S5–S6.
4. Association S. Sphere Handbook: *Humanitarian Charter and Minimum Standards in Humanitarian Response*: PRACTICAL ACTION, 2018. Available at: https://spherestandards.org/wp-content/uploads/Sphere-Handbook-2018-EN.pdf
5. Integrating palliative care and symptom relief into responses to humanitarian emergencies and crises: a WHO guide: World Health Organization; 2018. Available at: https://apps.who.int/iris/handle/10665/274565
6. Phillips SJ, Knebel A, Roberts M, et al. *Mass Medical Care with Scarce Resources. A Community Planning Guide*. 2007. Available at: https://www ahrq gov/research/mce/mceguide pdf
7. Karunakara U, Stevenson F. Ending neglect of older people in the response to humanitarian emergencies. *PLoS Med* 2012; 9(12): e1001357.
8. Stanke C, Murray V, Amlôt R, Nurse J, Williams R. The effects of flooding on mental health: Outcomes and recommendations from a review of the literature. *PLoS Curr* 2012; 4: e4f9f1fa9c3cae.
9. Fernandez A, Black J, Jones M, et al. Flooding and mental health: a systematic mapping review. *PloS One* 2015; 10(4): e0119929.
10. Norris FH, Perilla JL, Riad JK, Kaniasty K, Lavizzo EA. Stability and change in stress, resources, and psychological distress following natural disaster: findings from Hurricane Andrew. *Anxiety, Stress & Coping* 1999; 12(4): 363–396.
11. Dar KA, Iqbal N, Prakash A, Paul MA. PTSD and depression in adult survivors of flood fury in Kashmir: the payoffs of social support. *Psychiatry Res* 2018; 261: 449–455.
12. World Health Organization (WHO). *Psychological First Aid: Guide for Field Workers*. 2011. Available at: https://www.who.int/publications/i/item/9789241548205
13. Shah A. Relief, rehabilitation and development: the case of Gujarat. *J Humanitarian Assistance* 2003:1–52.
14. Burbeck R, Candy B, Low J, Rees R. Understanding the role of the volunteer in specialist palliative care: a systematic review and thematic synthesis of qualitative studies. *BMC Palliat Care* 2014; 13(1): 1–12.
15. Burbeck R, Low J, Sampson EL, et al. Volunteers in specialist palliative care: a survey of adult services in the United Kingdom. *J Palliat Med* 2014; 17(5): 568–574.
16. Sallnow L, Kumar S, Numpeli M. Home-based palliative care in Kerala, India: the neighbourhood network in palliative care. *Prog Palliat Care* 2010; 18(1): 14–17.
17. Sallnow L, Smith R, Ahmedzai SH, et al. Report of the Lancet Commission on the Value of Death: bringing death back into life. *Lancet* 2022; 399(10327): 837–884.
18. Kelly M, Mitchell I, Walker I, Mears J, Scholz B. End-of-life care in natural disasters including epidemics and pandemics: a systematic review. *BMJ Support Palliat Care* 2023; 13(1): 1–14.

CASE

38 Spiritual Care

Sarah Maan and Alice Gray

Expert: Andrew Goodhead

Case history

Rose, a 66-year-old retired nurse, had a background of interstitial lung disease. She was admitted to the inpatient unit of her local hospice with shortness of breath and deteriorating mobility. Already dependent on oxygen 24 hours a day, her breathlessness had led to multiple hospital admissions in the preceding 12 months. During her most recent hospital admission, the respiratory team felt a palliative approach was most appropriate and referred her to the hospice team for symptom control and advance care planning.

A delayed diagnosis of a right leg deep vein thrombosis (DVT) during a previous inpatient spell, led to some mistrust of healthcare professionals and a desire to avoid further hospital admissions. Despite this, the idea of being admitted to a hospice was met with some resistance, 'but I'm not dying' she told the community palliative nurse who visited her at home and suggested the admission. After persuasion by the community team, she agreed to hospice admission.

Expert Comment

The spiritual and religious aspects of a patient's life are possibly the most 'knotty' to begin to explore and understand. Spirituality is undoubtedly unique to every person. Even two people who share the same religious faith may understand and express that faith and how it relates to everyday life differently. Clinicians naturally shy away from entering areas of a person's life which are considered private. Yet, the approach a person takes to their faith or spiritual outlook on life can significantly affect decisions they make around treatments and interventions.

Learning Point What is Spirituality?

Spirituality has been defined as the way individuals seek and express meaning and purpose, and the way they experience their connectedness to the moment, to self, to others, to nature, and to the significant or sacred. It may include religion but also embodies more general ways of expressing these experiences, e.g. relationships with others/nature/arts.[1]

Spiritual well-being can be described as feeling 'at peace'. Conversely spiritual distress/pain can occur when people are unable to find sources of meaning, purpose, or connection and is often seen in terminal illness. Spiritual pain is a component of 'total pain',[2] a concept coined by Dame Cicely Saunders. See Figure 38.1.

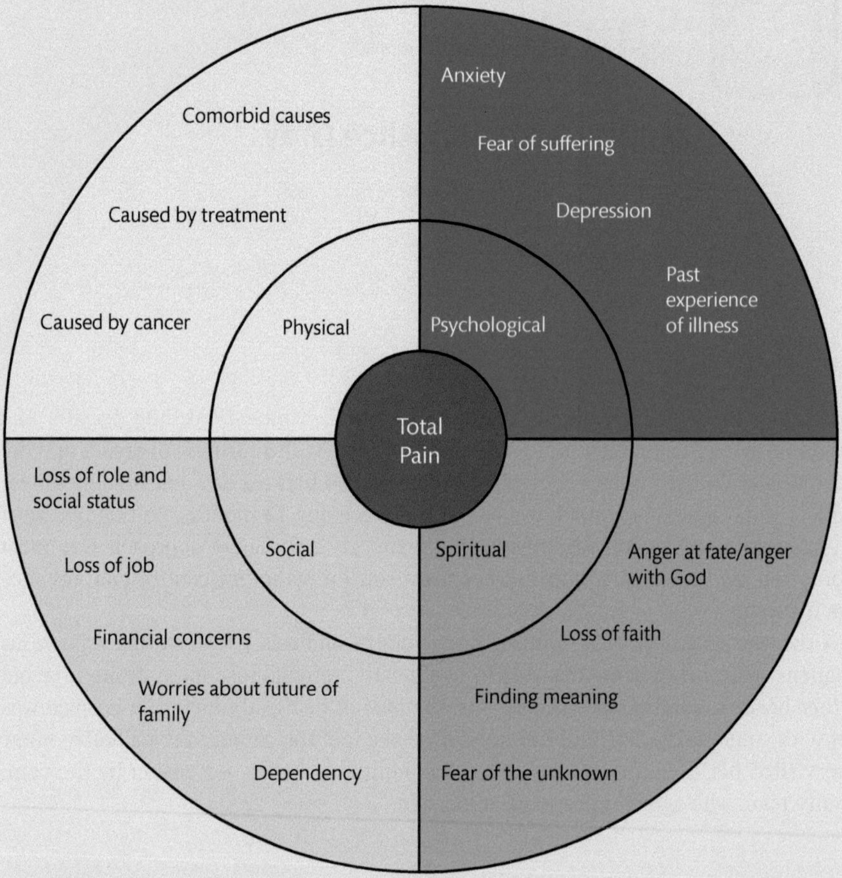

Figure 38.1 Total pain dimensions.

Reproduced with permission from Franklin, A.E., Lovell, M.R. (2019). Pain and Pain Management. In: MacLeod, R., Van den Block, L. (eds) *Textbook of Palliative Care*. Springer, Cham. https://doi.org/10.1007/978-3-319-77740-5_10

Saunders met a dying man who would have a profound effect on her life. David Tasma, a Polish Jewish refugee, who had fled the Warsaw Ghetto, worked as a waiter and, at the age of 40, felt he had achieved little in life. He and Saunders developed an intense friendship during the weeks he spent in Archway Hospital. She was moved by his loss of hope in approaching the end of his life with a struggle to find meaning. It was this experience, where the idea of developing a dedicated home for the dying first germinated and which she discussed with David. He left her £500, and the prophecy, 'I'll be a window in your home'. Some argue that this was Saunders's first interaction with someone in 'spiritual pain'. 'Tasma told me of the difficulties of laying down a life that felt incomplete and unfulfilled'.[3,4]

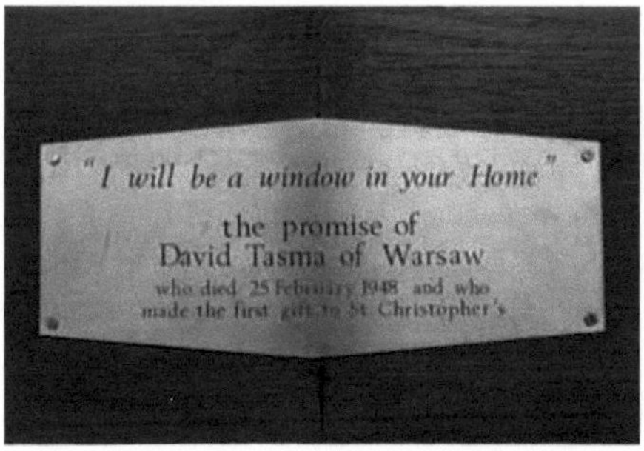

Figure 38.2 Plaque found in St. Christopher's hospice to commemorate the first donation that began the modern-day hospice movement.

> **Evidence Base Why Do We Do Spiritual Care? Research on Whether Patients Want Us To Talk About It**
>
> Whilst the biomedical model of healthcare has resulted in advances in physical health, it doesn't allow space or time for acknowledging spiritual, social, and cultural health. Clinicians are not given the training they require to address these needs and are often left feeling unable to tackle them. However, research demonstrates that patients not only want us to acknowledge them but also to address them.[5] When left unaddressed, there is an association, 'with poor quality of life, dissatisfaction with care, less hospice utilization, more aggressive treatment, and increased costs, particularly among ethnic minority groups and patients with high levels of religious coping'. However, when confronted and intervention offered, the benefits are reported across ages, patient groups, and disease profiles, including organ failure and dementia.[6]

> **Evidence Base Who Should Ask About Spirituality**
>
> A systematic review by Best et al. in 2015 looked at 54 studies that reported spirituality discussions within a medical consultation.[7] They found that up to 70% of patients felt it was appropriate for their doctor to enquire about their spiritual needs. Anatole Broyard, an American writer who wrote about watching his father die of cancer famously said 'I'd like my doctor ... to grope for my spirit as well as my prostate'.[8] Palliative care teaches us the importance of seeing patients as a whole person, and this includes their spirituality.

Rose was originally from Tanzania but had lived the majority of her life in the UK and identified as Pentecostal Christian. She lived in a bungalow with her husband and had four adult children. She had no carers or any equipment at home. As her disease progressed, she began to struggle with daily activities. She was no longer able to cook and host family members as she once had and found herself relying heavily on her husband to help with even the most mundane tasks. This served as a devastating realization for her, as she had always been the head caretaker of her large extended family. She was a pillar in her community, respected by many, and a regular volunteer at church gatherings. Her faith was very important to her and provided her with a strong sense of belonging. The huge contrast in who she had been and who she was now because of her condition, became a great source of distress. She felt her disease was robbing her identity and sense of purpose.

As an inpatient, she engaged well with breathing techniques, working with the hospice physiotherapist who she had connected with on arrival. After a 2-day trial, she began to decline immediate release morphine solution for breathlessness, saying it made her feel like she couldn't breathe and that she worried it was going to kill her. Discordance began to arise between the patient and the medical team when advance care planning was introduced. The patient reiterated that she wasn't dying and didn't feel she needed to think about death. She acknowledged that she was unwell and that maybe her condition would eventually kill her, but she was not ready to make decisions about dying and instead took offence at the question being asked.

Expert Comment

In this case study, Rose presented her clinicians with the symptoms of a chronic respiratory condition. Their expertise lies in the diagnosis and treatment of this. Underneath the physical aspects of her presentation are the cultural, religious, and spiritual aspects of what makes Rose a whole person. It is very likely that through her life religious and spiritual values have guided decisions. Now, faced with an unexpected diagnosis, she is struggling to understand what her life means and how it can have purpose. The clinician's role in meeting with her is to understand what principles will guide her choices around treatment and conversations around care planning and even dying and death.

Clinical Tip How to Conduct a Spiritual Assessment

The Integrated Palliative care Outcome Scale (IPOS)[9] is a validated tool used to measure physical, psychological, social, and spiritual symptoms in palliative care settings. It was developed as conventional outcome measures such as morbidity and mortality were unhelpful in the palliative population, and was designed to capture the holistic nature of palliative care. The IPOS asks 'Have you felt at peace?'; the response to this question can then be explored further to attain a more comprehensive spiritual assessment.

Other phrases which can be used to broach spirituality with patients include:

- What helps you get through a tough day?
- How do you enjoy spending your time? Has your health affected this?
- How do you make sense of what is happening to you?

Detailed to follow are two common assessment tools that can be used as aide memoires to help assess spiritual needs. They are designed to help screen for spiritual distress and identify patients who may require support in this area. Spiritual assessments should ideally be integrated into daily practice to assess how spiritual needs are evolving.

HOPE[10]

- What are your sources of Hope/comfort/strength?
- Do you have organized religion/faith?
- What do you do to give you a sense of purpose?
- Effects—has being unwell stopped you from doing things that give you meaning/purpose?

FICA[11]

- Faith/beliefs
- Importance/Influence
- Community
- Address—how would you like me to address these issues in your healthcare

After almost a month at home, Rose's symptoms began to considerably worsen and her family had called the ambulance multiple times in distress. She was readmitted to the hospice for what the staff suspected was terminal care. She had built up a relationship with one of the hospice physiotherapists on a previous admission and had found the breathing techniques relieved a lot of her symptom burden and asked to see her again, despite not being well enough for formalized therapy. During one of their sessions, it became clear that Rose had not told her relatives in Tanzania how unwell she was as they had been praying for her healing. The staff in the hospice began to recognize that her faith in the ability of God to cure her was still strong and that outwardly acknowledging the thought of dying would undermine this strongly held belief that was giving her hope. Following a multidisciplinary team meeting, staff recognized their conflict in wanting Rose to have open conversations, versus her desire to hang on to the hope of a miracle, and so the focus of ward rounds was modified. Now, the physiotherapist would lead with one of the junior doctors, exploring non-opioid strategies for managing her breathlessness. The team involved her church pastor to help her join church meetings via video conference from her hospice bed so she could still feel part of the community. This shift resulted in an improvement in her iPOS score and less discordance between her and the clinical team. This allowed Rose to feel heard, and she subsequently deteriorated and died peacefully in the hospice.

Expert Comment

The most important 'task' for any person who meets with a patient such as Rose is the ability to remain open and enquiring. There is clearly a dichotomy between information given by clinicians and information she is sharing with family. It is very easy to see this as a challenge to medical information and advice—around treatment decisions (either starting a course of treatment or stopping a course of treatment). It is better to understand that there is a partnership between clinicians and patient, and that Rose is 'planning for the worst and hoping for the best'. Her belief is the underpinning of her life and her understanding that 'Christ is the Great Healer' is the lens through which she comprehends her illness. The approach of the hospice staff, developing a partnership with her pastor to enable her to continue being part of the life of her church, enabled them to engage with her and was supportive of her faith and spiritual life.

Learning Point How Do We Do Spiritual Care?

A significant part of spirituality is about relationships and so it is crucial professionals build up a relationship with their patient. However, we are aware that in relationships, each participant holds perspectives and beliefs that will help shape that interaction. It is therefore important that clinicians explore their own spirituality and engage with their worldview in order that they not confuse their own spirituality with their patients'. This enables clinicians to differentiate between perspectives and avoid conflict by acknowledging the patient experience and how they are formulating their decisions. This does not mean that clinicians have to align their worldview with their patients, but helps them navigate towards a mutually agreed path forward, recognizing the truth when Anais Nin said, 'We don't see things as they are, we see things as we are'.

There must also be space for patients and their loved ones to hold on to hope, even when confronted with bad test results and news. Elisabeth Kubler-Ross found in her research that patients had the most confidence in the clinicians that had allowed them to continue to hope, in spite of the bad news they were receiving.[12] This may also be important for patients' relatives who need to maintain hope in the midst of pain, not forgetting that they are spending more time just being with the patient than our shorter and often more functional interactions. This does not mean that we paint a different picture when breaking bad news, and still encourage patients to 'prepare for the worst whilst hoping for the best'.

With time constraints and pressures, sometimes spiritual care can appear like a luxury that health services cannot afford. It can therefore be a helpful place to start with some practical steps that are

Clinical Tip How Do We Do Spiritual Care?

Exploring spirituality is often easier to do in someone's own home or hospice, but with the input of the patient, their relatives and spiritual leaders, an ordinary room can be transformed into a 'sacred space', creating an 'anywhere' space into a 'somewhere' space. This is another means of spiritual care.[14]

realistic in all settings. Pulchalski lists some really helpful and relevant starting points for clinicians looking to give compassionate spiritual care.[13]

- Practising compassionate presence—i.e. being fully present and attentive to their patients and being supportive of them in all of their suffering
- Listening to patients' fears, hopes, pain, and dreams
- Obtaining a spiritual history
- Being attentive to all dimensions of patients and their families: body, mind, and spirit
- Incorporating spiritual practices as appropriate
- Involving chaplains as members of the interdisciplinary healthcare team

One case on this topic is insufficient to cover the breadth of ways to support a patient's spirituality. But taking steps towards a patient in this manner will begin to open doors that can then be navigated with the help of spiritual leads and are epitome of patient-centred care.

Future Advances

The model of total pain has helped in the vast improvement of managing patients' symptoms in a holistic manner. However there appears to be a hierarchy of the different components, with spiritual care often getting the least attention and is therefore the least researched and developed.

Societies in the West are becoming less formally religious and there remains a spectrum of beliefs and values amongst healthcare staff and patients. Despite the lack of formalized religion, research shows that spirituality still remains a crucial aspect to be addressed in patient care and so research must reflect the ever-evolving beliefs of our patient population.[15]

Discussion

Patients will not come to us and say, 'I have spiritual pain'. Therefore, we have a duty to recognize spiritual needs, religious or otherwise. It is our job to assess for any distress and acknowledge that often there is no quick fix to existential pain, forcing us to challenge our natural inclination to medicalize and 'treat' this distress. Avoiding assumptions about someone's religion or background and being open to cues and opportunities to learn more about them as an individual, will enable us the privilege of walking alongside our patients on their spiritual journey.

A Final Word from the Expert

Attention is a vital tool in enabling a person to feel comfortable and confident in expressing what matters to them. This may sit in the model which Viktor Frankl described around how meaning is made, or found, in the most difficult circumstance. This may be how a person's faith supports their life now or has led to a loss of faith. Here, the clinician is often asked 'why am I being punished?' or a similar questioning. Offering attention; listening carefully, holding eye contact, and not rushing to move onto the next patient is the most important way spirituality has 'space to breathe'. The patient does not expect answers, but does expect an empathic listener. It is from the initial conversations with a patient that a referral to a chaplaincy team, or to alternative forms of support e.g. cognitive behavioural therapy, Social Work or an art/music based therapeutic intervention, can be implemented. The expression of spirituality is as diverse as the patients clinicians meet day to day.

References

1. Puchalski C, Ferrell B, Virani R, et al. Improving the quality of spiritual care as a dimension of palliative care: the report of the consensus conference. *J Palliat Care* 2009; 12: 885–904.
2. Franklin AE, Lovell MR. Pain and pain management. In: MacLeod R, Van den Block L (eds). *Textbook of Palliative Care*. Cham: Springer, 2018, pp. 149–177.
3. Saunders C. Hospice—a meeting place for religion and science. In: Clark D (ed.). *Cicely Saunders: Selected Writings 1958–2004*. Oxford: Oxford University Press, 1989, pp. 263–276.
4. SYDENHAM: Dame Cicely—a revolutionary woman. News Shopper, Buckinghamshire, UK. c2001–2022. Available at: https://www.newsshopper.co.uk/news/4998520.sydenham-dame-cicely-a-revolutionary-woman/
5. Speck P. Culture and spirituality: essential components of palliative care. *Postgrad Med J* 2016; 92: 341–345.
6. Gijsberts MHE, Liefbroer AI, Otten R, Olsman E. Spiritual care in palliative care: a systematic review of the recent European literature. *Med Sci (Basel)* 2019; 7(2): 25.
7. Best M, Butow P, Olver I. Do patients want doctors to talk about spirituality? A systematic literature review. *Patient Educ Couns* 2015; 98(11): 1320–1328.
8. Broyard A. *Intoxicated By My Illness*. New York: Fawcett Books, 1993.
9. Murtagh FE, Ramsenthaler C, Firth A, et al. A brief, patient- and proxy-reported outcome measure in advanced illness: validity, reliability and responsiveness of the Integrated Palliative care Outcome Scale (IPOS). *Palliat Med* 2019; 33(8): 1045–1057.
10. Anandarajah G, Hight E. Spirituality and medical practice: using the HOPE questions as a practical tool for spiritual assessment. *Am Fam Physician* 2001; 63(1): 81–88.
11. Borneman T, Ferrell B, Puchalski C. Evaluation of the FICA tool for spiritual assessment. *J Pain Sympt Manage* 2010; 40(2): 163–173.
12. Kübler-Ross E, Wessler S, Avioli V. On death and dying. *J Am Med Assoc* 1972; 221(2): 174–179.
13. Puchalski CM. The role of spirituality in health care. *Proc (Bayl Univ Med Cent)* 2001; 14(4), 352–357.
14. English G. 'This is it!' An approach to spirituality. In: Parker J, Aranda S (eds). *Palliative Care: Explorations and Challenges*. Rosebery, Sydney: Macleannan & Petty, 1998.
15. Voetmann S, Hvidt NC, Viftrup DT. Verbalizing spiritual needs in palliative care: a qualitative interview study on verbal and non-verbal communication in two Danish hospices. *BMC Palliat Care* 2022; 21(3). doi.org/10.1186/s12904-021-00886-0.

CASE

39 Cultural Care

Max Charles

Expert: Jonathan Koffman

Case history

Nadim, a 72-year-old gentleman, presented to the Emergency Department at his local District General Hospital following a sudden collapse at home. He had a Glasgow Coma Scale (GCS) of 9 and remained unconscious. A CT scan showed an extensive intracerebral haemorrhage, thought to be due to Nadim's long-standing, poorly controlled hypertension. There was no surgical intervention possible and Nadim was therefore expected to deteriorate and die. Nadim had appeared agitated over the preceding days and due to his low consciousness level, it was unclear to the medical team if this was due to pain, agitation, or both. His family were present in the medical admissions unit and were shocked and traumatized by this acute event, as well as the impending death of their relative. The family raised several concerns about the treatment plan that the medical team were proposing.

Nadim was born in Pakistan and moved to the UK in the 1970s. He and his family were of Muslim faith. His children were born in the UK and whilst they all spoke fluent English, the medical team perceived a cultural mismatch when they were attempting to discuss Nadim's care needs with the family.

Clinical Tip Interpreters

Communication can be challenging and, in some instances, overwhelming for the patient, their family and healthcare professionals (HCP), particularly when the former does not speak English as their first language. Professionally trained interpreters' knowledge of the culture, the nuance associated with particular words, and appropriate behaviours help HCPs provide appropriate individualized patient-centred care.[1, 4–6] Discussion with the interpreter before the clinical consultation is useful for the HCP to gain cultural insight into how that patient and their family may wish to proceed. This is also helpful for the interpreter, to increase awareness of likely medical terminology, discussion topics, and potentially emotive issues. Such preparation allows for accurate translation.[5] We need to be cognizant that the interaction may be distressing for the interpreter, so adequate, accessible, and timely support should be available to them.

Wherever possible, family members should not be used for interpretations.[1] Relatives may not accurately translate the conversation, through a lack of understanding of medical concepts, or purposeful editing/filtering of the information they believe the patient should not know. Some topics around illness can be intimate and either party may not want to discuss certain issues which are personal or potentially embarrassing.[1]

Evidence Base Migration

There has been increasing migration across the globe,[1,2] leading to considerably greater cultural diversity in the United Kingdom.[2] Both patients and physicians bring with them their languages, religion, respective understandings of illness, and how they attribute meaning to symptoms, suffering, dying, and grief.[2,3]

The conflict that arose between Nadim's family and the medical team led to the involvement of the Imam for the hospital and the Hospital Palliative Care team, to try to address the concerns and questions the family had about Nadim's end of life care.

Clinical Tip Assumptions on Cultural Impacts on End of life Care

HCPs need to ensure they do not make assumptions about a person's wishes, beliefs, and preferences solely based on which ethnicity, culture, or religious faith they are labelled as coming from. Stereotyping can lead HCPs to think patients from a supposed subtype will all understand their illness or symptoms in the same way, wish for the same level of involvement in treatment decisions and want the same type of care.[2,7,8] This may inadvertently result in aggressive medical interventions that the patient would not want or the rejection of potentially beneficial therapies[1,8] leaving them at risk of health inequity.

Assuming the patient has mental capacity, it is imperative to ask a patient what is important to them personally to ensure the care they receive is following their wishes and beliefs.

Clinical Tip The Clinician's Culture

Clinicians need to be aware of their own cultural identity as it represents an 'amalgam' or 'recipe for living in the world'. It comprises multiple complex ingredients; for example, where we grew up geographically, our social class, education, our medical training, ethical and religious beliefs, as well as our respective histories, experiences as a clinician, personally and institutionally.[8-10] All, or some of these ingredients, come to bear in the way we communicate and behave with others. Consequently, HCPs' perspectives and beliefs may be very different to those of patients and families. Unless we have insight into our own beliefs surrounding 'a good death', HCPs may attempt to inadvertently and inappropriately impose their priorities and goals on the patient and their family. This may not meet or respect their needs.

Nadim was not taking in any food or drink due to his low consciousness level. His family thought the lack of fluids might make him feel thirsty and unwell and hasten his death. Intravenous fluids (IV) were therefore started at the family's request. However, over the next few days, he started to develop peripheral oedema and retained secretions, potentially due to the fluids, requiring the use of hyoscine butylbromide and intravenous furosemide.

Learning Point Truth-telling Ethics

Palliative care in the United Kingdom is founded on the ideals of patient choice and the right to patient autonomy.[1,2,6,11,12] Legislation and the General Medical Council support this, stating that all patients should be informed of their prognosis unless they are at risk of serious harm.[1,11,12] Autonomy should therefore be respected, unless the person lacks decision-making capacity.

HCPs from a western background tend to promote autonomy by ensuring a patient understands their illness and potential interventions, enabling them to make decisions about medical interventions, including potentially life-prolonging treatments. This is based on the belief that without adequate and accessible information patients cannot make an informed decision about their goals of care, and plans for their future and highlight their wishes and preferences based on their value system.

This need for clinicians to tell the 'truth' fits into the models of healthcare provided in the UK and is felt to be part of the duty of care. A lack of 'truth-telling' may lead to feelings of discomfort and dissatisfaction and potentially moral injury. However, in many cultures, this is not the cultural norm[2,6,10,13] and can be actively rejected when it comes to life-limiting diagnoses and end of life care.[1] Instead, greater emphasis is placed on protecting the patient from harm. Talking about death, especially prognostication can be seen as harmful to the individual and socially incongruous, leading to greater family distress.[6,10,13] It can also be seen to remove hope, even if the hope is not based on realistic options.[10] Moreover, many cultures feel that prognosis and decisions about death are governed by their deity[10] and that people may be required to prove their faith by enduring rather than avoiding suffering.[10] If HCPs are not careful, our need to tell the 'truth' to our patients is more about servicing our own needs rather than supporting the patient alongside their beliefs and illness behaviours. Consequently, whilst our intentions may be grounded in non-maleficence, we may cause moral harm and distress to the patients, their families, and possibly those who care for them.

Nadim deteriorated further, becoming agitated. The medical team were concerned he was in pain. The family became very distressed when the medical team suggested stopping the IV fluids and introducing a syringe pump of morphine and midazolam for symptom control. Nadim's family believed this treatment plan would hasten his death and were adamant this should be dictated only by Allah. The tension between them and the health team looking after Nadim rapidly escalated, requiring negotiation of an agreed care plan.

Expert Comment Mistrust

People from different cultural backgrounds or countries may have no previous experiences with the health system in which they are being cared for, the provision of palliative care, including the drugs used to manage symptoms and the medico-legal system under which decision-making is governed.[1,6,8,10] Moreover, patients may have faced previous direct discrimination through racism and racial prejudice. This, together with poverty, political unrest, or conflict within their own culture may have been associated with poor healthcare encounters in the past. This legacy may present as mistrusting the intentions and goals associated with western-centric palliative care.[1,13,14] HCPs must ensure they are sensitive to these issues and work to gain trust through honest and open discourse; and not presume that they automatically have the trust of patients and their families, which may be more present and explicit in western society.

Learning Point Information Level Assumptions

As clinicians, delivering information is often accompanied by an agenda of what we believe warrants discussion.[12] This presumes we know what information patients want and this may not be the case.[4, 15] Too much information or information shared in the wrong way may lead to heightened levels of distress and a potential breakdown in relationships with HCPs.[15,16]

Before delivering information, consider asking the patient:

- Is this the right setting for sharing information, including privacy?
- Is now the right time and are the right people present to support the patient?
- How much information would they want to know?
- Would they want to know about their situation, even if the news was 'bad news'?

If they do not wish to receive the news:

- Sensitively and non-judgementally explore why they do not want to know; do not just take it at face value.
- If the patient does not want to know, is there someone else who might want to know on the patient's behalf? What is their relationship to that individual?

Learning Point Do Not Attempt Cardiopulmonary Resuscitation (DNACPR)

In some countries, medical decisions and discussions, for example, DNACPR, are perceived to be for the doctor to decide and are not shared, participatory decisions.[8] As a result, HCPs trained elsewhere may have different repertoires for engaging in end of life care decision-making and discussions.[8,10,14]

Evidence Base Diversity in Patterns of Advanced Disease

There is growing evidence that inequities are present concerning ethnicity and health. This is also evident in access to palliative care, chronic disease, mental health, cancer care, and pain management.[1,14]

Expert Comment Misuse of Concepts

Identity is multifaceted and is a composition of a person's race, religion, ethnicity, and culture. These terms are often used interchangeably and incorrectly combined with a person's social class and education to try to define an individual or group of people.[1,9,14]

Race

This has a long and dishonourable history. It relies on an erroneous belief that people can be categorized according to shared physical and biological characteristics such as skin colour, facial features, and other hereditary traits. This framework for categorizing people has been largely discredited, with a clear demonstration that genetic variations between racial groups are small, inconsequential, inaccurate, and misleading. Instead, race can be viewed as a social representation created to devise groupings to create and maintain a power hierarchy between groups and enforce systems of privilege.

Population

Designated groups that have adapted in a similar advantageous way genetically, physiologically, and ecologically to a particular environment.[4]

Ethnicity

This can be viewed as a collective with a putative, common ancestry that shares cultural symbols and practices, including language, dress, diet, religion, values, and norms. This conceptualization of culture also accommodates the possibility that an individual's values and norms are neither static nor intrinsic entities.[1,4,14]

Culture

Culture is a way of life and interpreting the world around someone. Making sense of health, illness, and death all fit within this structure.[1,4,7,9,10,14] Culture is dynamic and if we acknowledge that, it is something that is always changing. We can never be truly 'culturally competent' apart from the culture in which we live. Thinking of culture in this way should allow us to enquire and learn[9,17] rather than relying heavily on a predetermined list of religious customs, beliefs, or values that categorize what different groups do (or do not). Cultural 'fact files' or 'recipe guides' are overly reductionist and do not capture the rich nuance and 'tapestry' associated with difference.[1,14]

Learning Point Communication Models

An effective confident clinician needs to be able to communicate with people from cultures that are different to his or her own about complex medical decisions. Ideally, the clinician and the patient need to come to a shared decision that encompasses their respective world views (Figure 39.1).

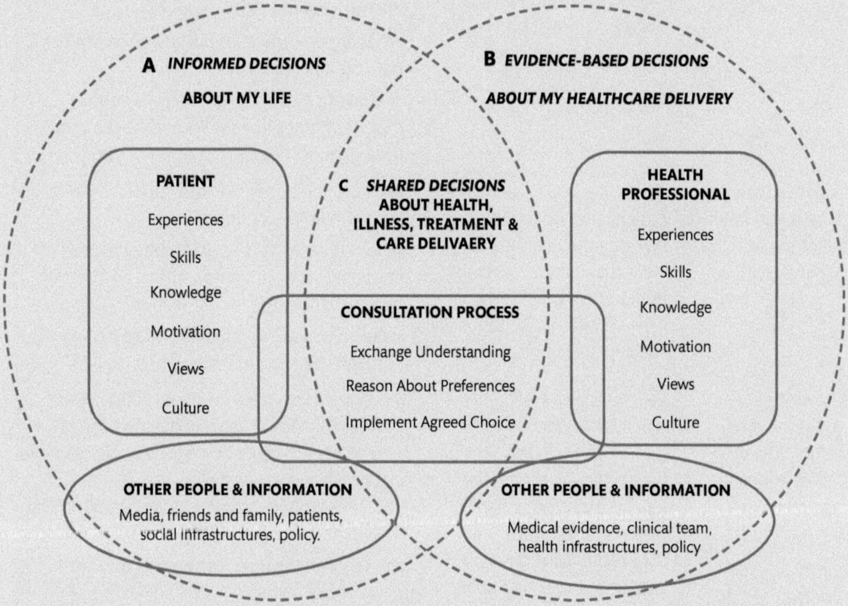

Figure 39.1 Shared decision support for the patient, the clinician and the consultation.[19]

Reproduced with permission from Breckenridge K, Bekker HL, Gibbons E, van der Veer SN, Abbott D, Briançon S, Cullen R, Garneata L, Jager KJ, Lønning K, Metcalfe W, Morton RL, Murtagh FE, Prutz K, Robertson S, Rychlik I, Schon S, Sharp L, Speyer E, Tentori F, Caskey FJ. How to routinely collect data on patient-reported outcome and experience measures in renal registries in Europe: an expert consensus meeting. *Nephrol Dial Transplant.* 2015 Oct;30(10):1605-14. doi: 10.1093/ndt/gfv209. Epub 2015 May 16. PMID: 25982327; PMCID: PMC4569391.

Clinical Tip Communication Models

Without appearing to make assumptions or stereotype the patient or their family. Skilled and empathetic communication is required. Various strategies have been proposed for cross-cultural communication. Two recommended strategies are presented in Tables 39.1 and 39.2. Clinicians should consider which one suits their personal style of consultation to allow authentic and genuine interactions to take place.[4,9,10]

Table 39.1 RISK Reduction Assessment to ascertain the level of cultural influence.[9] A structure to enable a patient's or family's place within their culture to be understood

	Relevant Information	Questions and Strategies
Resources for patients and families	Tangible resources that the family can draw on, such as: level of education, socioeconomic status (including insurance), social support networks, in-language social service agencies, transportation, grocery shopping, etc.	'What kind of assistance is available to you in your community that might be helpful during this time?' 'Do you know others in your community who have faced similar difficulties?'
Individual identity and acculturation/ assimilation	Questions about the patient, the context of his or her life, and individual circumstances, including place of birth, refugee, or immigration status, languages spoken, and degree of integration within the ethnic community.	'Where were you born and raised?' When did you emigrate to the US and how has your experience been coming to a new country?' 'What languages do you speak and in which are you most comfortable talking?' 'What are your most important concerns now that you have this illness?' Life history assessment: 'What were other important times in your life and how might these experiences help us to know you?'
Skills available to the patient and family to adapt to the disease requirements	The actual ability of the patient and the family to navigate the healthcare system and cope with the demands of the disease itself—emotionally, physically, socially, and spiritually.	'Who are the people in your support system that are helpful or harmful?' 'Who is there to help you with physical care, emotional support, transportation, and care of loved ones?' 'Who do you see or talk with, where do you go for religious or spiritual strength, or solace?'
Knowledge about the ethnic group's health beliefs, values, practices, and cultural communication etiquette	Beliefs, values, and practices associated with communication etiquette and health, including attitudes toward truth-telling, family-centred vs. individual-centred decision-making style, historical, social, and political issues that might affect relationships between the patient and elements of the dominant culture.	The clinician knows the dominant ethnic groups in his or her practice. Reads about the different cultures. Attends continuing education programmes about each culture—the beliefs, values, and practices surrounding health, including truth-telling_ What is the symbolic meaning of the disease? Learns about the usual community and family practices surrounding death and dying; Does the patient/family adhere to any of these beliefs and practices? How are decisions made in this cultural group? Who is the head of the household? Does this family adhere to traditional cultural guidelines or do they adhere more to the Western model?

Reproduced with permission from Kagawa-Singer M, Shaheen KL. A Strategy to Reduce Cross-cultural Miscommunication and Increase the Likelihood of Improving Health Outcomes. *Academic Medicine*: June 2003; 78: 6: 577–587.

Table 39.2 Unpeeling layers of cultural influence. This method suggests topics and example questions that can be interwoven into a sensitive conversation about a patient's culture, their illness, and associated symptoms[4,18,20]

Embracing patient and family-centred care, healthcare providers prioritize the needs, preferences, and perspectives of both the patient and their family, ensuring a holistic and collaborative approach to treatment and decision-making	Understanding the attitudes towards truth-telling requires a patient-centred approach, considering the cultural background, personal values, and communication style of the individual patient and their family. Some individuals may prefer direct and transparent information, appreciating a straightforward discussion of diagnosis and prognosis. Others may value a more nuanced approach, where information is shared gradually or through a trusted intermediary.	It is essential to expand your understanding of the cultural beliefs and values prevalent among the ethnic groups most encountered in your practice. By doing so, you can gain insights into the attitudes and perspectives that your patients and their families may hold. This endeavour involves delving into the symbolic interpretations attached to the disease or condition.
Adopting a patient and family-centred approach that incorporates the patient's beliefs, healthcare providers strive to provide personalized care that respects and integrates their cultural, spiritual, and personal values, fostering a meaningful and supportive healthcare experience.	Understanding the patient's and family's religious and spiritual beliefs can guide healthcare professionals in tailoring their approach to end of life care and discussions surrounding prognosis. It enables the healthcare team to respect and support the patient's cultural and spiritual needs, while also providing appropriate emotional and psychological support during difficult times.	Recognize that spirituality and religion often serve as sources of solace and support for individuals during challenging times. Inquiring about a patient's faith or spiritual needs and offering support can contribute to their overall well-being and coping mechanisms. Some helpful questions to ask include: 'How can we support your specific spiritual needs and practices during this time?' 'What aspects of your faith or spirituality are important for us to understand to provide the best care at this time?' 'From where do you find the strength to navigate this experience and discover meaning in it?' These open-ended questions allow the patient to reflect on their personal sources of strength and resilience. They acknowledge that everyone has unique coping mechanisms and perspectives when confronted with difficult situations. By actively listening to their response, healthcare providers can gain valuable insights into the patient's worldview and identify potential avenues for support.

Exploring the historical and socio-political backdrop of their lives, including their place of birth, refugee or immigration status, poverty, experiences of discrimination or limited access to care, languages spoken, and level of integration within their ethnic community.	Exploring the historical and political context of a patient's life can provide valuable insights into their unique experiences, including factors such as place of birth, refugee or immigration status, poverty, discrimination, access to care, languages spoken, and level of integration within their ethnic community. Asking appropriate questions sensitively can help healthcare providers understand the patient's background and tailor their care accordingly. Consider asking the following questions: • 'Can you share with me some details about your place of birth and any significant experiences related to your upbringing?' Understanding the patient's place of birth and upbringing can shed light on their cultural heritage and the factors that may have influenced their worldview. • 'Could you tell me about your refugee or immigration status and any challenges or opportunities that have arisen from your migration experience?' • Inquiring about the patient's refugee or immigration status acknowledges the potential difficulties they may have faced during the migration process and enables healthcare providers to better understand their journey and resilience. • 'Have you encountered any challenges accessing healthcare services due to discrimination or other barriers?' This question highlights the importance of equity in healthcare and encourages patients to share any experiences they may have had with discrimination or limited access to care. Understanding these challenges can help healthcare providers address any barriers and ensure appropriate support.	Religious and community organizations can be valuable resources for obtaining general information about a particular ethnic or cultural group. However, to gather specific information and better understand an individual patient's background, it is important to engage in thoughtful and respectful conversations. Asking the following questions can help facilitate this process: • 'Where were you born and raised?' This question allows the patient to share their place of origin, which can provide insights into their cultural background and upbringing. It helps in understanding the influences that shape their beliefs, values, and healthcare expectations. • 'When did you immigrate to this country? Inquiring about the patient's immigration history and their experiences of adapting to a new country fosters a deeper understanding of their unique journey. It acknowledges the challenges they may have faced and their potential acculturation process. • 'How has your life changed since you became unwell?' Asking about the changes in the patient's life helps to understand the impact of migration and cultural adjustment on their overall well-being. This question opens up a dialogue about potential shifts in lifestyle, social connections, and support networks. • 'What language would you feel most comfortable speaking to discuss your health concerns?' Inquiring about the patient's preferred language for discussing their health concerns is essential for effective communication. It demonstrates respect for their linguistic and cultural needs, ensuring that they can fully express themselves and understand important medical information.

	• 'What languages do you speak, and which language would you prefer to use when discussing your health concerns?' Inquiring about the patient's language proficiency and their preferred language for medical discussions ensures effective communication and patient-centred care. It demonstrates respect for their linguistic needs and facilitates a more accurate exchange of information. • 'To what extent do you feel integrated within your ethnic community or the broader society?' Understanding the patient's degree of integration can provide insights into their social support networks, community resources, and potential cultural influences on their health beliefs and behaviours. This information helps healthcare providers offer culturally sensitive care. Approaching these questions with sensitivity and cultural humility is crucial. Patients should feel comfortable sharing their experiences, and healthcare providers should actively listen, respect confidentiality, and adapt their approach based on the patient's responses. By gaining a deeper understanding of the patient's historical and political context, healthcare providers can deliver more comprehensive and patient-centred care that addresses their unique needs and experiences	These questions provide a foundation for building rapport, establishing cultural competency, and tailoring healthcare services to meet the individual patient's needs. Remember to approach these conversations with sensitivity, actively listen to the patient's responses, and adapt your approach accordingly to ensure a patient-centred and culturally responsive healthcare experience.
The decision-making style prevalent within the group, as well as the preferences of the individual patient and their family, can significantly impact the approach to healthcare, with considerations given to whether it is more individual-centric or family-oriented.	What styles of decision-making are commonly embraced by the group, as well as by the individual patient and their family? Does the cultural inclination lean towards emphasizing the individual patient's autonomy in making decisions, or does the approach prioritize a family-centred dynamic?	Acquire knowledge about the prevalent ethnic groups encountered in your practice: How do decision-making processes unfold within this cultural group? Who assumes the role of the household leader? To what extent does this family adhere to traditional and cultural norms and guidelines?

Consider the influence of the environment on the patient's well-being, considering factors such as their physical surroundings, social dynamics, and cultural context, as these elements can significantly impact their overall health and healthcare experience.	Utilize available resources to help the interpretation of cultural dimensions central to the patient and their family, such as translators, healthcare workers from the same community, religious leaders, and family members. These individuals can provide valuable insights.	Identify religious and community organizations affiliated with the ethnic groups frequently encountered in your practice. Collaborate with hospital social workers chaplains and faith-based leaders, as they can provide valuable assistance.

Source: data from Koenig B. A. and Gates-Williams J. (1995). Understanding Cultural Difference In Caring For Dying Patients. *West J Med*. 163(3): 244. PMC1303047; and Kagawa-Singer M. and Blackhall L. J. (2001). Negotiating Cross-Cultural Issues At The End Of Life. *JAMA*. 286(23):2993–3001. DOI: 10.1001/jama.286.23.2993.

Learning Point Cultural Vulnerability

As the cultural needs of the population evolve and expand, there is a drive within medicine to become culturally astute and 'literate'. Although increased awareness is needed, a clinician cannot be expected to be fluent in all the cultures within their patient population in a way that does not ultimately become superficial and tokenistic. This may risk reifying a culture by viewing it as a completed object, a 'thing' that all members share equally rather than its reality, a complex aggregate of processes in which different people participate to a greater or lesser extent.[4, 17] This may lead to a breakdown of trust and ultimately poor patient and family experiences and outcomes of care.

Clinicians can find not being proficient or having enough knowledge when caring for their patients unsettling. The fear of coming across as racist, non-caring or causing offence may lead to a retreat to a 'place of safety' with potentially negative repercussions for all parties. Instead, perhaps there is a place to be 'culturally vulnerable'[6, 17] highlighting that culture is a varied, ultimately fascinating, and very personal concept. In the meantime, clinicians must attempt to improve their skills when communicating with patients about what they believe, why it matters, and what they want in an open, non-judgemental manner.[4]

Nadim died in the medical admissions unit two days later, receiving a low volume infusion of subcutaneous fluids and a syringe pump of hyoscine butylbromide and midazolam. The nurses were asked to use the ABBEY pain scale to assess for any potential pain and use extra medication to take as needed. He died peacefully with his family present and feeling more supported, listened to, and importantly trusting of the medical team's intentions.

A Final Word from the Expert

It is important to be aware of differences in culture when interacting with patients. For example, referring to someone merely as a '72-year-old Muslim gentleman' denies that individual their unique identity, beliefs, values, culture, and language, or which may have a bearing on his wishes and preferences for care and treatment received. We must strive to learn the skills required to sensitively and empathically, explore the person's culture with an authentic curiosity to best serve them during this ultimately unrehearsed and unrepeatable moment in their lives.

It has been suggested that working in ethnically different clinical encounters 'conjures up a sense of danger'. We need to ask the patient about what is important to them, what their goals and wishes are, and what makes their life have meaning, particularly as their illness progresses. If we avoid working through a series of tick-box exercises[13] and openly ask questions, avoid assumptions, and a generalist approach to culture.[4] We can promote better care and avoid conflict, distress, and potential offence. This will allow us to listen to the patient, their families, and their histories to allow truly individualized care at the end of their lives. It needs to add value to the patient and their community, not just to the clinician's sense of doing a 'good job'.

We also need to take steps to create faithful and trustworthy community partnerships to allow people from other cultures to understand what palliative care services can do to enrich the dying experiences of those we help[6] and start to close the gaps for inequity in health and palliative care currently experienced by many in society.[1, 6, 14]

References

1. Koffman J. Servicing multi-cultural needs at the end of life. *J Ren Care* 2014; 40 (1): 6–15.
2. Brown E.A. Ethnic and cultural challenges at the end of life: setting the scene. *J Ren Care* 2014; 40 (s1): 2–5.
3. Kagawa-Singer M, Leslie J. Negotiating cross-cultural issues at the end of life: 'You got to go where he lives'. *JAMA* 2001; 286: 2993–3001.
4. Cain CL, PhD. Surbone A, et al. Culture and palliative care: preferences, communication, meaning, and mutual decision making. *J Pain Symptom Manage* 2018; 55(5), 1408–1419.
5. Silva MD, Genoff M, Zaballa A et al. Interpreting at the end of life: a systematic review of the impact of interpreters on the delivery of palliative care services to cancer patients with limited English proficiency. *J Pain Symptom Manage* 2016; 51(3): 569–580.
6. Johnson MRD. End of life care in ethnic minorities. *BMJ* 2009; 338: a2989.
7. Gysels M, Evans N, Meñaca A, *et al.* Culture and end of life care: a scoping exercise in seven european countries. *PLoS One* 2012; 7(4): e34188.
8. Gibbs AJO, Malyon AC, Fritz ZB. Themes and variations: an exploratory international investigation into resuscitation decision-making. *Resuscitation* 2016; 103: 75–81.
9. Kagawa-Singer M, Shaheen KL. A strategy to reduce cross-cultural miscommunication and increase the likelihood of improving health outcomes. *Acad Med* 2003; 78(6): 577–587.
10. Brown EA, Bekker HL, Davison SN, Koffman J, Schell JO. Supportive care: communication strategies to improve cultural competence in shared decision making. *Clin J Am Soc Nephrol* 2016; 11: 1902–1908.
11. General Medical Council. Treatment and care towards the end of life: good practice in decision making. GMC, 2022.
12. Collis E, Sleeman KE. Do patients need to know they are terminally ill? Yes. *BMJ* 2013; 346: f2589.
13. Sallnow L, Smith R, Ahmedzai SH, et al. Report of the Lancet Commission on the value of death: bringing death back into life. Lancet 2022; 399(10327): 837–884.
14. Hussain JA, Koffman J, Bajwah S. Racism in palliative care. Palliat Med 2021: 35(5): 810-813.
15. Back AL, Arnold RM. Discussing prognosis: 'how much do you want to know?'. Talking to patients who do not want information or who are ambivalent. *J Clin Oncol* 2006; 24(25): 4214–4217.
16. Baile WF, Buckman R, Lenzi R, Glober G, Beale EA, Kudelka AP. SPIKES—a six-step protocol for delivering bad news: application to the patient with cancer. *Oncologist* 2000; 5 (4): 302–311.
17. Gunaratnam Y. Cultural vulnerability: a narrative approach to intercultural care. *Qualitative Social Work* 2011; 12(2). doi.org/10.1177/1473325011420323.
18. Kagawa-Singer M, Blackhall L.J. Negotiating cross-cultural issues at the end of life. *JAMA* 2001; 286: 2993–3001
19. Breckenridge K, Bekker HL, Gibbons E, et al: How to routinely collect data on patient-reported outcome and experience measures in renal registries in Europe: An expert consensus meeting. *Nephrol Dial Transplant* 2015; 30: 1605–1614.
20. Koenig BA, Gates-Williams J. Understanding cultural difference in caring for dying patients. *West J Med* 1995; 163: 244

CASE 40 Supportive Care and Survivorship

Lara Datta-Paulin and Mark Warren

Expert: Richard Berman

Case history

Sarah, a 47-year-old female patient, presented to the supportive care clinic having been referred by her oncologist for management of chronic pain, following curative cancer treatment. The supportive care clinic (also called supportive oncology clinic in some centres) is based in a tertiary oncology centre, led by a supportive and palliative care consultant, with assistance from palliative care specialist nurses and specialty trainees. The focus of this clinic is to provide early access to supportive care for patients at all stages of illness from diagnosis onwards, regardless of treatment intent, including cancer survivors.

Three years previously, Sarah had been diagnosed with stage 3 endometrial adenocarcinoma, treated surgically with a hysterectomy and bilateral salpingo-oopherectomy, which was uncomplicated. She then underwent adjuvant chemotherapy, which comprised six cycles of Carboplatin and Paclitaxel, followed by 24 fractions of external-beam radiotherapy to the pelvis. Following adjuvant chemotherapy Sarah had developed right hip pain. This was investigated and was diagnosed as post-chemotherapy rheumatism, for which she was started on opioids; initially as required immediate-release oxycodone, later changed to an increasing dose of transdermal buprenorphine. She then commenced adjuvant radiotherapy to the pelvis, which was completed a year after her surgery. During radiotherapy Sarah developed abdominal cramping, nausea, diarrhoea, and weight loss, which were presumed to be side effects from the treatment. After radiotherapy was completed the abdominal pain persisted, alongside diarrhoea, tenesmus, mucus in stools, urgency, and urinary symptoms. Imaging was undertaken to exclude disease recurrence, which was negative, and Sarah was diagnosed with likely pelvic radiation disease. Sarah's opioid doses escalated rapidly from this point in order to achieve pain control, although this was only partially effective. She was also treated with multiple other agents to manage her symptoms including dexamethasone, hyoscine butylbromide, levomepromazine, ondansetron, amitriptyline, and fentanyl nasal spray. Repeated imaging did not reveal any recurrent disease, nor any other cause for her presentation. However, Sarah's symptoms continued to be poorly controlled for a period of almost two years.

Learning Point Post-chemotherapy Rheumatism

Post-chemotherapy rheumatism, or arthropathy, is a syndrome of pain, stiffness, swelling, and tenderness affecting a variety of joints. Symptoms can be migratory in nature and affect both large and small joints. It tends to occur in the months following initiation of chemotherapy and duration is variable, with some patients reporting spontaneous resolution within months to a year, whereas some have ongoing symptoms. Post-chemotherapy rheumatism has been reported in patients with a variety of cancers and chemotherapeutic regimens.[1]

Expert Comment

The Evidence Base for post-chemotherapy rheumatism is weak, comprising mostly small case series and case reports.

These retrospective studies have suggested that non-steroidal anti-inflammatory drugs and disease-modifying antirheumatic drugs such as sulfasalazine, methotrexate, and corticosteroids can improve symptom severity.[1] However, more robust evidence is required before specific recommendations can be given.

Expert Comment

Late or long-term effects of pelvic radiotherapy can be termed 'pelvic radiation disease' (PRD). PRD can involve the bladder, with urinary incontinence, urgency, dysuria, and haematuria; the bowel with altered bowel habit, incontinence and pain; and the reproductive organs, leading to sexual dysfunction. Treatment is supportive and symptom led, with referral to appropriate specialists and multidisciplinary input. Endoscopic treatment, for example of haematuria or rectal bleeding, is sometimes considered. The nature and long duration of symptoms can cause significant distress so psychological support is an essential part of treatment.[3]

Sarah presented to the supportive care clinic three years after her initial diagnosis. She reported severe colicky abdominal pain, nausea, generalized pruritus, night sweats, and tiredness. She had also developed an atonic bladder, which required her to perform intermittent self-catheterization. Sarah was frustrated at the impact her ongoing symptoms were having on her quality of life and was emotionally drained. She had found it difficult to access help as she felt her symptoms were not taken seriously and that in some cases she was dismissed by the healthcare professionals she had seen. Her medications comprised: fentanyl transdermal patch 62 microgram/hour (she had been on this dose for more than 18 months) and oxycodone immediate-release 5 mg, fentanyl nasal spray 100 micrograms, and ondansetron 4 mg all as required. On examination, Sarah was thin and pale. There were no overt signs of opioid toxicity. Her abdomen was generally tender throughout, but there were no palpable masses. Bowel sounds were of normal pitch but scanty. Abdominal X-ray (Figure 40.1) showed faecal loading throughout the colon. A recent CT scan remained free of evidence of cancer. A diagnosis of narcotic bowel syndrome, in addition to other side effects from long-term opioid use, was made.

Clinical Tip Side Effects of Radiotherapy

The side effects of radiotherapy will vary widely depending on the location and size of the radiation field. Most side effects tend to begin during, or in the weeks after, treatment and can continue for a number of weeks to months. Common side effects of pelvic radiotherapy include: diarrhoea, abdominal pain, nausea and vomiting, urinary symptoms, local skin irritation and hair loss, fatigue, sexual dysfunction, and infertility.[2]

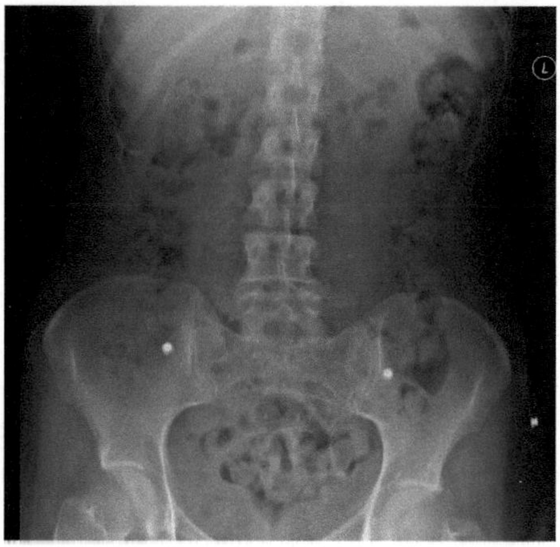

Figure 40.1 Abdominal XR demonstrating faecal loading of the colon.

Clinical Tip Opioid Side Effects

Common opioid side effects include nausea and vomiting, constipation, dry mouth, dizziness, sedation, or delirium. Less commonly seen are neurotoxicity, sweating, urinary retention, postural hypotension, pruritus, and sphincter of oddi dysfunction.[4] There is also an increased risk of falls and fractures, particularly amongst older patients.[5]

Learning Point Long-term Harms Associated with Opioids

In addition to the commonly observed side effects of opioid therapy, there are problems occurring in association with prolonged use.[6] These include:

- Endocrinopathy: effects on the hypothalamic-pituitary-adrenal and hypothalamic-pituitary-gonadal axes lead to hypogonadism and adrenal insufficiency. Symptoms include sexual dysfunction, infertility, depression, and fatigue.

- Immune-modulation: animal and human studies have shown that opioids have regulatory effects on the immune system with some evidence of immune suppression leading to increased risk of infection. There may be some impact on cancer cell growth and spread but the clinical relevance of these effects is unclear.[7]
- Opioid-induced hyperalgesia: characterized by a paradoxical increase in pain, which may be diffuse and of a different quality, with associated allodynia.

Expert Comment

The pathophysiology of opioid-induced hyperalgesia is not clearly defined but proposed mechanisms include[8]:

- Increased glutamate-associated activation of NMDA receptors, leading to spinal neurone sensitization.
- Release of pronociceptive excitatory neuropeptides secondary to raised levels of spinal dynorphins.
- Descending facilitation of pain signals from the rostral ventral medulla.
- Reduced opioid receptor responsiveness due to changes in G-protein activity.
- Peripheral mechanisms including activation of serotonergic receptors and substance P, changes to cytokine production, calcium channels, and nitric oxide synthase.

Learning Point Narcotic Bowel Syndrome

Narcotic bowel syndrome (NBS) is characterized by opioid-induced hyperalgesia in the gut, which causes a paradoxical increase in abdominal pain despite escalating opioid doses. The pathophysiology is thought to be similar to other forms of opioid-induced hyperalgesia.

Diagnosis can be made using the ROME IV criteria.[9] In addition to pain, patients report other symptoms of delayed gastrointestinal motility. Commonly significant faecal retention or sometimes signs of ileus or pseudo-obstruction are seen on investigation.[10]

Pharmacological management involves a gradual taper of the opioids. Concomitant medications can be used to manage withdrawal symptoms, anxiety, and hyperalgesia. Examples include a tricyclic antidepressant or serotonin-noradrenergic reuptake inhibitor for general well-being and pain/hyperalgesia, benzodiazepines for anxiety, laxatives and peripheral opioid antagonists for constipation, and clonidine for autonomic symptoms of opioid withdrawal and functional bowel symptoms. Nutritional support may be required if oral intake is significantly reduced due to symptoms. Psychological approaches to self-management of pain and anxiety may also be helpful. In terms of outcomes one observational study reported an 89.7% success rate with an inpatient detoxification programme, which was associated with a 35% reduction in abdominal pain.[11]

Expert Comment

NBS is estimated to affect around 5% of those using opioids on a long-term basis,[12] although it may well be under-recognized. Often patients will have had multiple other investigations without a cause for the pain being found, although NBS can coexist with structural abdominal disease in which case diagnosis may be more complex. It is not unusual for patients to present to multiple services with difficult to manage pain before a diagnosis is made, and so gaining the patient's trust and agreeing a mutually acceptable management plan is vital.

A plan was agreed with Sarah for gradual reduction of opioids and addition of a neuropathic agent (pregabalin) for management of hyperalgesia. Sarah's constipation, due to OIBD, was treated with traditional laxatives and later the addition of naloxegol (a peripheral opioid-antagonist) as the former were ineffective. Referral to complementary therapy, psych-oncology, and dietetics also occurred. After two months of gradual opioid reduction, Sarah's symptoms began to improve with a reduction in colic and nausea. At this point, she was using a fentanyl 37 microgram/hour patch and had stopped all other opioids. Opioid reduction continued in a patient-led manner with regular review and support from the supportive care team. After a total of five months, Sarah was able to stop all opioids. She experienced some brief withdrawal symptoms with removal of her last fentanyl 12 microgram/hour patch, but these were short-lived and did not require any pharmacological intervention. She was also able to reduce the dose of her pregabalin with a view to stopping that as well. Sarah continued under the follow-up of the supportive care team.

Learning Point Opioid-induced Bowel Dysfunction

Opioid-induced bowel dysfunction (OIBD) describes a spectrum of symptoms occurring due to activation of opioid receptors within the enteric nervous system, which leads to reduced motility, impaired fluid secretion, and sphincter dysfunction. Symptoms include gastro-oesophageal reflux, nausea, vomiting, bloating, colic, incomplete evacuation, and opioid-induced constipation (OIC). OIC is the most common symptom, occurring in 51–87% of patients receiving opioids for cancer pain.[13]

Treatment of OIBD involves management of the associated symptoms. General measures include lifestyle and dietary advice, and review of other medications. Laxatives, which stimulate motility and/or fluid secretion, can be used in the initial prevention and management of constipation. If these laxatives are ineffective then use of a peripherally acting μ-opioid receptor antagonist (PAMORA) should be considered. PAMORAs work by blocking the opioid receptors in the enteric nervous system whilst preserving analgesic effect. Examples of PAMORAs include naloxegol, methylnaltrexone, and naldemedine. Both naloxegol and naldemedine are recommended by NICE for the management of OIC. Third line options include specialist laxatives such as prucalopride and linaclotide. There is evidence of efficacy for both drugs in OIC,[13] although their use would be off-label so guidance suggests they are used under specialist/secondary care.

Evidence Base 'μ-opioid Antagonists for Opioid-induced Bowel Dysfunction in People With Cancer and People Receiving Palliative Care' (Cochrane Review)

The review[14] was published in 2022 and included ten trials of methylnaltrexone, naldemedine, and naloxone (alone or in combination with oxycodone). Primary outcomes were laxation, effect on analgesia and adverse events.

The review found moderate-quality evidence that naldemedine increased spontaneous laxation over 2 weeks compared to placebo (Risk Ratio (RR) 2.00). There was moderate-quality evidence of increased adverse events (RR 1.49), the most common of which was diarrhoea. There was little to no impact on the risk of serious adverse events.

In the trials of naloxone laxation was not assessed and so no conclusions could be drawn.

Methylnaltrexone had low-quality evidence of increased spontaneous laxation within 24 hours (RR 2.97) and moderate-quality evidence of increased spontaneous laxation over 2 weeks (RR 8.15) compared to placebo. There was low-quality evidence that there was no increased risk of serious adverse events, but an increased risk of non-serious adverse events (RR1.17) including abdominal pain, nausea, vomiting and flatulence.

There was low to very low-quality evidence that naldemedine and methylnaltrexone had no effect on analgesia or opioid withdrawal symptoms.

Expert Comment

Naloxegol was not included in the Cochrane review due to a lack of data in the relevant populations at the time. However, is it recommended by NICE following evidence from large phase III trials in non-cancer patients with OIC. In these trials naloxegol significantly increased response compared to placebo.[15] Frequently reported adverse events were diarrhoea, abdominal pain, nausea, and flatulence. Observational data from recently published real-world studies support the use of naloxegol in patients with cancer pain and OIC.[16]

Discussion

In summary this is a case of a young female patient who had curative treatment for a stage 3 endometrial carcinoma. She developed treatment-related side effects during adjuvant chemotherapy and radiotherapy and it was during these treatments that she was commenced on opioids. Her symptoms were difficult to control both throughout and following her treatment, and as a result, the dose of her opioid medication was escalated, alongside addition of numerous adjunctive therapies. In hindsight, escalation of opioids was not an effective management strategy in this case and Sarah began to develop symptoms consistent with opioid side effects and specifically NBS, which is most commonly seen in young female patients.[17] Her symptoms remained unmanaged for some time before the diagnosis was made, which had a significant effect on her quality of life and psychological well-being.

When Sarah presented to the supportive care clinic she was three years post-cancer diagnosis. NBS was diagnosed based on her symptoms, medication history, and radiological investigations. She was highly motivated to engage with an opioid reduction, which was undertaken slowly as an outpatient. This was appropriate, as she was relatively well and able to cope at home. However, there is also some evidence to support inpatient detoxification if required, which can be undertaken over a shorter time frame.[17] Sarah was commenced on other supportive medications including adjunctive analgesia and laxatives to aid this process. Her symptoms improved significantly as the dose of her opioids reduced and over a period of 5 months, she was able to stop opioids completely. The vast majority of her symptoms resolved, although constipation did remain problematic.

In addition to pharmacological management, multidisciplinary support is an important aspect of treatment of NBS. Sarah found complementary therapy particularly helpful, but other services such as psychology and dietetics may be required. An outcome trial of patients with NBS reports that approximately half will return to using opioids within three months,[11] and so ongoing follow-up will be important to ensure continued support.

Future Advances Supportive Care

Supportive care is defined by MASCC (The Multinational Association of Supportive Care in Cancer) as 'the prevention and management of the adverse effects of cancer and it's treatment. This includes management of physical and psychological symptoms and side effects across the continuum of the cancer experience from diagnosis through treatment to post-treatment care. Supportive care aims to improve the quality of rehabilitation, secondary cancer prevention, survivorship, and end of life care'.[18] The potential benefits of supportive care include decreased morbidity, improved quality of life, reduced usage of healthcare resources and improved treatment outcomes with a potential to decrease mortality.[19]

As part of the development of wider supportive care services, the provision of 'enhanced supportive care' (ESC) through existing palliative care services has been established in both cancer centres and district general hospitals across the UK. ESC encompasses many of the values of supportive care in providing coordinated care between oncology and supportive services throughout the cancer journey, and has been recognized nationally by NHS England, receiving a national QiC (Quality in Care) patient care pathway award in February 2016. However, the format of supportive care services across the UK remains variable, as is the patient cohort and the interventions offered. In the future a national strategy, alongside investment and research funding, will be required to standardize supportive care services in relevant settings and ensure equity of care for all cancer patients, irrespective of their diagnosis or stage.

A Final Word from the Expert

This case demonstrates just a few of the problems that patients can face during or after their cancer treatment, and the importance of comprehensive and holistic ongoing care.

Supportive care in cancer (also called supportive oncology) aims to reduce the adverse effects of cancer and cancer treatments and spans the entire cancer spectrum. 'The advent of new cancer therapies, alongside expected growth and ageing of the population, better survival rates, and associated costs of care, is uncovering a need to more clearly define and integrate supportive care services'.[19] Optimal supportive care of cancer patients requires input from a range of specialties outside of oncology (Figure 40.2) to assist in accurate diagnosis and management and ultimately improve outcomes. Palliative care clinicians, who have expertise in managing the adverse effects of cancer towards the end of life, have an important role to play in supportive care. Improvements in cancer treatments mean that there are growing cohorts of cancer survivors, those on curative treatment pathways, and those who are incurable but treatable. Some palliative care physicians have adapted their approach to also provide care in these other parts of the cancer continuum (as in this case). This is particularly relevant, as we enter an era where chemotherapy is progressively less used, and new areas for supportive care are emerging. In the twenty-first century, the focus is increasingly on living with cancer. Whilst there is growing evidence demonstrating the benefit of supportive care in cancer, it is much less well established in non-cancer illnesses, though this is likely to become an area of future interest.

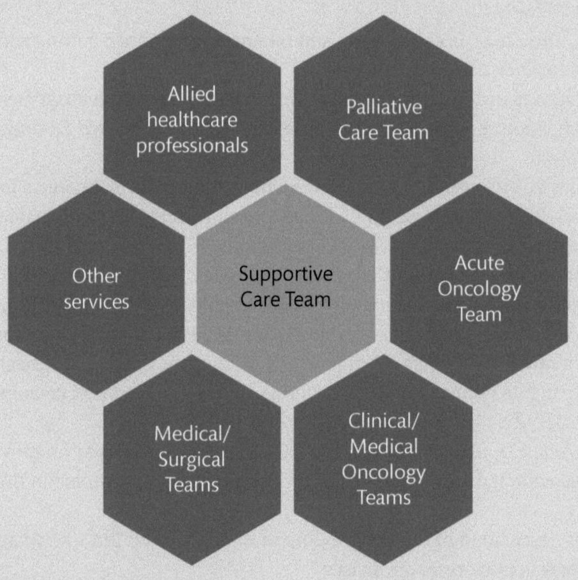

Figure 40.2 The extended supportive care team.

Reproduced with permission from Berman R, Davies A, Cooksley T, et al. Supportive Care: An Indispensable Component of Modern Oncology. *Clinical Oncology*. Elsevier (2020). 32:781–788.

References

1. Kim MJ, Ye YM, Park HS, Suh CH. Chemotherapy-related arthropathy. *J Rheumatol* 2006; 33(7): 1364–1368.
2. National Cancer Institute. Radiation therapy side effects. 2022. Available at: https://www.cancer.gov/about-cancer/treatment/types/radiation-therapy/side-effects
3. Dalsania M, Shah K, Stotsky-himelfarb E, Hoffe S, Willingham FF. Management of long-term toxicity from pelvic radiation therapy. *Am Soc Clin Oncol Educ* 2021; 41: 147–157.
4. Wilcock A, Howard P, Charlesworth S. *Palliative Care Formulary*, 7th ed. London: Pharmaceutical Press, 2020.

5. Yoshikawa A, Ramirez G, Smith ML, et al. Opioid use and the risk of falls, fall injuries and fractures among older adults: a systematic review and meta-analysis. *J Gerontol A Biol Sci Med Sci* 2020; 75(10): 1989–1995.
6. Faculty of Pain Medicine. Long term harms of opioids. Available at: https://www.fpm.ac.uk/opioids-aware-clinical-use-opioids/long-term-harms-opioids
7. Boland JW, McWilliams K, Ahmedzai SH, Pockley AG. Effects of opioids on immunologic parameters that are relevant to anti-tumour immune potential in patients with cancer: a systematic literature review. *Br J Cancer* 2014; 111(5): 866–873.
8. Velayudhan A, Bellingham G, Morley-Forster P. Opioid-induced hyperalgesia. *Cont Educ Anaesth Crit Care Pain* 2014; 14(3): 125–129.
9. Keefer L, Drossman DA, Guthrie E, et al. Centrally mediated disorders of gastrointestinal pain. *Gastroenterology* 2016; 150(6): 1408–1419.
10. Grunkemeier DM, Cassara JE, Dalton CB, Drossman DA. The narcotic bowel syndrome: clinical features, pathophysiology, and management. *Clin Gastroenterol Hepatol* 2007; 5(10): 1126–1139.
11. Drossman DA, Morris CB, Edwards H, et al. Diagnosis, characterization, and 3-month outcome after detoxification of 39 patients with narcotic bowel syndrome. *Am J Gastroenterol* 2012; 107(9): 1426–1440.
12. Kurlander JE, Drossman DA. Diagnosis and treatment of narcotic bowel syndrome. *Nat Rev Gastroenterol Hepatol* 2014; 11(7): 410–418.
13. Farmer AD, Drewes AM, Chiarioni G, et al. Pathophysiology and management of opioid-induced constipation: European expert consensus statement. *United European Gastroenterol J* 2019; 7(1): 7–20.
14. Candy B, Jones L, Vickerstaff V, Larkin PJ, Stone P. Mu-opioid antagonists for opioid-induced bowel dysfunction in people with cancer and people receiving palliative care. Cochrane Database Syst Rev 2022; 9: CD006332.
15. National Institute for Health and Care Excellence (NICE). Naloxegol for treating opioid-induced constipation. Technology appraisal guidance [TA345]. 2015. Available at: https://www.nice.org.uk/guidance/ta345/chapter/3-the-companys-submission.
16. Lemaire A, Pointreau Y, Narciso B, Piloquet FX, Braniste V, Sabaté JM. Effectiveness of naloxegol in patients with cancer pain suffering from opioid-induced constipation. *Support Care Cancer* 2021; 29(12): 7577–7586.
17. Kilgallon E, Vasant D, Shields P, Paine PA. OC-050 A national survey on prevalence, diagnosis, management and service provision for narcotic bowel syndrome in the UK. *Gut* 2017; 66: A26.
18. Multinational Association of Supportive Care in Cancer. About MASCC. Available at: https://www.mascc.org/about-mascc
19. Berman R, Davies A, Cooksley T, et al. Supportive care: an indispensable component of modern oncology. *Clin Oncol* 2020; 32: 781–788.

CASE

41 Specific Challenges: Homelessness

Toni Mortimer

Expert: Caroline Shulman

Case history

Kieran, a 41-year-old man, was referred by a hepatobiliary oncology clinical nurse specialist (CNS) to community palliative care (CPCT) following a new diagnosis of liver cancer. Two weeks prior to referral he had attended the emergency department (ED) with severe abdominal pain. He was admitted, his ascites drained, and he was treated for alcohol withdrawal. He was already established on methadone for opioid addiction and this was prescribed once his maintenance dose was confirmed. Cross-sectional imaging was convincing for a multifocal hepatocellular carcinoma with no distant metastases. He appeared agitated on the ward and self-discharged 48 hours later. He did not attend oncology follow-up.

Treatment options were discussed at the oncology multidisciplinary team meeting (MDM). The consensus was for best supportive care (in view of advanced cirrhosis and poor performance status) and the CNS was tasked with referring the patient to CPCT and relaying the MDM outcome.

The oncology CNS could not reach Kieran by phone and so contacted his general practitioner (GP). Kieran lived in a homeless hostel and with the support of its manager, the GP arranged a visit. The GP reviewed Kieran with the oncology CNS (by phone) and relayed the diagnosis. Though Kieran ended the conversation abruptly the GP gained consent to share information with the hostel staff and CPCT.

Hostel staff had noted Kieran's deteriorating condition. He had recently become more reclusive and was drinking less alcohol. When he had self-discharged from hospital they had tried, unsuccessfully, to persuade him to return.

A doctor and social worker (SW) from the CPCT attended and first met the hostel manager, who expressed her fear at Kieran remaining there. She cited the limited staffing and (not being a care home) the difficulty in supporting someone with health or care needs and medication. The CPCT said they would explore alternative places of care with Kieran.

Though initially reluctant to see the CPCT as he wanted to be 'left in peace', Kieran's key worker persuaded him to meet with them.

Learning Point Forms of Homelessness

There is no universal definition of homelessness, but common definitions include living on the street, squatting, 'sofa-surfing', living in homeless hostels, or in temporary or emergency accommodation.[1]

Expert Comment About UK Hostels

Hostels for homeless people are designed to provide short-term accommodation (usually for up to 2 years). There is great variation in hostel provision, depending on who they are commissioned to provide support for. Many people with a history of rough sleeping and support needs, such as addictions or mental health difficulties, are in hostels. Most have key workers whose remit is to support people into recovery, e.g. through engagement with addiction and health services and to

Expert Comment

Hostel staff often struggle to get a package of care for their residents, particularly when there are concurrent substance misuse issues, so may need support advocating for this.

Expert Comment

Many hostels do not have ground-floor accessible accommodation. Fire officers can often advise as to access and safety on a case-by-case basis.

develop skills to enable independent living. Only some hostels provide food and most have shared facilities. Key workers are not trained in health or social care, and even 'high support' need hostels (for people with complex needs) would not have trained health or social care staff on site. Considering the complexity of residents, staff-to-client ratios can be low (such as one member of staff to ten residents) with just a concierge at night.

Since leaving hospital Kieran had mainly stayed in bed and had paid friends to buy him alcohol. He continued to experience abdominal pain, leg swelling, nausea, diarrhoea, and fatigue. He disclosed a mistrust of health professionals owing to previous negative experiences and feeling unwelcome in healthcare settings. He had self-discharged from hospital due to feeling unkindly treated, including delays in receiving his methadone.

Kieran's understanding was explored: he knew his liver condition was worsening and staying in hospital to see more doctors was recommended but he didn't see the point. He had been treated for hepatitis C and knew he had cirrhosis. The CPCT doctor reiterated the diagnosis of an untreatable cancer, and explained they wanted to ensure he got the necessary support and was as comfortable as possible. They suggested an admission to the hospice while finding somewhere more appropriate for Kieran to live. Kieran refused this, saying people were always trying to move him on and he just wanted to stay where he finally felt at home. Despite signs of mild encephalopathy, the doctor determined he had capacity to make decisions regarding place of care.

The doctor and SW relayed the conversation to the hostel manager and explored what support would enable Kieran to stay there. This included NHS-funded carers, a clear emergency care plan, some training from the hospice, and assurance of ongoing support. The manager reluctantly agreed to him remaining, cautioning that if she felt the situation was untenable, he would need to be transferred elsewhere.

An MDT was organized at the hostel, led by the CPCT, comprising a palliative care doctor, CNS and SW, the hostel manager, hostel psychologist, GP, and a key worker from the addictions team.

An emergency care plan was prepared with instructions for hostel staff. It was agreed that if Kieran became acutely unwell, with an emergency such as bleeding or seizures, he would have to be transferred to hospital or a hospice. Kieran accepted this and was also aware he could change his mind about remaining at the hostel. The care plan was shared electronically and an alert added to the hospice records. Hostel staff suggested a move to a ground-floor room.

Learning Point Hepatitis C

There is an increased prevalence of hepatitis C infection in underserved populations including people experiencing homelessness. Injecting drug use is the main risk factor in the UK.[2] Oral antivirals are usually highly effective at curing the virus, but their success depends on access to screening and adherence to treatment programmes. Approaches such as peer-led models have shown promise for increasing engagement with treatment, but patients with cirrhosis in underserved populations may still miss out on the recommended six-monthly surveillance for hepatocellular carcinoma.[3, 4]

Future Advances Joint-Working Examples

A range of different approaches have been helpful in supporting the homeless population. In-reach primary care is really valuable. However, due to growing awareness of the inequity of palliative care support, several projects across the United Kingdom are aiming to improve access to high-quality palliative care and support by providing in-reach into homeless hostels and training for frontline staff. Some projects have been instigated by homelessness services (e.g. St Mungo's palliative care coordinator) with others by palliative or primary care services.[5–7]

Evidence Base Frailty and Multiple Long-Term Conditions

Hostel populations have high levels of unmet needs. In a recent study, a geriatrician undertook frailty and holistic needs assessments with hostel residents. Their mean chronological age was 55, however, frailty scores were equivalent to people in their late 80s.[8] Chronic conditions normally associated with older age were highly prevalent, with high rates of cognitive impairment, urinary incontinence, falls, and poor mobility. All residents had multiple-long-term-conditions, with the average number of conditions per resident being seven.

See Case 31 for more details on frailty and multiple-long-term conditions.

Over subsequent visits from the CPCT Kieran shared some of his personal history. He was born in Manchester and was placed in care aged 7 years, when his mother was hospitalized with paranoid schizophrenia. He was separated from his younger sister when she was separately adopted. At school he was labelled as 'hyperactive' and repeatedly excluded, leaving aged 15. He moved between multiple care settings until he was 18. He started drinking alcohol from the age of 14, drinking more heavily after a dramatic decline in his mental health provoked by his mother's death by suicide when he was 17. He was first street homeless around age 20 and began injecting drugs after meeting other users in a squat. He had difficulty trusting people and maintaining relationships.

Expert Comment Adverse Childhood Experiences/Complex Trauma

Homelessness is associated with a high prevalence of trauma, including adverse childhood experiences (ACEs).[9] ACEs include abuse, neglect, domestic violence, and parental separation. ACEs may impair the development of stable attachments, which can have profound long-lasting effects. People may view the world as fundamentally unsafe or others as untrustworthy. They may struggle to understand others' perspectives, or their own emotions. Emotional arousal can thus escalate quickly, but without effective self-soothing skills, can lead to conflict with others, self-directed harm, or substance misuse as a means of coping. Working with traumatized individuals requires compassion, understanding, and trauma-informed care. Exploration of trauma is not needed, in order to provide trauma informed care and it can be retraumatising for people to retell their story.

The CPCT CNS and SW explored with Kieran what was important to him and what he considered as 'living well'. He recognized his deteriorating condition but avoided any discussion of prognosis. He did not believe he was dying since he had been told for years that if he continued drinking, he would die within months. He wanted to stay at the hostel, where he had been resident for longer than anywhere since childhood.

He was adamant that he would not give up alcohol as without it he was haunted by intrusive thoughts and memories. At this point he was only drinking two cans of strong lager a day.

The palliative care SW noted Kieran had drawings up in his room from a past hostel project. He felt art was one thing he was good at. The SW sourced him some further art materials as he was too unwell to attend the hospice day centre.

Kieran had always hoped to reconnect with his sister. He accepted the SW's offer to try to reach her. He chose a specific drawing and they prepared a message for her.

Clinical Tip Managing Controlled Drugs in a Hostel

Hostels are not CQC registered, and it is rarely possible for controlled drugs to be kept in a resident's room, or for staff to assist with administration or storage of medications. As in this case a lockbox managed by community nursing may be a solution to storing medications on site. Where there is a danger of breakthrough pain, a lockbox could be placed in the patient's room, containing one dose of medication, which they could access themselves.

Expert Comment Discussing Advance Care Planning (ACP)

People experiencing homelessness frequently die young, and yet rarely get referred to palliative care services. Most deaths are unplanned, crisis-led, and undignified. The reasons for this are relevant when considering ACP and include[10, 11]:

1. Prognostic uncertainty in conditions prevalent within the population, e.g. advanced liver disease, respiratory disease, frailty, etc., making it harder to identify those needing referral.
2. Many people experiencing homelessness lack trust in healthcare services and feel stigmatized, resulting in significant barriers or delays in accessing support.
3. Hostel staff frequently struggle to get adequate support from health or social care providers and are left to support unwell residents alone.
4. A lack of choices around place of care for people who are young with complex needs such as addictions and mental health difficulties.
5. Very reasonable concerns about not removing hope from already fragile and traumatized people, who may use substances to blank out past experiences.

ACP should therefore focus more on exploring people's insights into their illness and what living well means to them. Discussing death and dying preferences may be delayed, particularly where prognosis is uncertain. Parallel planning, hoping for the best while planning for the worst, is a useful approach. Crucially, the focus of the ACP should be connecting with the person where they are, in a person-centred and trauma-informed way. It may take repeated meetings to develop trust and to establish insights, wishes, and preferences.

Pain management for Kieran was complicated by his liver impairment and substance use disorder. He had previously worked hard in reducing to 30 milligrams of methadone daily and was anxious that using other opioids for pain could precipitate, or be interpreted as, relapse. Difficulties storing medications at the hostel led to a decision to use fentanyl patches, in addition to his regular methadone (see Case 4 for further learning on pain in people with drug dependence). An arrangement was made for a single patch to be issued at a time, which was collected by a district nurse who supervised the patch being changed. Though this arrangement generally worked, there were some challenges: where the patch was displaced, a delay in replacing it, or staff did not have the capacity to collect new patches. Injectable medications were kept in a lockbox in the hostel reception room, only accessed by clinical staff.

When Kieran's ascites became symptomatic again, the CPCT liaised with the local hospice for a planned day attendance for paracentesis. The hospice noted his ongoing alcohol use and were concerned about intoxication and safety. They were reassured that he would only have access to the amount of alcohol he needed to prevent withdrawal. Kieran also needed reassurance that he wouldn't be denied alcohol but that his intake would be managed by the hospice staff. He was warned that should he deteriorate, there was a possibility he may need to stay at the hospice.

Four weeks after being first referred, Kieran was found by his morning carer breathless and in distress. An ambulance was called. He repeated his preference to remain at the hostel and the CPCT CNS referenced his electronic ACP to support their discussions with the paramedic and hostel staff. Subcutaneous medication (morphine sulphate 2.5 mg and midazolam 2.5 mg) was given by the paramedic under the direction of CPCT, who visited the patient urgently. The injection helped temporarily and Kieran agreed with hospice admission to commence a continuous infusion (as this could not be safely managed at the hostel). Admission was arranged for the following day but unfortunately Kieran died before transfer.

A debrief was held with hostel staff by the SW and a CNS from CPCT. The hostel staff recognized they had helped meet Kieran's wishes but were angry that he had been distressed before he died and not been transferred to the hospice in time. The events also had a significant impact on other residents. The CPCT supported the hostel manager to hold a gathering to remember Kieran, where some of Kieran's art was celebrated. Sadly, his sister could not be traced.

Expert Comment
Bereavement

Recognition of the impact of a bereavement on frontline staff and residents of a hostel, and marking or celebrating a life is important. This can be an opportunity for residents to reflect on what's important to them but also serves to validate the importance of their own lives. Hostel residents/peers should be involved in the planning of celebrations.

Discussion

This case describes the last weeks of life of a patient with hepatocellular carcinoma, secondary to cirrhosis from hepatitis C and alcohol. His young age, frailty, substance use history, and fractured childhood are common for people who become homeless. He has experienced stigma and faced barriers to accessing health and social care. What is atypical is that he received palliative care and was able to remain in the hostel towards the end of his life. For this to be achieved required intensive support from the community palliative care team and careful communication with other professionals and, most importantly, hostel staff.

Such cases can be challenging for palliative care teams because they can be resource intensive for often overstretched services. A lack of understanding and apprehension can impact the confidence of palliative care teams in supporting homeless patients. Twinning palliative care services with hostels (to develop relationships and provide regular in-reach) can help both sides provide this essential support.[6]

This case also touches on the impact deaths, which are frequent, can have on these communities. Acknowledging their impact and supporting hostel staff and residents can have lasting benefits.

A Final Word from the Expert

People experiencing homelessness die young and rarely receive high-quality care at the end of their lives. This case shows what can happen when people work together to support someone with complex needs to die in a place that he considered home. This was successful due to the recognition that one professional group cannot achieve this in isolation. The joined-up support from the palliative care, district nursing, and primary care team, together with the addiction services and those providing frontline support for Kieran supported person-centred trauma-informed care. Hostel and other frontline homelessness staff are often the equivalent of next of kin and should be supported as such. Many people experiencing homelessness have experienced loss, so considering the impact of bereavement on other residents and staff, and the potential need for further support, is vital.

References

1. FEANTSA. About homelessness. 2022. Available at: https://www.feantsa.org/en/about-us/faq
2. Harris HE, Costella A, Mandal S, et al. *Hepatitis C in England*. London: UK Health Security Agency, 2022, p. 9.
3. Surey J, Menezes D, Francis M, et al. From peer-based to peer-led: redefining the role of peers across the hepatitis C care pathway: HepCare Europe. *J Antimicrob Chemother* 2019; 74(Suppl 5): v17–v23.
4. National Institute for Health and Care Excellence. *Quality Statement 4: Surveillance for Hepatocellular Carcinoma*. London: NICE; 2017, p. 19.

5. Tackling Inequalities in End of Life Care for Minority Groups VCSE Health and Wellbeing Alliance Project Group. *Care Committed to Me*. London: Hospice UK, 2018, pp. 14–26. Available at: https://professionals.hospiceuk.org/docs/default-source/Policy-and-Campaigns/briefings-and-consultations-documents-and-files/care_committed_to_me_web.pdf?sfvrsn = 0
6. Armstrong M, Shulman C, Hudson B, et al. The benefits and challenges of embedding specialist palliative care teams within homeless hostels to enhance support and learning: Perspectives from palliative care teams and hostel staff. *Palliat Med* 2021; 35(6): 1202–1214.
7. Care Quality Commission and The Faculty for Homeless and Inclusion Help. A second class ending: exploring the barriers and championing outstanding end of life care for people who are homeless. 2017, pp. 8–18. Available at: http://cqc.org.uk/sites/default/files/20171031_a_second_class_ending.pdf
8. Rogans-Watson R, Shulman C, Lewer D, et al. Premature frailty, geriatric conditions and multimorbidity among people experiencing homelessness: a cross-sectional observational study in a London hostel. *Housing, Care and Support* 2020; 23(3/4): 77–91.
9. FEANTSA. FEANTSA Position: recognising the link between trauma and homelessness. Brussels, 2017, pp. 2–3. Available at: https://www.feantsa.org/download/feantsa_traumaandhomelessness03073471219052946810738.pdf
10. Shulman C, Hudson B, Low J. End-of-life care for homeless people: a qualitative analysis exploring the challenges to access and provision of palliative care. *Palliat Med* 2017; 32(1): 36–45.
11. Hudson BF, Shulman C, Low J, et al. Challenges to discussing palliative care with people experiencing homelessness: a qualitative study. *BMJ Open* 2017; 7: e017502.

CASE

42 Transition from Children's to Adult Palliative Care

Gurpreet Gupta

Expert: Jo Elverson

Case history

Simran, an 18-year-old girl, and her family were referred to adult palliative care services by the GP. The request was for support with advance care planning, having been discharged from paediatric services. As a newborn, she had developed an intraventricular haemorrhage and as a result had a learning disability, epilepsy, and spasticity. She lived with her father and eight-year-old brother. Her father had taken leave from work to provide care and her brother attended primary school. Simran's aunt and cousin also helped with her care. Simran had been attending school supported by a special educational needs coordinator. Although her verbal communication was limited, she was able to express her likes and dislikes and follow two-step instructions. She was able to mobilize but fatigued easily and had an adapted wheelchair for use outdoors. She was able to feed herself but needed assistance with personal care. At 12 years old she developed a benign brain tumour and underwent several resections. At age 16 the tumour transformed and became malignant. Despite treatments the tumour progressed, and she experienced increasing debility.

Three months prior to the referral to adult palliative services Simran was admitted to hospital with severe headaches and an MRI scan demonstrated a new brain haemorrhage. Her case was discussed at the neurosurgical and oncology MDM and surgical input was not deemed possible or appropriate. The family were informed that Simran was approaching the end of her life. She was discharged from oncology follow-up but maintained contact with neurology services for management of the epilepsy. She was on antiepileptic medications that had required regular adjustment due to refractory symptoms.

At the point of referral, Simran had had several episodes of status epilepticus requiring transfer to the emergency department. Her mobility and coordination had deteriorated such that she was now limited to bed, and carers were attending her home four times a day.

Clinical Tip Approach to Rare Conditions

Patients transitioning from paediatric to adult palliative care services have a wide range of conditions and symptoms that may be less familiar to adult palliative medicine clinicians.[1] Rather than aiming to become an expert in each condition, palliative clinicians should utilize their expertise in holistic care and multidisciplinary working to manage symptoms, address psychosocial needs, and coordinate care more broadly. It is essential to involve other specialist teams to ensure appropriate medical management. Ideally, the transition to adult services should involve a handover period where the new team is introduced to the young person and their family by the paediatric team.[2] This supports continuity of care and builds trust and rapport with the new team.

Learning Point Psychosocial Assessment

Assessing the psychosocial context of a young person (age 16–25) is an essential part of providing developmentally appropriate care. The HEEADSSS tool[3, 4] was developed to support psychosocial screening at every adolescent healthcare interaction. Asking these potentially difficult questions gives the young person permission to share any concerns they have and highlights the influence of their psychological and social well-being on their health.

With some adaptation, this mnemonic can give a helpful structure for assessment of young people with evolving palliative care needs with questions for both the young person, their family, and the other teams supporting them. For example:

Home: *Who is at home? Who is involved in giving care? What support do family carers need (are there any young carers)? Is the right equipment in place? Are you using residential care or short-breaks, and can this continue with changing physical needs?*
Education/Employment: *What do you like/dislike about work/school/college? Is school/college able to support changes in physical needs? If you have an Education Health and Care Plan (England), is the health section up to date? What emotional/bereavement support is available for friends and classmates?*
Eating: *What food/drink do you enjoy? Are there any concerns about swallowing, nutrition, or weight? Is poor nutrition or oral health contributing to any symptoms?*
Activities: *What activities/gaming/music/TV help to entertain, calm, or distract you? Are there ways you can continue to access the activities and social groups you enjoy?*
Drink/Drugs: *Are you drinking/using any substances that could impact physical symptoms or interact with medication? Are there any risks to safety?*
Sex and relationships: *Who is important to you? Have you had/are you in a relationship? Do you need private space and time alone or with a partner? Is any information or support needed around safe sex, consent, or birth control?*
Self-harm (depression): *Do you feel low or sad a lot of the time? What do you do to feel better? Have you thought about hurting yourself? NB: It may be appropriate to explore carers' emotional health and risk of self-harm as well.*
Safety: *Do you feel safe? Is there anyone in your life that you feel unsafe around? Have the answers to any other section triggered safeguarding concerns for the young person or a family member?*

Expert Comment

As well as tailoring holistic care to the young person, the HEEADSSS assessment enables clinicians to identify who else may need additional support, and to understand what support structures they may already have in place. Parents and siblings often take on a large proportion of physical and personal care provision as well as the emotional burden of the young person's illness. This can have an impact on the physical, psychological, and financial well-being of the whole family.

Simran's father was keen to maintain her care at home and avoid hospital readmission. Simran was unable to understand the nuances of her health conditions and lacked mental capacity to make informed decisions about the ongoing management of these. Her father and the palliative care consultant collaborated on an advance care plan in her best interests.

Clinical Tip Making Decisions

Care planning and decision-making with young people and their families may require several meetings and take more overall time when compared with adult patients. For young people with complex conditions, plans often need to be made in collaboration with other specialists. Advance care planning can be a helpful way to ensure all clinical teams know which interventions are likely to be effective, as well as communicating any treatments that are not appropriate or desired.

In all situations, it is essential that the young person is supported to participate as much as they are able. Their preferences and priorities must remain in the foreground, even if they are unable to make decisions themselves.

Parents may not be aware about the way their role in decision-making changes when their child reaches adulthood. This is particularly significant if the young person does not have mental capacity to make their own decisions about health or care. Alongside clear information, families should be reassured about their ongoing valued role as an advocate for the young person in best interest decisions, even if they have not applied for formal recognition of this through deputyship (or regional/national equivalent).

The outcomes of the planning conversations were:

- A detailed seizure management plan in event of status epilepticus recurring. Guidance on this was sought from the neurology team. The local hospital emergency department were also consulted and made aware of the plan in case of acute attendance.
- Simran's father was taught how to administer subcutaneous injections in the event that district nurses were unable to attend quickly.
- Provision of 'just in case' medications to manage anticipated symptoms at the end of life.

Learning Tip Involving Parents

As a young person develops their independence, it is important to encourage their autonomy and ability to manage their own health. Readiness for independence, however, develops over time and varies between individuals. Parents often continue to have an important role in helping the young person navigate systems and process information. Appropriate parental involvement[5] recognizes that the interdependence of the young person with their parents is dynamic and may extend far beyond the age that they reach adulthood. Clinicians need a flexible approach which recognizes the parent's role and expertise in their young person's condition and care while encouraging the young person's emerging autonomy.

Where a young person has a learning disability, complex health needs, or has not previously had opportunity to make or communicate healthcare decisions, they may need additional support to understand their condition and to express their own preferences or concerns.

Expert Comment

Identifying all professionals who are involved in supporting the young person early is key to planning and providing ongoing care. Education and social care providers bring helpful insights alongside primary and secondary healthcare teams, learning disability services, and paediatric medical and nursing teams. Good communication between teams creates a supportive network around the young person and their family.

Clinical Tip Communication

Clinicians may need to adapt their practice and communication to ensure that while the young person is empowered to speak for themselves, the parent is also included and involved appropriately.

Some helpful tips include[6]:

- Introduce yourself to the young person first and address the conversation to them.
- Check they are happy for you to ask the parent about their perspective.
- Routinely offer the young person time to speak to you on their own.
- Reassure about confidentiality.
- Ensure letters are addressed to the young person.

It may also be helpful to speak to the parent alone, as they may have concerns that they do not feel able to share when their child is present.

Expert Comment

When prescribing for young people with complex conditions, standard 'adult' doses may not be appropriate. Consider factors such as low weight, delayed physical development, altered drug absorption or metabolism, and the effects of polypharmacy. A paediatric formulary can guide dosing by weight and age however pharmacy advice is essential to support safe and effective prescribing in more complex situations.

Simran continued to deteriorate. She developed dysphagia to solids and liquids, which made administration of oral medications challenging. She developed increasing spasticity and was requiring frequent repositioning. Her communication became harder to understand and carers relied on her father to interpret her vocalizations and body language. During this time, a bed was set up on the floor of Simran's bedroom. Her father and aunt stayed by her all day, often single-handedly repositioning her many times an hour. The occupational therapy team were consulted, however the family felt that their setup served Simran's needs adequately. A syringe driver was commenced to manage headaches, spasticity, and seizures.

Clinical Tip Assessing Distress

If a young person has limited communication, and symptoms are unstable, tools such as the Distress and Discomfort Assessment Tool (DisDAT)[7] may help the family and carers to keep a record of the young person's distress and communicate it to professionals. This will enable better assessment of any reversible causes of distress, as well as appropriate titration of medication.

Clinical Point Bereavement

When preparing for death and offering bereavement support, consider the needs of siblings and friends as well as parents. If a young person has been living in a residential setting, other residents and support staff may also need bereavement support.

Expert Comment

For some young people with complex physical or behavioural needs, it can be difficult to recreate an acceptable environment for care in an in-patient setting. Families may find ways to provide physical care at home that would not be encouraged in a healthcare environment due to risks to themselves or the patient. In this context, supporting the decision to remain at home and offer care in a 'suboptimal' way may make healthcare professionals feel vulnerable and uncomfortable. A team approach should be taken to support the patient and family with safe and appropriate person-centred care in a consistent way, while addressing any significant risks and considering and planning for governance or safeguarding concerns.

Simran was assigned a community palliative care clinical nurse specialist and she was also supported by the palliative care consultant and specialist trainee. Simran's father had scheduled daily contact with palliative care professionals in the final month of her life. The district nurses also sought regular input from the palliative care team.

Frequent questions were asked about:

- The process of dying.
- Whether expertise had been sought from other teams.
- The impact of medications.
- Planning for all eventualities, even if unlikely.

Simran died at home and her father expressed gratitude for the palliative care input provided.

Expert Comment

Teams who are not accustomed to providing end of life care for young adults can find their role carries a high emotional burden. This may be due to the intensity of involvement with the young person and their family, along with unfamiliarity with clinical and practical aspects of working with this age-group. A debrief meeting can be a supportive way for professionals to reflect on the emotional impact as well as identifying any learning opportunities. Where possible, involving the whole 'team around the young person' in the debrief can also build constructive relationships between teams and services.

Evidence Base

Adolescents and young adults are increasingly recognized as a distinct population with specific healthcare needs.[8] These needs are brought into greater focus when the person has a complex or life-limiting condition. Fraser[9] and Jarvis[10] demonstrate not only the growing population of young adults with complex or life-limiting conditions, but also the changes in morbidity for this population as they transition to adult services. It is essential that all adult services are well prepared to give coordinated, developmentally appropriate care.

Recent studies and guidance[2,11–14] have highlighted the aspects of good practice in transition that have been shown to improve patient experience including:

- Beginning transition planning from 14 years, developing a clear cross-agency plan.
- Preparing the young person and parents for adulthood including self-managing their condition.
- Increasing GP involvement as the young person's 'lifelong practitioner'.
- Meeting the adult team(s) before transfer of care.
- All services trained to offer developmentally appropriate healthcare.
- Appropriate parental involvement.
- A named lead professional to oversee transition.
- Use of health passports to aid information-sharing between teams.

Unfortunately, services often struggle to embed these principles consistently for all young people, particularly if they are supported by several different specialties or when there is no adult specialty offering an equivalent service to the paediatric one.

A Final Word from the Expert

This case highlights the challenges in supporting a young adult where the transition process did not include preparation for a significant deterioration in health. The palliative care team rapidly needed to assimilate the wider medical and social context of the patient and to establish rapport with the patient and family in order to develop complex care plans at a time of crisis. As has been shown, a patient-centred approach that recognized the role of parents and collaborated with other teams was essential to achieve this. The learning from this case can be applied to young people with and without a learning disability. By adopting a developmentally appropriate approach the clinician will be able to adapt their practice to support the individual and their family.

When health is unstable or deterioration is anticipated, pre-emptive involvement of the adult palliative care team can give time to build relationships with the young person and family, connect with the established healthcare team, and to plan care at a time that the young person may be well enough to participate in decision-making.

While many adult palliative care services are unable to replicate the service model of a children's hospice or palliative care team, it remains essential that adult palliative professionals are equipped to support young adults appropriately, particularly where there is a need for a specialist, holistic approach to symptom management, advance care planning, or end-of-life care.

References

1. Hain R, Devins M, Hastings R, Noyes J. Paediatric palliative care: development and pilot study of a 'Directory' of life-limiting conditions. *BMC Palliat Care* 2013; 12(1): 43.
2. Colver A, McConachie H, Le Couteur A, et al. A longitudinal, observational study of the features of transitional healthcare associated with better outcomes for young people with long-term conditions. *BMC Med* 2018; 16(1): 111.
3. Goldenring JM, Rosen DS. Getting into adolescent heads: an essential update. *Contemporary Pediatrics* 2004; 21(1): 64–92.
4. Doukrou M, Segal TY Fifteen-minute consultation: Communicating with young people—how to use HEEADSSS, a psychosocial interview for adolescents. *Arch Dis Child Educ Pract* 2018; 103: 15–19.
5. Heath G, Farre A, Shaw K. Parenting a child with chronic illness as they transition into adulthood: a systematic review and thematic synthesis of parents' experiences. *Patient Educ Couns* 2017; 100(1): 76–92.
6. White B, Viner RM. Improving communication with adolescents. *Arch Dis Child Educ Pract* 2012; 97: 93–97.
7. Regnard C, Reynolds J, Watson B, Matthews D, Gibson L, Clarke C (2007). Understanding distress in people with severe communication difficulties: developing and assessing the Disability Distress Assessment Tool (DisDAT). *J Intellect Disabil Res* 51(4): 277–292.
8. Lee L, Upadhya KK, Matson PA, Adger H, Trent ME. The status of adolescent medicine: building a global adolescent workforce. *Int J Adolesc Med Health* 2016; 28(3): 233–243.

9. Fraser LK, Gibson-Smith D, Jarvis S, Norman P, Parslow RC. Estimating the current and future prevalence of life-limiting conditions in children in England. *Palliat Med* 2021; 35(9): 1641–1651.
10. Jarvis SW, Roberts D, Flemming K, Richardson G, Fraser LK. Transition of children with life-limiting conditions to adult care and healthcare use: a systematic review. *Pediatr Res* 2021; 90(6): 1120–1131.
11. National Institute for Health and Care and Excellence (NICE). Disabled children and young people up to 25 with severe complex needs: integrated service delivery and organisation across health, social care and education. NICE Guideline 213. 2022. Available at: https://www.nice.org.uk/guidance/ng213
12. National Institute for Health and Care and Excellence (NICE). Transition from children's to adults' services for young people using health or social care services. NICE Guideline 43. 2016. Available at: https://www.nice.org.uk/guidance/ng43
13. Care Quality Commission. *From the Pond Into The Sea: Children's Transition To Adult Health Services*. Gallowgate: CQC, 2014.
14. The National Confidential Enquiry into Patient Outcome and Death. '*The Inbetweeners*' 2023. London.

CASE

43 Developing Compassionate Communities

Joseph Sawyer

Expert: Libby Sallnow

Case history

Theresa, an 82-year-old lady with Alzheimer's dementia, was referred to the community palliative care team by her GP who was concerned she was in the last weeks of life. She was diagnosed with dementia 10 years previously and has been progressively declining over that time. Theresa had three daughters and two sons. Lauren, her youngest daughter, had moved back into the family home to support her mother two years ago, whilst continuing to work as a recruitment manager.

Prior to referral, Theresa was requiring continuous care and support. She was able to communicate through facial expression and non-verbal sounds and to eat a normal diet with assistance. Theresa could initiate movements but needed support to transfer. She had been going out of the house but only when pushed in a wheelchair. Two weeks ago, Theresa's mobility deteriorated, and her oral intake significantly reduced; she was now cared for in bed. Lauren remained the main carer with some support from the rest of the family. There was no advanced decision to refuse treatment or lasting power of attorney, so a best interest's decision was made for her to be cared for at home rather than being admitted to hospital. The GP had discussed resuscitation with Lauren and the wider family. Following this, a 'do not attempt resuscitation' recommendation form had been left at the house and the decision recorded in Theresa's primary care record.

> **Learning Point Recognizing the End of Life as a Spiritual and Social process**
>
> Within a compassionate community and the social, ecological, and healthcare systems that contribute to it, there is a recognition that death is principally a relational and spiritual process rather than purely a physiological event.[1,2] Death therefore is not characterized simply by the absence of life and the social vacuum this brings. Rather, death is understood as being 'full of life' through the interpersonal experiences that the process of dying, caring, and bereavement brings. Because of this, the balance of care changes and relationships are made central to care and support during the dying or grieving process. This is true in all settings, from care homes and hospitals to people's homes. Relationships between healthcare professionals and patients shifts from being transactional in nature towards a relationship based on connection and compassion.

The community palliative care clinical nurse specialist (CNS) decided to visit Theresa at home to assess the situation. She found her lying in her bed upstairs, with her daughter Lauren present. Theresa was restless, grasping at things that didn't appear to be there. Lauren had not slept much in the last two weeks as Theresa has been groaning and calling out at night, but without indicating what may be wrong. Lauren appeared exhausted and admitted to feeling isolated, out of her depth, feeling that she could no longer cope. She had not told her siblings as she felt that they were unable to support her more than they already did.

Clinical Tip Mapping Social Networks to Understand Social Capital and Hidden Resource

Social networks and social capital are seen as a target for public health interventions that seek to build supportive networks in anticipation of the practical and emotional challenges to end of life care. There are multiple definitions of social capital. One perspective is to understand it as an asset-based approach realized through connections between people.[3] A three-tier system is generally described[4]:

(i) Bonded social capital: relationships between people with characteristics in common
(ii) Bridged social capital: relationships between people with different characteristics
(iii) Linked social capital: relationships taking place across power gradients

New public health approaches to palliative care seek to operationalize social capital. On a case-by-case basis this can mean mapping out someone's social networks to help uncover hidden resource.

Evidence Base How do Social Networks Help?

The evidence base for social networks stems from work that has demonstrated the value of relationships in shaping positive outcomes relating to mortality, smoking cessation, and obesity.[5-7] In relation to palliative care, caregiving at the end of life has been shown to contribute to the acquisition of social capital and community development.[8] The role for social networks and social capital in dementia has also been reviewed.[9] Here social capital was found to influence how people transition from early to advanced dementia, influencing key outcomes relating to transitions in the care environment and how caregiving is experienced.

Expert Opinion The Complexity of Social Capital and the Implications For Its Operationalization

Compassionate communities are inextricably linked to the concept of social capital. However, it is important for clinicians to understand such concepts are highly nuanced. For example, whilst bonded ties might bring access to support and resource, they may also bring damaging relationships and caregiving roles may be subject to gender, cultural, and economic bias. Where individual ties are strong and multiple, a collective culture may form that holds specific values. The strength of such networks may bar outsiders, especially if they hold a different perspective to the collective norm.[3] Whilst there is a growing evidence base to suggest that caregiving at the end of life can build social capital and improve equity and access to care, there is also value in the support of people outside the immediate network, allowing access to bridging or linking social capital. The intersection between formal and informal networks, within which clinicians work, is therefore crucial to the coordination of care.

Future Advances Understanding the Role of Social Capital in Community-led Care

Whether enhanced social capital is desirable, or useful, is therefore very much dependent on the context. Balancing the social nature of dying alongside the intimacy of such processes is not straightforward. This has been shown in research that demonstrates older people may actively withdraw from, or resist, community support.[10] For social capital to be successfully operationalized at the end of life, an approach that appreciates cultural and social context is essential. This accommodates new relationships in a way that means 'community' is not something that is produced for people, in the way a service may be, but created together in a way that allows individuality to work alongside collective principles.

The CNS explored relationships that were important to Lauren and Theresa. Lauren commented that she had no time for friends and she had been off work for the last two weeks to care for her mother, doubting whether she would be able to return. Lauren commented that they used to go to a dementia café run by a local charity, but she felt that her mother was no longer well enough to attend. Lauren felt it would be inappropriate to have paid carers, or even volunteers, as her mother had always been a very proud and private person and would be embarrassed and ashamed of her current state. This had left her struggling to know what to do for the best.

Clinical Tip Balancing Personhood, Autonomy, and Paternalism in the Context of Dementia

Personhood and person-centred care have come to define good quality care. However, how these concepts are understood at the end of life in advanced dementia can be conflicting. For example, working to preserve an identity that has now changed may invoke feelings of failure and cause moral distress when it comes to decision making. Sometimes it may help to reframe questions, asking what the person may think now, knowing the reality of the situation, and its effects on all those involved. This can lead to more context appropriate conversations whilst accommodating a range of opinions.

As Lauren talked about important relationships, the CNS identified areas that could translate to a supportive resource, including Theresa's neighbour, whom she had known for over 20 years, the dementia café, and the local church where Theresa had been a long-term parishioner.

Evidence Base Understanding Communities as Independent Agents of Care

Caring relationships can exist beyond genealogical ties and have been shown to create a sense of social identity.[8, 10–12] The evidence for this has led to work that develops community capacity by identifying local end of life needs and meeting them through community resource.[13]
Using in-depth interviews and focus groups, researchers have examined carers' experience of home-based dying with reference to supportive networks during this time. Here it was shown that people are often reluctant to ask for or accept help from informal networks, despite an apparent need. A willingness of such networks to provide support was limited by uncertainty in what to offer and the possibility of infringing on people's privacy. The study highlights the idea that deeply engrained social norms need to change if communities are to function as independent agents of care.

Expert Comment Tensions Within the Model

Attempting to conceptualize death in a way that unifies and mobilizes entire communities is a process fraught with complications. For example, where society is trained to foster self-optimization, independence, and autonomy, proposing an alternative paradigm that revolves around vulnerability, interdependency, and death can cause confusion and may be resisted. Such complexities preclude the rollout of large-scale, standardized 'one size fits all' community-based interventions. New public health measures in palliative care seek a more contextual and culturally appropriate approach. Evidencing this phenomenon in 'scientific terms' is perhaps a challenge and relates to the need for innovative and creative research methodologies.[14]

The CNS made a plan to investigate for and treat Theresa's possible delirium within the home setting, whilst acknowledging that she could deteriorate further and die despite this. At the same time, the CNS tried to support Lauren to rekindle some of the supportive relationships important to Lauren, Theresa, and the family. She offered to write to Lauren's employer explaining the situation and the need for amended duties whilst helping to coordinate a family meeting to discuss the challenges of care in an open and honest way.

Expert Opinion The Intersection Between Public, Professional, and Lay Services, and the Implications for Responsibility of Care

Research has sought to better understand how formal and informal care providers work together at the end of life. It was found that formal care providers are often aware and supportive of informal networks yet this does not translate into meaningful actions that establish, support, or maintain them.[15] Indeed, formal care is often provided from the 'service provider as expert' position rather than a partnership or a community development position. Such work suggests there is a need to reframe how professionals engage with citizens. The term 'asset-based community development' has been used to describe how community resource may be developed from 'within' by starting with what is strong and building outwards.[16] Within this concept, and interdependent upon it, is nestled the idea of a compassionate community.[15] In its broadest sense, a compassionate community is conceptualized as sharing some responsibility for end of life care, whilst the specifics of what it is responsible for, and how this is held between networks will vary. Perhaps there is a need to be more fluid with the idea of responsibility, and the sharing of roles may need to be more common in a compassionate community model. Traditionally described in the biomedical literature as a source of burden and distress, the sharing of roles can also be perceived as a fulfilling and rewarding process.[8]

The CNS visited Theresa and Lauren the following week and heard that the situation had improved. Lauren was starting to feel that she had a network of support, and whilst recognizing there will be challenging times to come, she felt better equipped to meet them. Theresa herself had also improved, was eating again, was showing some improvement in her mobility and was less disturbed at night.

Clinical Tip Manging Uncertainty and Unknown In The Context of Human Suffering

Caring for people with advanced dementia is a challenge. Prognostication is difficult whilst detecting symptoms, delineating their origin, and successfully treating them requires patience and an acceptance that you may not necessarily succeed. This is representative of wider questions that relate to the very purpose, aims, and objectives of end of life care in this context. The literature relating to new public health approaches to palliative care suggests the fundamental purpose to the work of care is to provide support and security at a time of great sadness and vulnerability. A large part of this relates to being present with people as they confront the uncertainty and loss of control inherent within the dying process. How this works alongside notions of control and autonomy inherent within the paradigm of a 'good death' requires careful consideration. The ideal of a good death can become problematic when there are elements of human suffering that cannot be remedied or prevented, despite access to resource. Ultimately this may be interpreted as a failure in care when the reality couldn't be further from this. A different approach is grounded in the idea that death, much like the life lived until that point, is an assortment of both joy and sadness. Such an approach recognizes that whilst the end of life can inflict pain, fear, and terrible sadness, there is also companionship, courage, strength, and love. To provide care at the end of life, people must accept, and accommodate, both the joy and pain the processes of dying and bereavement can bring. Working *with* rather than *against* the suffering that comes with death can mean it is experienced in a healthy way so that individuals and communities can transition through such processes and develop from the experience it brings.[17]

A Final Word from the Expert

Bringing the conceptual components of a new public health approach to palliative care alongside a practical action plan is Kellehear's theoretical framework for compassionate communities.[18]

Examples of such practice exist from across the world, with many taking reference from the model of care developed in the Indian state of Kerala. Here, through a series of paradigm shifts, there has been a complete system change in relation to end of life care.[1] A community-led response has garnered support from other institutions that has ultimately resulted in a new state palliative care policy. Today, there are over 1600 institutions working together to deliver palliative care in what has become a beacon of hope for low-cost, equitable, and participatory end of life care. This model has been established in the UK and internationally, yet success in this approach is not guaranteed. Significant tensions remain in adopting a social approach to death and dying. Learning from past examples, whilst recognizing compassionate communities do not conform to a neatly packaged intervention amenable to scientific evaluation, are important steps in progressing knowledge in this area. Understanding compassionate communities as a lens through which people might evaluate their own actions, helping to build trust, membership and 'know how' to develop community capacity in real terms is perhaps a useful first step and something we can all integrate into our daily practice.

References

1. Sallnow L, Smith R, Ahmedzai SH, et al. Report of the Lancet Commission on the value of death: bringing death back into life. *Lancet* 2022; 399(10327): 837–884.
2. Sawyer JM, Higgs P, Porter JD, Sampson EL. New public health approaches to palliative care, a brave new horizon or an impractical ideal? An integrative literature review with thematic synthesis. *Palliat Care Soc Pract* 2021; 15: 26323524211032984.
3. Portes A. Social capital: its origins and applications in modern sociology. *Ann Rev Sociol* 1998; 24(1): 1–24.
4. Kawachi I, Kim D, Coutts A, Subramanian SV. Commentary: reconciling the three accounts of social capital. *Int J Epidemiol* 2004; 33(4): 682–690.
5. Holt-Lunstad J, Smith TB, Layton JB. Social relationships and mortality risk: a meta-analytic review. *PLoS Med* 2010; 7(7): e1000316.
6. Christakis NA, Fowler JH. The collective dynamics of smoking in a large social network. *N Engl J Med* 2008; 358(21): 2249–2258.
7. Christakis NA, Fowler JH. The spread of obesity in a large social network over 32 years. *N Engl J Med* 2007; 357(4): 370–379.
8. Horsfall D, Noonan K, Leonard R. Bringing our dying home: How caring for someone at end of life builds social capital and develops compassionate communities. *Health Sociol Rev* 2012; 21(4): 373–382.
9. Sawyer JM, Sallnow L, Kupeli N, Stone P, Sampson EL. Social networks, social capital and end-of-life care for people with dementia: a realist review. *BMJ Open* 2019; 9(12): e030703.
10. Gott M, Wiles J, Moeke-Maxwell T, et al. What is the role of community at the end of life for people dying in advanced age? A qualitative study with bereaved family carers. *Palliat Med* 2018; 32(1): 268–275.
11. Leonard R, Horsfall D, Noonan K. Models of caring from India and Australia and their relationship to social capital. *NJPG* 2010; 26(3): 15–25.
12. Leonard R, Horsfall D, Noonan K. Identifying changes in the support networks of end-of-life carers using social network analysis. *BMJ Support Palliat Care* 2015; 5(2): 153–159.

13. Grindrod A, Rumbold B. Healthy End of Life Project (HELP): a progress report on implementing community guidance on public health palliative care initiatives in Australia. *Ann Palliat Med* 2018; 7(Suppl 2): S73–S83.
14. Sawyer JM, Sallnow L. The evidence for the effectiveness of a public health palliative care approach. In: Abel J, Kellehear A (eds). *Oxford Textbook of Public Health Palliative Care*. London: Oxford University Press; 2022, pp. 221–232.
15. Horsfall D, Leonard R, Noonan K, Rosenberg J. Working together–apart: exploring the relationships between formal and informal care networks for people dying at home. *Prog Palliat Care* 2013; 21(6): 331–336.
16. Mathie A, Cunningham G. From clients to citizens: Asset-based community development as a strategy for community-driven development. *Dev Pract* 2003; 13(5): 474–486.
17. Kellehear A. Compassionate cities: global significance and meaning for palliative care. *Prog Palliat Care* 2020; 28(2): 115–119.
18. Abel J, Kellehear A. Palliative care reimagined: a needed shift. *BMJ Support Palliat Care* 2016; 6(1): 21–26.

CASE

44 Grief and Bereavement

Charlotte Chamberlain

Expert: Lucy Selman

Case history

Julia Baptiste is a 44-year-old British-Caribbean nutritionist and mother of three (ages 12, 8, and 6) with progressive metastatic rectal cancer. She has been a sociable member of her community in the past. More recently, Julia has stopped participating in her book club or cooking, activities she used to enjoy, and describes struggling with social relationships since learning of her poor prognosis. She talks to her oncology nurse about a series of losses: activities she can no longer do or enjoy, from driving the children to school, to attending her church group. She does not like to talk about the future.

Clinical Tip

Grief can occur with either an abrupt or a more gradual succession of losses to someone's capability and functioning, resulting in impaired well-being and sense of self. Grief does not only occur in those who are bereaved but can occur in our patients.

Evidence Base Models of Normal Grief

A number of theoretically derived models of grief have been proposed and evolved over time. The most publicized 'five-stages' model originated with Kubler-Ross.[1] The stages of Denial, Anger, Bargaining, Depression, and Acceptance have been frequently misinterpreted as phases that everyone needed to transition through, in a linear order, as part of the grieving process. While some empirical evidence supports a different staged model including, 'shock-numbness, yearning-searching, disorganization, and reorganization' (Bowlby and Parkes),[2] grief has also been described as 'tasks' rather than stages. For example, Worden outlines the griever's tasks of accepting the reality of loss, processing the pain of grief, adjusting to the world without the deceased, and finding an enduring connection with the deceased while continuing to engage in new relationships.[1] An alternative dominant model of grief is the dual process model (Stroebe),[3] which describes instead an oscillation between loss-oriented activities characterized by behaviours involving attending to the grief, and restoration-oriented behaviours focused on avoiding or seeking respite from the grief. This model sees healthy grieving not as linear but as a dynamic process, oscillating between loss-oriented and restoration-oriented coping.

Learning Point Identifying Anticipatory Grief

'Anticipatory grief' describes grief that occurs prior to a loss. It can include elements of mourning, coping, and proactive planning.[1] In the clinical case, Julia is exhibiting some signs of distress, withdrawing from activities she enjoyed. She is likely grieving already from her losses to date, but Julia as well as her close family members may also be experiencing anticipatory grief for her approaching death.

Anticipatory grief is important for several reasons. Firstly, anticipatory grief is modifiable. Poor communication, high caregiver burden, and inadequate preparation for death are associated with worse anticipatory grief in patients with advanced cancer.[4] In this case, Julia had declined involvement in advance care planning discussions. Health professionals' recognition of anticipatory grief amongst patients and their loved ones may improve shared decision-making and quality of

Clinical Tip

It's appropriate to ask sensitively about a culture that is not your own to understand how it impacts on the person and their families' experience of advanced illness.

care.[5] Secondly, among caregivers greater pre-death grief has been identified as a key predictor of post-death complicated grief.[6] Prolonged or complicated grief can lead to depression and other mental health distress and ill-health, which impacts relationships, activities of daily living, and risk of substance misuse.[7] Interventions to reduce burden and stress in dementia caregivers can decrease levels of post-death depression and complicated grief.[8]

Julia's mother has attended hospital with her and is helping Julia to 'stay positive'. Julia is an only child and her mother is widowed, with her close support network in Trinidad.

Learning Point The Impact of Culture on Grief and Bereavement

Julia's and her mother's close ties with Caribbean culture may influence their experience of grief and bereavement. Experiences of grief and bereavement, particularly mourning, funeral and memorialization practices, are inherently shaped by culture and religion (e.g. the wake of Nine-Nights in the Caribbean, or Shiva, the Jewish mourning ritual). These cultural, social, and religious norms impact on health, health-seeking behaviour, and coping. Current research addressing interventions to support bereaved people is almost exclusively conducted in high- and middle-income countries and in a limited range of cultural contexts.[9] Therefore, extrapolating these results to different cultural contexts is often inappropriate. Experiences of 'cultural incongruity' in death and mourning, where the beliefs and expectations in someone's culture of origin differ from those in the setting in which they live or die, can 'contribute to detachment, estrangement, and distrust'—which can exacerbate prolonged grief disorder (PGD) and other negative outcomes following bereavement.[10]

In a palliative care setting, individualizing care such that cultural and social differences are recognized and minimizing cultural cognitive dissonance, which may impact on grief, mourning, and future life-opportunities for surviving carers, is the clinical goal. Given variation in individual needs and preferences after a bereavement, clinicians can play a key role in signposting bereaved people to a diverse range of support options—from peer-to-peer support groups and online services to one-to-one counselling. Since most bereaved people cope through the support of family, friends, and community, rather than solely through traditional health service structures, community empowerment, working with third-sector and community groups familiar with the social and cultural needs which are often poorly addressed within the dominant cultural practice is essential.[11]

Expert Comment Barriers and Inequities in Accessing Support

Bereaved people often experience problems getting the right support. In a UK survey of 711 people bereaved during the COVID-19 pandemic (median 5 months post-bereavement), most respondents had not sought support from bereavement services (59%) or their GP (60%).[9] Of those who had sought support, over half experienced difficulties accessing bereavement services (56%) and GP support (52%). Overall, half (51%) reported high or severe vulnerability in grief, and three-quarters of this group were not accessing formal bereavement or mental health support. Signposting and information provision were poor, with 51% of bereaved respondents reporting that they had not been given any information about bereavement services from healthcare providers, either at the time of death or during follow-up. There are also known, persistent inequities in accessing mental health and bereavement services. These include a lack of information and knowledge of what support is available and how to access it, and discomfort or reluctance to seek help from services. Particular barriers for minoritized ethnic communities include limited outreach by bereavement services and a lack of culturally competent services.[12] Meeting a population's needs for bereavement support is likely to require integrated statutory, voluntary, and community-level services designed to meet the needs of diverse communities, with healthcare providers playing a crucial role in signposting to services as well as providing generalist bereavement support.

Clinical Tip

An estimated 10%[13] of bereaved people are diagnosed as having PGD[14]: pervasive preoccupation with the dead person for at least six months, with intense emotional pain and substantially impaired functioning. In PGD, grief persists beyond the norms for the person's social, cultural, or religious context, and becomes increasingly debilitating over time.[13] In this instance, targeted specialist mental health support in the form of individual or group psychotherapy is recommended.[15]

Tracey, the oncology specialist nurse, has updated you about Julia and her family. She stayed late yesterday to talk to Julia's family and has recognized she is finding it difficult to 'hold' the family distress. Tracey hasn't shared her worries with anyone else. It is 'part of the job'. She admits that she was very distracted at work today and couldn't sleep last night.

Learning Point Professional Grief

Julia is young, with a young family. Tracey and her clinical team may identify with her and therefore may struggle to identify or communicate that she is dying given the length of their clinical relationship. Growing research investigating oncologist experiences of grief resulting from patient loss have described compartmentalization or dissociation coping strategies, which resulted in distraction while seeing patients and affected their personal lives. A systematic review of distress among oncologists revealed high burnout (32%), high psychiatric morbidity (27%), and evidence of unhealthy behaviours (up to 30% drink alcohol in a problematic way), with evidence that patient death is implicated in these reactions.[16] Historically, grief in health professionals has often been described as disenfranchised grief: any grief that goes unacknowledged or unvalidated by social norms, and is hence associated with a lack of understanding and support, making it particularly hard to process. Since the COVID-19 pandemic has highlighted a common experience of shared grief amongst health professionals,[17] organizations are increasingly recognizing the burden of grief amongst staff and encouraging informal debriefing, Schwartz rounds, and signposting to formal counselling when needed. Disenfranchised grief is also common when the importance of a relationship is not properly or openly recognized (e.g. some LGTBQ+ relationships) or when a bereavement is stigmatized (e.g. death due to suicide or addiction).

Julia's disease has rapidly progressed on the latest imaging. Julia's CT scan has identified a colovesical fistula with a collection in the pelvis that is poorly responding to antibiotics. The oncology team feel that Julia is now approaching the last weeks of life. Her husband, Terence, has a history of anxiety and depression. He experienced a close bereavement (his mother) as a child. He is struggling to come to terms with Julia's disease progression.

Learning Point Risk Factors for Poor Bereavement Outcomes

There are a number of recognized risk factors for poor grief experiences and outcomes, such as trauma, depression, anxiety, and previous PGD. For *caregivers*, these risk factors include gender (female), age (older), low educational attainment, low socioeconomic status, and low levels of social support.[18] Therefore, the most marginalized in societies are more at risk of prolonged grief. In addition to the personal characteristics predicting risk of prolonged grief, other determinants are relational, such as the relationship to the deceased (close), family conflict at the end of life, insecure attachment styles, and childhood adversity, as well as the mode of death (with increased PGD in traumatic deaths), among other factors.[18] Other factors potentially protect against PGD: hospice involvement addressing death anxiety, palliative care involvement more generally, and pre-bereavement spirituality.[19] According to these risk factors, Julia's husband and mother in the clinical case may have an increased risk of PGD.

Clinical Tip Tools to Recognize Risk Factors for Prolonged Grief

Several tools have been developed to identify those at high risk of bereavement-related grief symptoms[20,21] which can be used in clinical settings to help ensure adequate bereavement support. Further research is needed to understand whether the tools can be used across different settings, whether their implementation leads to improved outcomes for those bereaved, and if meaningful, how we can best implement these tools in everyday practice.

Clinical Tip Signposting and Referral

It is particularly important for specialist palliative care, primary care, and intensive care health professionals to be aware of what bereavement support services (including informal community groups and resources) are available for those grieving in their locality and ensure signposting and referral are consistent. Available services, resources, and waiting lists differ widely region by region and country by country. Organizations are frequently charitably funded, rather than part of core universal healthcare. The UK has a wide range of bereavement services (see https://www.thegoodgrieftrust.org and https://www.ataloss.org), with services generally accessed through primary care general practitioners, self-referral, or, for those patients known to the local hospice, through the hospice bereavement networks.

Julia's children know that their mummy is unwell but do not know how seriously. Although the children's' school is aware Julia has cancer, the school is not yet providing any additional formal supervision or support.

Learning Point Bereavement in Children

While each family circumstance is unique, the general guidance health professionals give to families is to give clear information in manageable amounts, appropriate to the child's age and level of understanding. This honesty allows time for the child to process and ask questions, with information being given at the rate dictated by the child. Schools should be notified of advanced illness in a family to better support children. It allows children to maintain some of their usual routine, but alerts staff to be aware of symptoms of distress. Increasingly, bespoke resources for parents guiding grieving children and for grieving children themselves, such as books, games, apps and websites are available (for example, Child Bereavement UK and Winston's Wish signpost to a number of resources). In this clinical case, the fact the school is informed of Julia's cancer is helpful to provide a layer of support and early detection for signs of distress for Julia's children.

Clinical Tip Memory Boxes

Memory boxes are frequently used in palliative and dementia care. Their design and contents may vary, but they share the sentiment that there should be a physical means to aid a loved one in remembering and processing their grief. In the palliative care setting they may include audio files, a fingerprint or handprint-making kit, a book supporting parents to talk to children about grief, or a pair of toys to be shared between the person that is dying and the surviving family member or loved one. To date there is limited evidence of their impact on the grieving process. Qualitative research in parents who have survived perinatal death and in adult intensive care provides the strongest evidence of their benefit,[22] but the best way to offer this support is unclear. Given Julia's difficulty engaging with advance care planning to date, identifying the best time and approach to introduce memory boxes, or even whether to introduce them at all, is not evidence-based, but judged by the clinical team on an individual, person-centred basis.

Discussion

Grief, the emotional process we go through when losing someone or something important to us, is a natural part of life, which we all eventually face. Ultimately, the experience of grief is a universal part of living, not in itself a pathology requiring medical intervention. But a close bereavement can also be one of the most challenging, intense, and disruptive life events. While many people suffer greatly in early bereavement, and adjustment can take many years, most bereaved people adapt well, integrating their grief into their lives. Fundamental to this adaptation is the support of social networks: friends, communities, and family members.[23] Peer-to-peer support (for example, group support from others with shared experiences) currently has incomplete evidence of its efficacy.[24] One-to-one support from trained bereavement counsellors and therapists, particularly if bereaved people are socially isolated, marginalized, or specifically where PGD has been identified has a growing evidence base.[15] Although bereavement can be associated with a number of serious medical, psychological, and social consequences including lost work or school days, social isolation and loneliness, and increased use of medication and health services,[25] it can also provide a new lens to view the world. It can lead to creative, practical, and inspirational works that are a positive legacy for those who have died and a source of strength for those who survive. There is an urgent need for more research into how best to support those grieving.

A Final Word from the Expert

In Julia's case there were clear indicators that she was experiencing anticipatory grief (withdrawing from activities and people she previously enjoyed) and that her husband and mother may be at risk of PGD, given their respective risk factors (Terence: depression, childhood trauma; Julia's mother: age, sex, limited support network). A tailored approach to supporting Julia's family members, identifying any specific cultural or religious needs, is essential.

References

1. PDQ Supportive and Palliative Care Editorial Board. Grief, bereavement, and coping with loss (PDQ(R)): health professional version. 2002. In: PDQ Cancer Information Summaries [Internet]. Bethesda (MD): National Cancer Institute (US); 2002.
2. Maciejewski PK, Zhang B, Block SD, Prigerson HG. An empirical examination of the stage theory of grief. *JAMA* 2007; 297(7): 716–723.
3. Stroebe M, Schut H. The dual process model of coping with bereavement: a decade on. *Omega (Westport)* 2010; 61(4): 273–289.
4. Yu W, Lu Q, Lu Y, et al. Anticipatory grief among chinese family caregivers of patients with advanced cancer: a cross-sectional study. *Asia Pac J Oncol Nurs* 2021; 8(4): 369–376.
5. Ainscough T, Fraser L, Taylor J, Beresford B, Booth A. Bereavement support effectiveness for parents of infants and children: a systematic review. *BMJ Support Palliat Care* 2022; 12(e5): e623–e631.
6. Schulz R, Boerner K, Shear K, Zhang S, Gitlin LN. Predictors of complicated grief among dementia caregivers: a prospective study of bereavement. *Am J Geriatr Psychiatry* 2006; 14(8): 650–658.
7. Parisi A, Sharma A, Howard MO, Blank Wilson A. The relationship between substance misuse and complicated grief: a systematic review. *J Subst Abuse Treat* 2019; 103: 43–57.
8. Hebert RS, Dang Q, Schulz R. Preparedness for the death of a loved one and mental health in bereaved caregivers of patients with dementia: findings from the REACH study. *J Palliat Med* 2006; 9(3): 683–693.
9. Harrop E, Morgan F, Longo M, et al. The impacts and effectiveness of support for people bereaved through advanced illness: a systematic review and thematic synthesis. *Palliat Med* 2020; 34(7): 871–888.
10. Smid GE, Groen S, de la Rie SM, Kooper S, Boelen PA. Toward cultural assessment of grief and grief-related psychopathology. *Psychiatr Serv* 2018; 69(10): 1050–1052.
11. Sallnow L, Smith R, Ahmedzai SH, et al. Report of the Lancet Commission on the value of death: bringing death back into life. *Lancet* 2022; 399(10327): 837–884.
12. Mayland CR, Powell RA, Clarke GC, Ebenso B, Allsop MJ. Bereavement care for ethnic minority communities: a systematic review of access to, models of, outcomes from, and satisfaction with, service provision. *PLoS One* 2021; 16(6): e0252188.

13. Lundorff M, Holmgren H, Zachariae R, Farver-Vestergaard I, O'Connor M. Prevalence of prolonged grief disorder in adult bereavement: a systematic review and meta-analysis. *J Affect Disord* 2017; 212: 138–149.
14. World Health Organization. *International Classification of Diseases For Mortality and Morbidity Statistics (11th Revision)*. 2018. Available at: https://icd.who.int/en
15. Shear MK, Reynolds CF, 3rd, Simon NM, et al. Optimizing treatment of complicated grief: a randomized clinical trial. *JAMA Psychiatry* 2016; 73(7): 685–694.
16. Medisauskaite A, Kamau C. Prevalence of oncologists in distress: systematic review and meta-analysis. *Psychooncology* 2017; 26(11): 1732–1740.
17. Selman L. Covid grief has cracked us open: how clinicians respond could reshape attitudes to bereavement—an essay by Lucy Selman. *BMJ* 2021; 374: n1803.
18. Lobb EA, Kristjanson LJ, Aoun SM, Monterosso L, Halkett GK, Davies A. Predictors of complicated grief: a systematic review of empirical studies. *Death Stud* 2010; 34(8): 673–698.
19. Mason TM, Tofthagen CS, Buck HG. Complicated grief: risk factors, protective factors, and interventions. *J Soc Work End Life Palliat Care* 2020; 16(2): 151–174.
20. Newsom C, Schut H, Stroebe MS, Wilson S, Birrell J. Initial validation of a comprehensive assessment instrument for bereavement-related grief symptoms and risk of complications: the indicator of bereavement adaptation-cruse Scotland (IBACS). *PLoS One* 2016; 11(10): e0164005.
21. Roberts K, Holland J, Prigerson HG, et al. Development of the Bereavement Risk Inventory and Screening Questionnaire (BRISQ): item generation and expert panel feedback. *Palliat Support Care* 2017; 15(1): 57–66.
22. Riegel M, Randall S, Buckley T. Memory making in end-of-life care in the adult intensive care unit: a scoping review of the research literature. *Aust Crit Care* 2019; 32(5): 442–447.
23. Aoun SM, Breen LJ, White I, Rumbold B, Kellehear A. What sources of bereavement support are perceived helpful by bereaved people and why? Empirical evidence for the compassionate communities approach. *Palliat Med* 2018; 32(8): 1378–1388.
24. Bartone PT, Bartone JV, Violanti JM, Gileno ZM. Peer support services for bereaved survivors: a systematic review. *Omega (Westport)* 2019; 80(1): 137–166.
25. Stroebe M, Schut H, Stroebe W. Health outcomes of bereavement. *Lancet* 2007; 370(9603): 1960–1973.

SECTION 7

Legal considerations

CASE

45 A Desire for Hastened Death

Rebecca Payne

Expert: Samantha Lund

Case history

Helen was a woman in her 60s who was admitted to a hospice for symptom control, shortly after receiving a new diagnosis of metastatic cancer. There were no anticancer treatment options available to her, and her prognosis was likely short months. She had no other relevant medical or psychiatric history.

Her main physical symptom was pain in her leg, causing her to avoid movement, and interfering with sleep.

Helen was very afraid of dying in pain and following conversations with friends about their experiences of death, she believed that this was an inevitable part of dying with cancer. She 'had no fear of death but was afraid of dying' and described feeling angry and frightened. Control over her life was important to her, and she equated suffering with losing control. She was horrified by the thought of lying helpless in bed for weeks, 'watched over by everyone' and wished she could have the option of a quicker death, which lasted only a few minutes and could be done in privacy.

On admission Helen revealed that she had made the decision to go abroad to end her life via physician-assisted suicide (PAS) and had completed the initial paperwork. She described her mood as 'okay' and felt it had improved since firmly deciding to seek PAS. Prior to receiving her terminal diagnosis, Helen did not have strong beliefs about PAS—her decision was made as she adapted to the news. A referral was made to the hospice counselling team, but Helen declined to meet them as she felt her psychological needs had been misunderstood because of her decisions around PAS. She maintained that her illness and short prognosis had no great psychological impact on her, though at times staff noticed that she was distressed. There were no concerns about the patient's capacity to make decisions.

Expert Comment Multidisciplinary Team Approach to Care

Team working is one of the key elements of effective palliative care. Following a thorough holistic assessment, multidisciplinary care for an individual patient involves using the knowledge, skills, and expert practice of health professionals from different disciplines to find solutions to complex problems.[1] In a multidisciplinary team (MDT) meeting, individual patients and their care are discussed, with the aim of the patient achieving their goals when possible.

MDT working is also an important means of sharing complex decision-making and of providing support in situations where difficult ethical and legal situations arise.

Clinical Tip Assessment of Mood

It is important to assess whether low mood or anxiety are contributing to a patient's desire to hasten death, as they are potentially treatable.

Both anxiety and depression may have somatic symptoms which overlap with common symptoms of many life-limiting illnesses.

As per National Institute for Health and Care Excellence (NICE) guidance, depression can be diagnosed based on whether a person has either one or both of the main criteria (persistent sadness/low mood, and anhedonia, which is a marked loss of interests or pleasure), as well as any of the associated somatic symptoms (altered sleep pattern, changed appetite, and/or weight, loss of energy, agitation, or slowing of movements, poor concentration), present for most of the day for at least two weeks.[2]

Expert Comment Control

It is not uncommon for individuals with any illness to feel a lack of control and this is often intensified in patients with a life-limiting illness. Uncertainty about how the illness will be experienced and what will happen in the future all heighten the feeling that control is being lost and this can lead to distress and anxiety. Individuals may seek to hasten their death as a means of regaining control, and it is known that amongst individuals seeking assisted suicide many cite 'losing autonomy' as their primary concern.[3] Whilst autonomy is a broader ethical concept than having control, the sense of self-rule can understandably feel threatened for individuals with a terminal diagnosis.

Whilst the unpredictability of a life-limiting illness means that it is not possible for the patient to regain their usual control over their life, there are ways of restoring some sense of control. Advance care planning (ACP) is an essential component of this, as is shared decision-making throughout the illness. Regular review and clear communication are critical so that patients are informed and can then effectively participate in ongoing decision-making.

Learning Point Law Regarding Patients Requesting Assisted Suicide

The following explains the current law in the United Kingdom (2022), and practitioners are advised to be clear about the law in the country in which they work and to contact their regulatory body or indemnifier if they have any concerns.

Under UK law, any form of assisted dying is illegal. The British Medical Association (BMA) guidance from 2019[4] covers the legal position for medical practitioners throughout the UK. Any action which may be perceived as assisting suicide may lead to prosecution.

The guidance stresses the importance of a compassionate approach to a request to hasten death.[4] When a patient has a terminal diagnosis, it is important that they do not feel abandoned and that they are reassured that there will be care and support available to them. If a patient requests help in ending their life, the General Medical Council (GMC) advises that a doctor should explain that it would be illegal to 'encourage or assist a person to commit or attempt suicide'.[5] The doctor should avoid giving specific medical advice that may allow a patient to end their own life, including guidance on how to seek suicide abroad. Medical reports should not be written to facilitate assisted suicide abroad. Patients and their carers should be made aware of their legal position. If a patient requests a copy of their medical records, the GMC advise that they are entitled to this under the General Data Protection Regulations, as this is considered 'too distant from the encouragement or assistance', even if the notes may be used in the process of requesting PAS.

Helen's pain was controlled effectively with a combination of lidocaine patches, ibuprofen gel, and small doses of background opioid.

Learning Point

The severity of any physical symptom may not equate with the desire to die. The WTHD may arise as a result of the fear of what is to come along with other psychological or existential needs. The appropriate management of any symptoms will help as this can allay the fear of symptoms being 'uncontrollable'.

Although Helen had repeatedly reiterated her desire to hasten her death, as she deteriorated, she seemed calmer and more accepting of being unable to control the timing and means of her death. This may have been due in part to her increasing physical and mental fatigue, but perhaps also due to a growing trust in the staff at the hospice, who worked with her to understand her specific wishes. Personal care was kept to the safe minimum, and she was left alone as much as possible to avoid 'being watched over' as she had feared. She died in the hospice.

Expert Comment Refusal of Treatment

Informed consent is critical in respecting patient autonomy.[6,7]

Some patients who wish to hasten their death will attempt to do so by refusal of food, fluids, or medication. Any refusal made by a capacious patient must be respected although this can be difficult for those involved in their care. In many cases such refusal will not necessarily bring death more quickly and may lead to increased symptoms. Sensitive communication is essential when explaining this to patients not only to facilitate shared decision-making and to balance a WTHD and symptom control but also to plan for care when the patient loses capacity. If the patient agrees, consultations should be held jointly with those important to the patient. In this case, Helen did not want to be 'watched over' which sometimes led to her refusing nursing care. Such refusal can be difficult for healthcare professionals to manage largely because this care is a core component of nursing.[8] It is important to understand why such a refusal has been made, whilst respecting the decision. As in this case careful negotiation is often required to balance professional responsibilities and the patient's right to refuse care without coercion especially at the point that the patient loses capacity.

Expert Comment Prognosis

Estimating how long a patient has left to live can be crucial for guiding decision-making for patients, their loved ones, and for healthcare professionals[9] but there is often uncertainty around this. Declining functional status has been shown to be associated with shorter prognosis[11] especially in patients with cancer. The most important thing when discussing prognosis with patients is the use of sensitive language and if time estimates are to be given using 'ballpark' estimates, for example days to weeks, weeks to months, and months to years.[10]

In this case, the patient seemed calmer and more able to adapt to her loss of control when death was imminent.

Expert Comment Team Support

Working in healthcare frequently exposes clinicians to highly stressful situations as they witness the psychological distress of those suffering from illness. In palliative care these situations also include daily exposure to death and the distress that often surrounds having a terminal diagnosis. In this case, the distress felt by healthcare professionals related both to the suffering expressed by the patient and, for some staff, to the feeling that an inability to alleviate the WTHD was a failure of care. Support for staff is crucial to promote and maintain mental health and well-being. Strategies may include personal and group reflection and clinical supervision, which has been shown to be an effective means of self-care.[12] Many healthcare organizations now participate in Schwartz Rounds© where the emotions of individual workers are voiced and there is a sharing and acknowledging of these feelings.[13]

Evidence Base

To clarify the definition of a 'wish to hasten death' a Delphi process in 2016 arrived at:

'The wish to hasten death (WTHD) is a reaction to suffering, in the context of a life-threatening condition, from which the patient can see no way out other than to accelerate his or her death. This wish may be expressed spontaneously or after being asked about it, but it must be distinguished from the acceptance of impending death or from a wish to die naturally, although preferably soon'.[14]

Between 1.5 to 38% of patients with a terminal diagnosis may wish to hasten their death.[15] This desire may fluctuate over time but, in its most severe expression, a patient may start to make concrete plans to end their life, and request PAS or euthanasia.

In a study comparing patients with similar functional and physical symptom levels, patients who had expressed a strong wish to hasten death were also found to have a worse Health Related Quality of Life score, particularly for the emotional aspects, including loss of dignity and a sense of dependence.[15] This study highlights that the wish to hasten death can arise from a global sense of despair and suffering, not just from distressing physical symptoms. Other studies have identified a correlation with the WTHD and depression, loss of meaning, and loss of control.[17, 18] A systematic review identified five themes underlying patients' expressions of a WTHD: loss of self, fear, a wish to live but 'not in this way', a way of ending suffering, and a sense of having some control.[16]

Discussion

Whilst a large proportion of patients in palliative care may have a WTHD, healthcare workers may worry about causing distress if they ask about it. A study addressing this question found up to 80% of patients did not find it upsetting to be asked, and most felt it was an important question.[19] The same study found that about a third of patients with a WTHD had not talked about it with anyone, therefore it can be important to ask the question in order to uncover a burden of hidden suffering.

When a patient does express a WTHD it is important to consider any underlying factors so that appropriate support may be provided, along with information about what to expect at the end of life. Working with the patient to maintain their sense of control may ameliorate the fear and sense of loss of control driving the wish.

Future Advances

As well as asking patients an unstructured, open question about whether they have a WTHD, two different scales can be used to assess for it: the Desire to Die Rating Scale (DDRS), and the Schedule of Attitudes towards Hastened Death (SAHD, and the short-form, SAHD-5). A study comparing both in the same population has suggested that the SAHD-5 could be used as an easy-to-administer initial screening tool, followed by the DDRS for more in-depth exploration of the 'intensity and significance' if a WTHD is identified.[20]

A Final Word from the Expert

This case is a good example of how a patient's desire for a hastened death can present. For Helen, the desire had motivated a detailed plan for PAS as a means of controlling the time and nature of death. Her case illustrates some of the recognized triggers for a wish to hasten death including fear of worsening and uncontrolled physical symptoms alongside an overwhelming feeling of loss of control. Thorough assessment and care, which is coordinated by different disciplines is essential to relieve suffering as much as possible. The effect on staff of such a case must not be underestimated and appropriate support should be put in place.

The law in the United Kingdom is clear about PAS. Helen understood this and did not ask the team to play any role in this, nor did she refuse food or drink or ask the team to hasten her death in any other way (such as inappropriate dosing of medication). However, these requests can and do arise and it is imperative that professional guidance and the law in the country of practice are followed.

References

1. NHS England. *Making it Happen: Multi-disciplinary Team (MDT) Working*. Available at: https://www.england.nhs.uk/publication/making-it-happen-multi-disciplinary-team-mdt-working
2. National Institute for Health and Care Excellence (NICE). Clinical Guideline 91: Depression in *Adults With A Chronic Physical Health Problem: Recognition And Management*. Available at: https://www.nice.org.uk/guidance/cg91
3. Ganzini L, Goy ER, Dobscha SK. Oregonians' reasons for requesting physician aid in dying. *Arch Intern Med* 2009; 169(5): 489–492.
4. British Medical Association. Responding to *Patient Requests For Assisted Dying—Guidance For Doctors*. Available at: https://www.bma.org.uk/media/1424/bma-guidance-on-responding-to-patient-requests-for-assisted-dying-for-doctors
5. General Medical Council. Guidance for the Investigation Committee and case examiners when considering allegations about a doctor's involvement in encouraging or assisting suicide. Available at: https://rcem.ac.uk/wp-content/uploads/2021/11/Guidance_for_Investigation-Committee_When_Considering_Allegations_About_a_-Doctor.pdf
6. General Medical Council. Guidance on professional standards and ethics for doctors. Decision Making and Consent. Available at: https://www.gmc-uk.org/-/media/documents/updated-decision-making-and-consent-guidance-english-09_11_20_pdf-84176092.pdf?la=en&hash=4FC9D08017C5DAAD20801F04E34E616BCE060AAF&msclkid=d06dfd23bb5f11ec980a223018ff0627
7. Nursing and Midwifery Council. The Code. Professional standards of practice and behaviour for nurses, midwives and nursing associates. Available at: https://www.nmc.org.uk/globalassets/sitedocuments/nmc-publications/nmc-code.pdf?msclkid=2b80d9d9bb6011eca166a32a0855b479
8. Aveyard H. The patient who refuses nursing care. *J Med Ethics* 2004; 30(4): 346–350.
9. Stone PC, Lund S. Predicting prognosis in patients with advanced cancer. *Annals of Oncology* 2007: 18(6): 971–976.
10. Chu C, White N, Stone PC. Prognostication in Palliative Care. *Clin Med* 2019; 19(4): 306310.
11. Cooper R, Kuh D, Hardy R. Objectively measured physical capability levels and mortality: systematic review and meta-analysis. *BMJ* 2010; 341: c4467.
12. Edmonds KP, Yeung HN, Onderdonk C, et al. Clinical supervision in the palliative care team setting: a concrete approach to team wellness. *J Palliat Med* 2014; 18(3): 1–4.
13. Dawson J, McCarthy I, Taylor C, et al. Effectiveness of a group intervention to reduce the psychological distress of healthcare staff: a pre-post quasi- experimental evaluation. *BMC Health Serv Res* 2021; 21: 392.
14. Balaguer A, Monforte-Royo C, Porta-Sales J, et al. An international consensus definition of the wish to hasten death and its related factors. *PLoS ONE* 2016; 11(1): e0146184.
15. Crespo I, Rodríguez-Prat A, Monforte-Royo C, Wilson KG, Porta-Sales J, Balaguer A. Health-related quality of life in patients with advanced cancer who express a wish to hasten death: a comparative study. *Palliat Med* 2020; 34(5): 630–638.
16. Monforte-Royo C, Villavicencio-Chávez C, Tomás-Sábado J, et al. What lies behind the desire to hasten death? A systematic review and meta-ethnography from the perspective of patients. *PLoS ONE* 2012; 7(5): e37117.
17. Breitbart W, Rosenfeld B, Pessin H, et al. Depression and hopelessness and desire for hastened death in terminally ill patients with cancer. *JAMA* 2000; 284(22): 2907–2911.
18. Robinson S, Kissane D, Brooker J, Hempton C, Burney S. The relationship between poor quality of life and desire to hasten death: a multiple mediation model examining the contributions of depression, demoralization, loss of control, and low self-worth. *J Pain Symptom Manage* 2017; 53(2): 243–249.

19. Porta-Sales J, Crespo I, Monforte-Royo C, Marín M, Abenia-Chavarria S, Balaguer A. The clinical evaluation of the wish to hasten death is not upsetting for advanced cancer patients: a cross-sectional study. *Pall Med* 2019; 33(6): 570–577.
20. Bellido-Pérez M, Crespo I, Wilson KG, Porta-Sales J, Balaguer A, Monforte-Royo C. Assessment of the wish to hasten death in patients with advanced cancer: a comparison of 2 different approaches. *Psycho-Oncology* 2018; 27: 1538–1544.

CASE

46 Treatment Escalation Plans

Gemma Lewis-Williams

Expert: Mark Taubert

Case history

Hamid, a 79-year-old widower, was referred to the palliative care clinic by the heart failure specialist nurse. The patient had a diagnosis of severe left ventricular systolic dysfunction (ejection fraction 15%, and an implantable cardiac defibrillator in place) and metastatic prostate cancer. He had bone marrow failure and was transfusion-dependent.

Hamid attended clinic in a wheelchair accompanied by his daughter. He was breathless at rest (New York Heart Association Class IV),[1] and had a Rookwood clinical frailty score of 7.[2] Hamid had become increasingly dependent on his daughter and son-in-law for help with activities of daily living and had been requiring blood transfusions every fortnight.

Hamid talked openly about his failing health, increasing care needs, reflecting on his life and how good it had been. Together, father and daughter talked about what would be important to him if the prognosis was limited, including dying at home.

Care at home at the end of life was discussed, along with cardiopulmonary resuscitation and treatment escalation plans, including further transfusions. Hamid's views regarding future hospital admissions were explored. Hamid was offered information resources, including videos and leaflets, to support the conversation and describe the balance of benefit of treatment and the harms and burdens of interventions, including cardiopulmonary resuscitation.

Hamid agreed with the medical decision to complete a DNACPR form having had time to consider his wishes and preferences regarding his future care and time to discuss further with the community palliative care team. Hamid and his family considered a TEP but found it difficult to navigate decisions about treating infections.

Hamid became acutely unwell two months later and was admitted to hospital with possible urosepsis. Despite a trial of intravenous antibiotics, he continued to deteriorate and died 4 days later in hospital with his daughter at his bedside.

Expert Comment

National guidance recommends that it is appropriate to identify individuals in whom CPR would not be appropriate, AND those who would refuse this treatment option.[6] Policies support consistent approaches to clinical practice, emphasize the importance of practitioners working within the law, and ensuring patients and those important to the patient are appraised of decision-making.[7, 8] Resources accompany policies to support patient and public understanding, these include information leaflets, videos, and websites. Some have been evaluated positively.[9] In UK law, CPR is a medical intervention. Patients may express their views but cannot insist on a treatment that the healthcare team consider inappropriate.[10]

Learning Point What is Cardiopulmonary Resuscitation?

Cardiopulmonary resuscitation (CPR) was first described in the medical literature in 1960: Kouwenhoven and colleagues described the novel technique of 'closed chest cardiac massage'.[3] CPR is an emergency medical intervention undertaken attempting to restore breathing and circulation following a respiratory or cardiorespiratory arrest. The intervention includes the administration of external chest compressions, artificial ventilation, electric shocks applied to the chest (known as defibrillation), the administration of medicines intravenously or intraosseously and attention to potentially reversible causes.

Learning Point Harms and Benefits

Fewer than 1 in 10 people survive an out-of-hospital cardiac arrest and of those, only 8% of people in whom resuscitation is attempted, survive to hospital discharge.[4] A population-based cohort study looking at the outcome of stage IV cancer patients receiving in-hospital cardiopulmonary resuscitation described a poor response, only 17% surviving to hospital discharge.[5]

Learning Point The Form and Process

Although not legally binding, a completed, signed, and dated DNACPR form is part/all of the clinical record that a first responder will review. The form along with a clinical assessment determines whether CPR should be commenced.

DNACPR forms are written and signed by clinicians. There is no requirement that the patient, or those important to the patient, consent to the clinical decision or sign the form. This is sometimes incorrectly portrayed in the press.[11]

Expert Comment

Legally it may be inferred that clinicians have the same duty to consult and/or inform patients, or those who can support patient's best interest decisions, about TEPs as they do for DNACPR decisions.

Clinical Tip

For tips on how to support end of life conversations with regard to DNA-CPR and advance care planning, go to www.talkcpr.com and www.wales.nhs.uk/AFCP.

Expert Commentary Important Cases in UK Law

There have been two significant legal challenges regarding DNACPR decisions in the past decade. Clinicians considering DNACPR decisions need to be aware of the law where they practice.

1. R (Tracey) v Cambridge. A DNACPR decision was made but the patient was not informed.[12] The judgement found that despite Mrs Tracey being very unwell following a road traffic collision and having advanced cancer she was well enough to be involved in discussions about clinical consideration of CPR.

The UK Court of Appeal agreed with Mrs Tracey's husband, following Mrs Tracey's death, that her rights under Article 8 of the European Convention of Human Rights (right to private and family life) were breached.

The court advised that where there is a realistic possibility that discussion of CPR would result in 'physical or psychological harm' to an individual a clinician my decide not to progress the discussion. Temporary distress or upset were felt to be a foreseeable consequence of the discussion and not a reason to avoid a discussion regarding CPR.

2. Winspear V Sunderland in 2015.[13] This case involved a young man, who had significant long-term medical problems and did not have capacity to be involved in discussions and decisions about his medical care. His mother was involved in decisions regarding his care. Following an emergency admission, a DNACPR decision was made, and the form completed. A written plan included the instruction that the in hours team discuss the decision-making with the patient's mother.

Mrs Winspear argued that making a DNACPR decision without discussing it with her represented a failure of her son's right to a private and family life (Art 8 of the European Convention of Human Rights).

The Mental Capacity Act 2005 for England and Wales and its code of practice sets out definitions for people who lack capacity, and a framework for how decision-specific capacity is assessed.[14] The Winspear ruling established that there is a duty to consult those identified in section 4 of the MCA, who will support best interest decision-making. The only exception to this duty would be where it is considered 'not practicable or appropriate to do so'.

Learning Point Treatment Escalation Plans

Treatment escalation plans (TEPs) are paper and/or electronic components of a patient's clinical record, that hold personalized recommendations for clinical care in emergency situations when a patient may not have capacity to be involved in decisions. They may include discussions and advisory decisions about readmission to acute care settings, the use of intravenous antibiotics, ventilation of the lungs (invasive and non-invasive), cardiopulmonary resuscitation, renal replacement therapy, among others. The TEP form should be identifiable and easily accessible.[15]

TEPs aim to address lack of continuity of care. Qualitative data shows that junior doctors undertaking clinical reviews for patients they do not know look at previous medical entries to guide decisions. Where the team leading care have not made a clear plan to guide others in the event of a patient deteriorating or failing to respond to a trial of therapy, clinicians are reluctant to de-escalate treatment, even if they think that might be the correct course of action.[16]

Current literature mainly reports inpatient use of TEPs.[17, 18] In Wales, a TEP offers guidance for one inpatient episode of care.[19] TEPs, are a *short-term* plan, whereas advance care plans, future care plans, and DNACPR forms are used to inform *longer-term* decision-making.[20]

A retrospective case note review demonstrated that the use of a TEP in addition to a DNACPR form was associated with a reduced frequency of harms, especially in patients judged to be nearing the end of life, compared to using DNACPR alone.[21] The use of TEPs can result in healthcare savings by minimizing non-beneficial or unwanted interventions.[22]

Future Advances

Paper-based forms carry significant risks. Therefore, it is important to plan for central electronic patient records and repositories, that hold information about DNACPR forms and other advance or future care planning statements and can highlight where a person has a lasting power of attorney for health and welfare. The electronic records need to be available as read versions for all providers, including paramedics, hospital staff, 999 or 111 call handlers, primary care, out-of-hours services, etc. They need to be editable, when, for instance, a patient's situation changes, or when a decision is revoked or temporarily suspended. The ability to audit records is essential.

A Final Word from the Expert

There is critique of decisions made in advance of an expected event (such as cardiac arrest) including the use of DNACPR forms, TEPs, and advance care plans. Morrison et al argue that that 'a substantial body of high-quality evidence exists to demonstrate that advance care planning fails to improve end of life care'. They conclude that efforts should shift from optimizing discussions in advance of medical decisions, to improving 'in-the-moment' decisions (i.e. when the emergency occurs).[23] Evidence found for this case suggests that the advocated shift toward improving in-the-moment decisions is not backed up by evidence. Therefore, both approaches, should be seen as co-existent or even complementary, and not mutually exclusive.

Future research must be adequately powered and judiciously designed to evaluate the best surrogate outcomes. But at present, if patient wishes and views are to be addressed and considered, then the evidence is more strongly weighted towards actively holding treatment escalation planning and treatment escalation discussions (well in advance), when patients are cognitively able to do so, even if these are hard conversations for some. Evidence towards a more public-health-centred approach also lends itself towards holding such conversations in advance. Abel et al.[24] suggest future ACP conversations focus on three main areas: 1) what matters most to you in life when you are well? 2) Which of these will become priorities when you become less well? 3) How can you gain access to support from your social network of support at a time when you become less well so that you can ensure the priorities you describe in #2?

References

1. New York Heart Failure Association Functional Classification. NYHA scale—Heart Failure Foundation. Available at: https://manual.jointcommission.org/releases/TJC2018A/DataElem0439.html
2. Rockwood Clinical Frailty Scale. Available at: https://www.england.nhs.uk/south/wp-content/uploads/sites/6/2022/02/rockwood-frailty-scale_.pdf
3. Kouwenhoven WB, Jude JR, Knickerbocker GG. Closed chest cardiac massage. *JAMA* 1960; 173: 106–147.
4. NICE. Cardiac arrest—out of hospital care: what is the prognosis? Available at: https://cks.nice.org.uk/topics/cardiac-arrest-out-of-hospital-care/background-information/prognosis/
5. Lee MR, Yu KL, Kuo HY, Liu TH, Ko JC, Tsai JS, Wang JY. Outcome of stage IV cancer patients receiving in-hospital cardiopulmonary resuscitation: a population-based cohort study. *Sci Rep* 2019; 9(1): 9478.

6. General Medical Council. Treatment and care towards the end of life. July 2010. Available at: https://cks.nice.org.uk/topics/cardiac-arrest-out-of-hospital-care/background-informat ion/prognosis/
7. Sharing and Involving—a clinical policy for Do Not Attempt Cardiopulmonary Resuscitation (DNA-CPR) for adults in Wales. Version 4. 2020. Available at: https://executive.nhs.wales/ networks/programmes/national-palliative-and-end-of-life-care-programme/resources-for-hea lth-care-professionals/dnacpr/
8. Do not attempt cardiopulmonary resuscitation (DNACPR)-integrated adult policy: guidance on decision making and communications policy in relation to NHS Scotland DNACPR policy. May 2010. Available at: https://executive.nhs.wales/networks/programmes/national-palliative-and-end-of-life-care-programme/resources-for-health-care-professionals/dnacpr/
9. Taubert M, Norris J, Edwards S, Snow V, Finlay IG. Talk CPR - a technology project to improve communication in do not attempt cardiopulmonary resuscitation decisions in palliative illness. *BMC Palliat Care* 2018; 17: 118.
10. Burke R (on the application of) v GMC & Ors [2005] EWCA Civ 1003.
11. Elderly patients feel pressured into signing 'do not resuscitate' forms and that their 'lives do not matter' amid coronavirus crisis, charities warn. *Daily Mail*. 2020. Available at: https:// www.dailymail.co.uk/news/article-8194965/Elderly-pressured-signing-Do-not-resuscitate-forms-charities-warn.html
12. Tracey V Cambridge NHS Trust [2012] EWHC 3670.
13. Winspear v City Hospitals Sunderland NHS Foundation Trust [2015] EWHC 3250 (QB).
14. Mental Capacity Act 2005. Available at: https://www.legislation.gov.uk/ukpga/2005/9/ contents
15. Obolensky L, Clark T, Matthew G, et al. A patient and relative centred evaluation of treatment escalation plans: a replacement for the do-not-resuscitate process. *J Med Ethics* 2010; 36: 518–520.
16. Reid C, Gibbins J, Bloor S, Burcombe M, McCoubrie R, Forbes K. Healthcare professionals' perspectives on delivering end-of-life care within acute hospital trusts: a qualitative study. *BMJ Support Palliat Care* 2015; 5: 490–495
17. Sayma M, Nowell G, O'Connor A, et al. Improving the use of treatment escalation plans: a quality improvement study. *Postgrad Med J* 2018; 94: 404–410.
18. Dahill M, Powter L, Garland L, et al. Improving documentation of treatment escalation decisions in acute care. BMJ *Open Quality* 2013; 2: u200617.w1077.
19. Taubert M, Bounds L. Advance and future care planning: strategic approaches in Wales. BMJ Support Palliat Care 2022 Feb 1:bmjspcare-2021-003498.
20. Fritz Z, Malyon A, Frankau JM, et al. The universal form of treatment options (UFTO) as an alternative to do not attempt cardiopulmonary resuscitation (DNACPR) orders: a mixed methods evaluation of the effects on clinical practice and patient care. *PLoS ONE* 2013; 8(9): e70977.
21. Lightbody CJ, Campbell JN, Herbison GP, Osborne HK, Radley A, Taylor DR. Impact of a treatment escalation plan/limitation plan on non-beneficial interventions and harms in patients during their last admission before in-hospital death, using the structured judgment method review. *BMJ Open* 2018; 8: e024264.
22. Boutell J, Gonzalez N, Geue C, Lightbody CJ, Taylor DR. Cost impact of introducing a treatment escalation/limitation plan during patients' last hospital admission before death. *Int J Qual Health Care* 2020; 32 (10), 694–700.
23. Morrison RS, Meier DE, Arnold RM. What's wrong with advance care planning? *JAMA* 2021; 326(16): 1575–1576.
24. Abel J, Kellehear A, Millington Sanders C, Taubert M, Kingston H. Advance care planning re-imagined: a needed shift for COVID times and beyond. *Palliat Care Soc Pract* 2020; 14: 2632352420934491.

CASE

47 Withdrawal of Treatment

Simeon Senders-Galloway

Expert: Anna Gorringe

Case history

A referral was received from a general practitioner requesting your input in the care of Jonathan, a 30-year-old diagnosed with prolonged disorder of consciousness (PDOC). His family requested that life-sustaining treatment (LST), in particular clinically assisted nutrition and hydration (CANH), be withdrawn (see Box 47.1 for key definitions).

Jonathan was diagnosed with PDOC following an anaphylactic reaction to shellfish and cardiac arrest with prolonged downtime. He had a long admission in intensive care with a diagnosis of a minimally conscious state secondary to hypoxic brain injury. Jonathan was successfully weaned off ventilatory support and discharged to a neurorehabilitation unit, receiving CANH via a percutaneous endoscopic gastrostomy (PEG) tube. He did not improve; two independent clinicians diagnosed a vegetative state. On discharge to a specialist nursing home, the clinical team and Jonathan's family decided to continue CANH.

Box 47.1 Key definitions

- Prolonged disorder of consciousness: A disorder of consciousness lasting at least four weeks following sudden onset brain injury. PDOC is further categorized into two states based on the patient's level of awareness:
- Vegetative state (VS): A wakeful state, with preserved sleep-wake cycle, but no awareness of self or one's environment. Movements only consist of reflexes and spontaneous purposeless movements.
- Minimally conscious state (MCS): a wakeful state with some, albeit few and inconsistent, responses demonstrating awareness and interaction with oneself and environment, e.g. localizing and pursuit eye movements.[1]
- Life-sustaining treatment: Any treatment that serves to prolong life without reversing the underlying medical condition, e.g. mechanical ventilation, antibiotics, and clinically assisted nutrition and hydration.[2]
- Clinically assisted nutrition and hydration: All forms of tube-feeding e.g. via nasogastric tube, percutaneous endoscopic gastrostomy (PEG) or parenteral nutrition. CANH does not include oral feeding, by cup, spoon, or any other method of delivering food or nutritional supplements into the patient's mouth,[3] this is considered basic care.

Evidence Base Legal Precedent—Withdrawing Clinically Assisted Nutrition and Hydration

This summary refers to UK case law. The law surrounding the withdrawal of CANH is likely to differ significantly by jurisdiction.

CANH is classified as a medical intervention, not basic care.[4]

In patients deemed to have capacity to make a decision about the use of CANH:

- A patient must be provided with CANH where it is considered necessary to maintain life, is not considered futile, and the patient wishes to receive it[5]
- An adult with capacity has the right to refuse LST[6]

In patients without capacity (as was the case with Jonathan):

- LST can be legally withdrawn or withheld if the treatment is deemed not to be in the patient's best interests[7]
- Healthcare professionals no longer require a court declaration to withdraw LST in patients with PDOC in certain circumstances.[8] A second opinion is advised[9]
- The decision to withdraw CANH should be based on the likelihood that the patient will regain a quality of life that is acceptable to them, and not solely based on the likelihood of regaining consciousness[10]

Expert Comment

Airedale NHS Trust v Bland [1993][4] established the status of CANH as a medical intervention rather than as basic care. Tony Bland was crushed in the Hillsborough Disaster, sustained a hypoxic brain injury, and was left in persistent VS. He received CANH. After three years his parents asked his doctors to allow him to die. The hospital trust applied to the court for permission to withdraw CANH. The court drew a clear distinction between withdrawing and withholding treatment on the basis that the treatment is not in the patient's best interests, which is legally acceptable, and withdrawing and withholding treatment *in order to* bring about death, which is considered murder. The classification of CANH as a medical treatment is significant as it follows that where a patient lacks capacity, medical treatments can be assessed as to whether it is in a patient's best interests to receive them. In contrast, basic care must always be offered.

Learning Point Key Legal Principles to Be Aware of In Those Lacking Capacity (in England and Wales Only)

Advanced decision to refuse treatment (ADRT): a person can record their wishes to refuse LST at a time when they have capacity. The ADRT is valid and applicable if capacity is lost and if the ADRT pertains to the specific clinical situation. If valid and applicable, it is legally binding.

Lasting power of attorney (LPA): Nomination of one or more persons to make decisions in your best interests regarding:

- Property and Affairs: Active, with permission of the donor, as soon as registered with the Office of the Public Guardian.
- Health and Welfare: Can include decisions on LST. Only active when the donor loses capacity.

Independent mental capacity advocate (IMCA): an independent person appointed to advocate for someone's best interests in the situation where they lack capacity for one or more decisions, and they do not have close family or friends who can advocate for them.

Expert Comment

An ADRT that refuses LST must be written and witnessed to be valid.

LPA documentation must be registered with the Office of the Public Guardian. If the donor wishes the donee to have power to make decisions regarding LST, this must be explicitly stated.

It is important to recognize the IMCAs are not decision-makers but have an important role in best-interests decision-making for adults who lack capacity and do not have close family or friends to represent their wishes.

Jonathan received CANH for five years. For several years he remained free of intercurrent illness, however in the past year he required three admissions to hospital for intravenous antibiotic treatment of community acquired pneumonia (CAP). On the most recent admission, Jonathan was reviewed by a nutritionist as staff suspected he was aspirating his PEG feed. The rate of feeding was reduced and metoclopramide, a prokinetic, commenced. Jonathan had three further episodes of CAP and two PEG site infections, all requiring antibiotics via his PEG tube in his nursing home.

Jonathan developed progressively worsening contractures of all four limbs in the nursing home. Physiotherapy and baclofen were of minimal benefit. Jonathan was cared for in a sleep pod and staff have been unable to transfer him safely to a chair for the past year. Jonathan developed reflex myoclonus on physical contact, was reviewed by a neurologist and commenced on gabapentin with some effect. Despite reassurance from the neurologist that Jonathan did not experience any suffering from the myoclonus, it caused distress to both his family and care staff.

Jonathan's family consisted of his 28-year-old fiancée, a younger brother, aged 24, his mother and father, and a grandmother who lived in Spain. Jonathan's brother had depression, first diagnosed 6 months after Jonathan's intensive care admission; he received antidepressants and counselling. Jonathan's fiancée had not visited him for the past year due to the distress that seeing him caused. She had not received any formal support.

Jonathan's deteriorating condition had prompted his family to reflect on his care. They felt that Jonathan was suffering and that he would not have wanted to be artificially kept alive in this situation. His parents told the GP that they thought that CANH should be withdrawn. Jonathan did not have a formal advance decision to refuse treatment, advance statement of his wishes, or power of attorney.

Learning Point Key Questions Surrounding the Withdrawal of Clinically Assisted Nutrition and Hydration in Jonathan

1. How often should the decision to continue CANH be routinely reviewed?
   Every six months, or more frequently if there is a change of situation. This can be increased to every 12 months where the situation has remained stable for an extended period. Reviews should be coordinated by the person with overall responsibility for the patient's care.[3]
2. What process should be followed when determining whether CANH should be withdrawn in this patient?
   Jonathan requires a formal capacity assessment followed by a best-interests decision-making process, as set out by the Mental Capacity Act (MCA) 2005.[11] In carrying out the capacity assessment, it was noted that Jonathan had a disorder of the mind (hypoxic brain damage) leading to PDOC and did not have capacity.
3. Who should be consulted in the best-interests process?
   As advised, MCA 2005, anyone engaged in caring for the patient or interested in his welfare should be involved.
   In Jonathan's case, this could include:
   - Family and friends.
   - Healthcare professionals who have cared for Jonathan, including his GP, neurology consultant, physiotherapist, occupational therapist, speech and language therapist, and members of the neurorehabilitation team.
   - Representatives from Jonathan's nursing home, such as the manager, lead nurse, and any carers who regularly care for Jonathan.

Where a decision involves the withdrawal of LST an independent second opinion should be sought, in this instance, from someone with specific training in diagnosing and managing patients with PDOC. It is also best practice to involve a clinical ethics committee where available. They are not a decision-making body but provide a critical overview of the decision-making process.

An application to the Court of Protection should be made if there is disagreement or uncertainty about what is in the patient's best interests.

4. What factors should be taken into account in making a best-interests decision?
   Information about Jonathan's diagnosis should be reviewed, including the likelihood of any meaningful recovery, his level of awareness, an estimated prognosis and expectations for Jonathan's health (with and without ongoing CANH), and how health needs will be met.
   It is vital to gather as much information about Jonathan's premorbid state and beliefs as possible. Important information could include Jonathan's premorbid health beliefs, his likes, dislikes, employment, and hobbies, any religious, spiritual or moral beliefs, and any spoken, written, or actioned evidence as to what he may want in this situation.

A clear picture of Jonathan's premorbid state emerged, that of a highly sociable man with a wide and long-standing network of good friends and a very close relationship with his immediate family. He met his fiancée in sixth form, had lived with her in the same town as his family for 5 years and was engaged to her for two years prior to his cardiac arrest.

Jonathan was a dedicated painter, leaving his job as an accountant to teach painting. He described this as 'the best decision' he had ever made. In his spare time, Jonathan had prioritized spending time with others, and loved being outdoors, choosing to spend most of his holidays trekking and mountain climbing.

Jonathan was first diagnosed with an anaphylactic reaction to shellfish at age 15. Whilst he recognized the life-threatening nature of this condition, he never expressed any wishes about LST in the event of being in a vegetative state, a state with dependence on others for activities of daily living, or a state of cognitive decline.

There was a clear opinion amongst Jonathan's immediate family that Jonathan, if able to make a decision, would object to the ongoing use of CANH in the circumstances. Jonathan's grandmother had a strong Roman Catholic faith, unlike Jonathan and the remainder of the family. The family initially did not discuss withdrawal of CANH with her due to fear she would object. On discussion however, she was also in full agreement.

A second opinion was requested from an independent clinician with expertise in PDOC, who confirmed a diagnosis of vegetative state. With the support of an external Ethics Committee, it was recognized that the following factors supported the withdrawal of CANH:

- The extent of deviation in Jonathan's life from what he most enjoyed and prioritized whilst healthy.
- Low probability of any significant improvement in either Jonathan's level of consciousness or quality of life.
- Evidence of deteriorating health.
- A prognosis possibly of years with continued CANH, however with the prospect of further deteriorating health with frequent infections (aspiration pneumonia and PEG site infections), worsening contractures, suboptimal nutrition, and the likely development of pressure lesions.
- Without CANH, Jonathan's prognosis would likely be that of weeks at most.

The best-interest decision was that the continuation of CANH would not be in Jonathan's best interests. A plan for symptom management and support for those close to Jonathan was developed and discussed with Jonathan's family. CANH was withdrawn. Jonathan died peacefully ten days after withdrawal of CANH, with his family present at his bedside.

Learning Point Justifications for Withholding or Withdrawing Treatment

1. Treatment will not be successful.
2. The patient does not consent to treatment or there is an ADRT available when the patient lacks capacity.
3. The treatment is clinically inappropriate or not in the patient's best interests where they lack capacity.

Learning Point Ethical and Legal Considerations in Withdrawing Life-sustaining Treatment

From an ethical and legal standpoint there is no distinction between withholding and withdrawing LST.[12] However, the withdrawal of treatment is frequently described as being more emotionally challenging for all parties involved. This is partly due to the withdrawal of LST being a direct act, as opposed to one of omission when withholding LST, and that death often proceeds comparatively more quickly after treatment is withdrawn than withheld (ICU study).[13]

Expert Comment

Patients and those important to them must be involved and supported in decision-making around withholding or withdrawing treatment. Where an adult lacks capacity to participate in discussions about withholding or withdrawing LST, the views of those close to the patient are important in representing the patient's values and wishes about treatment. Clinicians must not make decisions about whether or not it is in a patient's best interests to receive a treatment based on their own assumptions about the quality of life that a patient would find acceptable, or make decisions which discriminate against particular groups e.g. people with learning disabilities.

Clinical Tip Withdrawing Other Forms of Life-sustaining Treatment

The withdrawal of CANH is often clinically and ethically complex, however the fundamental principles are the same when deciding whether to withdraw any form of LST:

- The capacity of a patient to make this decision for themselves must be determined
- Where a patient lacks capacity, a best-interests decision-making process must be followed[11]
- Potential benefits and potential harms of withdrawing or continuing treatment must be considered and balanced
- Disagreement between parties can usually be resolved with effective communication. Where conflict persists, the following should be considered:
  - a second opinion
  - mediation
  - discussion at a clinical ethics committee
  - input from the legal team
  - an application to the Court of Protection
- Prior to LST being withdrawn a plan should be developed to rationalize medication, prescribe anticipatory medicines to manage expected symptoms, review interventions and place of care, agree a plan for emergency review and agree review timeframes for regular ongoing care.

Clinical Tip Religious Perspective on Withdrawing LST

Some people may oppose the withdrawal of LST on religious grounds. The reasoning behind this opposition differs between, and often within, religions.[14] When making a decision regarding the withdrawal of LST where significant religious views are held, the input of a chaplain and faith leaders can be valuable.

Expert Comment

A healthcare practitioner can withdraw from providing care if their religious, moral or other personal beliefs about providing life-prolonging treatment lead them to object to complying with a patient's decision to refuse treatment or a decision that providing treatment is not of overall benefit (if the patient lacks capacity)[1]. They must first ensure that arrangements have been made for another healthcare practitioner to take over their role.[1, 9]

A Final Word from the Expert

This case is a good example of the complexity surrounding decisions to withhold or withdraw life-sustaining treatment. These cases can encompass significant clinical, ethical, legal, emotional, and practical challenges. Thorough clinical assessment, including obtaining second opinions where necessary, as well as a sound understanding of the relevant ethical aspects, law, and professional guidance are essential to good management. Equally essential is effective communication with the patient and those important to them, and amongst the clinical team, which can help to avoid and resolve conflict and facilitate high quality decision-making. Future research to build a stronger evidence base for managing symptoms after withdrawal of CANH would aid clinicians in delivering high-quality care to patients with PDOC.

References

1. Royal College of Physicians. Prolonged disorders of consciousness following sudden onset brain injury: national clinical guidelines. 2020. Available at: https://www.rcplondon.ac.uk/guidelines-policy/prolonged-disorders-consciousness-following-sudden-onset-brain-injury-national-clinical-guidelines
2. Anonymous. Virtual mentor. *J Ethics* 2013; 15(12): 1038–1040.

3. British Medical Association and Royal College of Physicians. Clinically assisted nutrition and hydration (CANH) and adults who lack the capacity to consent. 2021. Available at: https://www.bma.org.uk/media/1161/bma-clinically-assisted-nutrition-hydration-canh-full-guidance.pdf
4. *Airedale NHS Trust v Bland* [1993] AC 789, 870.
5. *Burke v General Medical Council* [2005] EWCA Civ 1003. 34.
6. *Re B* (Adult: Refusal of Medical Treatment) [2002] 2 All ER 449.
7. *Airedale NHS Trust v Bland* [1993] AC 789, 866.
8. *An NHS Trust v Y* [2018] UKSC 46.
9. General Medical Council. *Treatment and Care Towards the End Of Life: Good Practice In Decision-Making*. GMC: London, 2010, p. 121.
10. Aintree University Hospitals NHS Foundation Trust v James. UKSC 67 (2013).
11. *Mental Capacity Act 2005, S4* [2005]. London: The Stationery Office.
12. Cherny NI. *Oxford Textbook of Palliative Medicine*, 5th ed. Oxford: Oxford University Press, 2015.
13. Sprung CL, Cohen SL, Sjokvist P. End-of-life practices in European intensive care units: the Ethicus Study. *JAMA* 2003; 290(6): 790–797.
14. Geppert CM, Andrews MR, Druyan ME. Ethical issues in artificial nutrition and hydration: a review. *JPEN J Parenter Enteral Nutr* 2010; 34(1): 79–88.

CASE

48 Autonomy in Children

Marie Claire Rooney

Expert: Joanna Laddie

Case history

A 15-year-old female, Rose (weighing 50 kg), with a known diagnosis of a mitochondrial cytopathy, was brought by her father to the emergency department with increased shortness of breath and abdominal discomfort. She was admitted under the paediatric metabolic team. Rose's mother and brother had the same mitochondrial cytopathy and died some years earlier from sequelae of the disease. Following her brother's presentation and diagnosis, genetic testing was carried out, and Rose and her mother were diagnosed. In Rose's case, symptoms did not manifest until she was 6 years old and consisted initially of neurological change. Subsequently Rose developed dilated cardiomyopathy—for which she was on diuretics—and mildly impaired renal function. Rose did not have a learning disability. Rose was able to express understanding of her condition and understood that her mother and brother had died from the same condition.

> **Clinical Tip Mitochondrial Cytopathy**
>
> Mitochondrial cytopathies may have different clinical pictures in different patients presenting across different timeframes. The same condition might present in infancy in one patient and in adulthood in another. While one patient might be severely affected by the condition, consequences for another patient might be minimal.

On admission, Rose had abdominal pain and evidence of cardiac decompensation requiring supplemental oxygen. During her admission Rose became notably more unwell. Both her cardiac and renal function began to deteriorate. She had periods of reduced consciousness. Rose's swallow deteriorated and she became confined to her bed.

The severity of her illness, guarded prognosis, and rapid deterioration were discussed with Rose's father. Proposed management included diuretics, urinary catheterization and nasogastric (NG) tube insertion to support safe administration of medications and feeding. These were commenced on discussion with Rose's father—Rose was not alert enough to engage in such discussions at that time. Of note, her father was keen for medications to prolong her life, while the medical team's focus was that of symptom management.

When Rose was more lucid, she expressed that she did not want any of these interventions: she pulled out her NG tube and catheter. Rose stated that she did not want to stay in hospital, and that she wanted to go home. While Rose displayed an understanding of her condition during her more lucid periods, the medical team thought that it was not in her best interest to withhold these interventions. Therefore, in order to improve symptom management they were pursued.

The acute crisis passed, but Rose was becoming frailer, and her condition deteriorated globally. The team offered discussions and Rose was keen to engage in discussions on her proposed ongoing management and likely disease trajectory. The medical team assessed that she had the ability to consent to undertake such discussions. Rose's father advised the team that he believed this would cause 'undue distress' for Rose and insisted that these discussions should not take place. A second opinion was sought from an adolescent psychiatrist, who agreed that Rose ought to be involved in these discussions. Rose requested that her father was not present during such discussions.

Rose was updated regarding what had happened since admission, on her current multiorgan failure and on the view of the medical team that she was at considerable risk of further deterioration and at risk of dying. She expressed her preferences not to go to ITU (Intensive Therapy Unit) and to go home as soon as possible (when symptoms were better managed). The medical team felt that a 'Do Not Attempt Cardiopulmonary Resuscitation' (DNACPR) decision was appropriate. Rose agreed, though her father disagreed. An ITU opinion was sought, they thought CPR would not be in keeping with Rose's best interests. Rose's father was still opposed to the decision. The discussion was referred to the in-house mediation committee, a team of accredited mediators who worked with Rose's father and the medical team to endeavour to create a mutual understanding of the issues and to seek an agreed way forward. While these teams are not available in every hospital, they are becoming more established, and aim to de-escalate to de-escalate disputes before they become litigious. The case was escalated to the ethical committee because an agreement was not secured. Despite extensive discussion with the ethical committee, Rose's father still disagreed with a DNACPR decision being recorded.

The case subsequently went to children's court. The court process took several months before ruling that it was not in Rose's best interest to undergo CPR and ITU admission. Rose's father was offered psychological support and over time came to accept the palliative nature of her disease. Rose died in hospital several months following her admission.

Learning Point Childhood

The Children Act 1989 (UK), an act of parliament which provides a framework for the safeguarding of a child, defines a child as 'a person under the age of 18' (section one, paragraph 16).[1] However, it can be argued that the definition of childhood is more complex than an arbitrary number of years lived.

The philosopher, Jean-Jacques Rosseau proposed five stages on the journey to adulthood:[2]

1. infancy—birth to age 2
2. the age of sensation—3 to 12
3. the age of ideas—13 to puberty
4. the age of sentiment—puberty to 20
5. the age of marriage and social responsibility—aged 20 onwards

Where UK law is concerned, persons under the age of 18 are subject to varying degrees of responsibility depending on their age. For example, from the age of 13 years children can carry out paid work for a limited number of hours, while those younger than 13 cannot carry out paid work.[3] Children under 10 years cannot be arrested, however those between 10 and 17 years can be taken to court if they have committed a crime.[4] When it comes to decisions surrounding management of children in the healthcare setting, where does the law stand? Can the child make decisions for themselves? Do parents hold legal authority? Is it the healthcare professionals who decide? Or is it the legal system?

There are three main concepts to consider when answering this question:

1. Parental Responsibility
2. Gillick Competence
3. Asymmetry of Consent

Learning Point Parental Responsibility

When considering the legalities surrounding decision-making in children or young persons, the child's parents (or those with parental responsibility) play a major role. This is referred to as 'parental responsibility', which is defined as 'all the rights, duties, powers, responsibilities and authority which by law a parent of a child has in relation to the child and his/her property'.[5] This includes the rights of parents in the consenting to—or the refusal of—medical interventions on their child's behalf. However, there are limits to what parents can decide: they cannot impose inappropriate treatments, nor can they refuse treatments which are felt to be in the child's best interests.[6]

In the case of Rose, the person with parental responsibility agreed with the specific interventions of diuretics, NG tube placement, and catheterization. This was important in order to proceed with the interventions. Given that the nature of Rose's preference was that of refusal (rather than that of granting consent), the team was not obliged to take Rose's refusal of these interventions into account. See learning point on 'Asymmetry of Consent'.

Expert Comment

Discussing the gravity of a child or young person's disease with them directly is often a contentious issue for parents, who want to protect their children from potentially distressing information. It is widely considered, however, to be helpful to provide the child or young person with information for the benefit of their mental well-being (it can be more distressing to be 'left in the dark') and to help build trust in the working relationship with the medical team (often children are aware of discussions happening without their involvement, which can be undermining and upsetting). Where parents are not in agreement with this despite efforts to explain the importance of engaging the child or young person in such discussions, it is best practice to seek a second opinion.

Learning Point Gillick Competence

Autonomy is a moral principle based on an individual's ability to govern oneself.[7] Consent is a legal expression of this moral principle.[8] When considering autonomy and consent in children, a central case is that of *Gillick v West Norfolk and Wisbech, England AHA*. This case involved a dispute over whether effective consent could be given by a teenage girl to receive contraception without the consent of her mother. The House of Lords stated that if her doctor was to decide that the girl had 'sufficient understanding and intelligence to enable her to understand fully what is proposed' then she would be considered able to give consent as effectively as an adult—that is, she would be considered 'Gillick competent'.[9]

Indeed 'Gillick competence' is now widely used beyond the issue of contraception, and can be applied when consenting children or young persons to most medical, surgical, and dental treatment.[10]

Factors considered in assessing whether a child or young person is 'Gillick competent' include—but are not limited to—the child's age, maturity, intelligence, and their ability to weigh up longer-term implications of their decision.[11]

Had Rose consented to the proposed specific interventions (diuretics, NG placement, catheterization), and displayed 'Gillick competency', even if her father was not in agreement, her consent would be valid and would over-rule the parental responsibility of her father.

Learning Point Asymmetry of Consent

Where a child or young person is considered able to give consent, their consent is valid. However, if this same, capable child or young person refuses an intervention, their refusal may be overridden. The apparent contradiction that a child or young person may have the ability to consent to but not have the ability to refuse treatment is often known as the 'asymmetry of consent'. Some deem this 'asymmetry' unjust. Culver and Gert argue that competence is derived from the ability of the person's cognitive processes and that this competence should not be retrospectively influenced by the outcome of the process.[12]

Expert Comment

When assessing Gillick competency, there is no defined lower age limit. It is at the discretion of the assessing clinician and is intervention-specific.

Expert Comment

While there is no explicit case law on the matter, experience from the expert author in clinical practice is such that while the court view is pending, legal advice given is to carry out routine care and emergency treatment that is essential to preserve life or prevent serious deterioration.[6] Therefore had Rose sustained a cardiac arrest while awaiting the court's decision, it would be advised that cardiopulmonary resuscitation be initiated.

Others argue that this 'asymmetry' can be justified when considering the welfare principle. The welfare principle stipulates that the paramount consideration is the *child's welfare* over and beyond other considerations, such as the child's consent. It is logical that a treating team would not offer a treatment that was felt to compromise a child's welfare, rather it would be offered to promote the welfare of the child. Therefore, for a child to refuse such an intervention may compromise their welfare, which is the consideration above all other considerations. Put simply, the law is devised to facilitate the medical team to provide treatment. Consent for such treatment must be attained from the Gillick competent child, or from those with parental responsibility, or from the court.[13]

Rose's refusal to consent to the use of diuretics, NG placement, urinary catheterization, and her refusal of cardiopulmonary resuscitation did not hold legal weight—as a Gillick competent child does not have the right to refuse treatment. However, Rose's wish to have a DNACPR decision in place was helpful when the case went to court.

Expert Comment

When presenting a case of this nature in court, a representative of the child or young person, the parents, the trust, and often an independent advocate are present. Should the parents lose the case in the High Court, they may wish to escalate to the Court of Appeal. From here, the case may be escalated to the Supreme Court. Following exhausting all domestic remedies, further escalation to the European Court of Human Rights may be pursued. At present, Brexit has not affected access to that court.[14]

Expert Comment

It is worth noting that communication breakdown is a recognized precursor to cases ending in conflict. Effective and consistent communication throughout is key. Over the last 10 years, particularly with the advance of social media, high-profile cases have played out in the media. This can exacerbate an already emotionally burdensome time for all parties involved. Furthermore, court cases of this nature can be financially burdensome. For these reasons, following efforts to optimize communication at a team level, early use of mediation and referral to ethics committees to reduce the need to go to court is advised to be best practice.

Future Advances

Use of mediation is increasingly encouraged as best practice to help prevent costly and strenuous court cases.[15] Indeed, NHS Resolution (known previously as NHS Litigation Authority) launched a five-year strategy in 2017 to engage in alternative dispute resolution (ADR), which aims to help reduce the number of claims going into formal litigation, thereby keeping patients and health practitioners out of court.[16] Not all trusts have these services and in such cases, mediation cannot be offered. Mediation committees charge trusts for their service. For trusts who do not have such facilities they may try to access another trust's ethics committee, which is a service that is free of charge. Mediation services may well be rolled out more extensively in the future.

A Final Word from the Expert

The care of paediatric patients is complex for many reasons. Children may present with uncommon clinical conditions that may not be found in the adult population. Medical interventions are often determined by size or age and maybe limited due to lack of adequate research within the paediatric population. Children may also present at different stages of both physical and cognitive maturity which can impact on their understanding of their condition and the implications of treatment decisions. The legal rights of both the child and their parents are dependent on the age of the child and assessments of their ability to consent to treatment and/or their capacity. Competence may fluctuate in time, for instance, dependent on their health status at that time, but is also dependent on the nature and complexity of the decision required. Furthermore, there may be disagreement between parents themselves or with the child or amongst the health care professionals regarding best interests decisions. Where possible health care professionals should maintain an open and clear line of communication with both parents and the child, and encourage shared decision making and involvement of the child where practical. Where disagreements do develop, the involvement of second opinions, mediation, ethics and court, can be helpful in finding a resolution.

References

1. Gov.uk. *The Children Act 1989.* Available at: https://www.legislation.gov.uk/ukpga/1989/41/data.pdf
2. Rosseau, J.-J. *Émile*, London: Dent, 1762.
3. Gov.uk. Child Employment. Available at: https://www.gov.uk/child-employment
4. Gov.uk. Age of Criminal Responsibility. Available at: https://www.gov.uk/age-of-criminal-responsibility)
5. Gov.uk. The Children Act 1989 Meaning of Parental Responsibility. Available at: https://www.legislation.gov.uk/ukpga/1989/41/section/3
6. BMA. *Parental Responsibility* 2008. Available at: https://www.bma.org.uk/media/1840/bma-parental-responsibility-oct-2008.pdf
7. Stanford Encyclopedia of Philosophy. Autonomy in Moral and Political Philosophy. Available at: https://plato.stanford.edu/entries/autonomy-moral/
8. Griffith R. What is Gillick competence? *Hum Vaccin Immunother* 2016; 12(1): 244–247.
9. Herring J. *Law Through the Life Course*. Bristol: Bristol University Press, 2021.
10. NSPCC Learning. Applying Gillick Competence and Fraser Guidelines. Available at: https://learning.nspcc.org.uk/child-protection-system/gillick-competence-fraser-guidelines
11. Larcher V, Hutchinson A. How should paediatricians assess Gillick competence? *Arch Dis Child* 2010; 95: 307–311.
12. Culver C, Gert B. The inadequacy of incompetence. *Millbank Q* 1990; 68: 619–620.
13. Gov.uk. The Children Act Welfare of A Child. Available at: https://www.legislation.gov.uk/ukpga/1989/41/section/1
14. Employers Perspectives. European Convention on Human Rights—*Still Relevant Post*-Brexit? Available at: https://www.employerperspectives.com/2022/03/european-convention-on-human-rights-still-relevant-post-brexit/#: ~ :text = Is%20the%20UK%20still%20committed,the%20EU%20and%20the%20UK
15. Yau CWH, Leigh B, Liberati E, Punch D, Dixon-Woods M, Draycott T. Clinical negligence costs: taking action to safeguard NHS sustainability. *BMJ* 2020; 368: m552.
16. Resolution.nhs.uk. Mediation in *Healthcare Claims—An Evaluation*. Available at: https://resolution.nhs.uk/wp-content/uploads/2020/02/NHS-Resolution-Mediation-in-healthcare-claims-an-evaluation.pdf

INDEX

Note: Tables and figures are indicated by an italic *t* and *f* following the page number.

B

E

N

O